Clinical Cytopathology of the Head and Neck

A Text and Atlas

Clinical Cytopathology of the Head and Neck

A Text and Atlas

Edited by

Gabrijela Kocjan MRCPath MBBS Spec. Clin. Cyt.
Senior Lecturer and Honorary Consultant in Cytopathology
University College
London, UK

GMM
LONDON ◦ SAN FRANCISCO

GREENWICH MEDICAL MEDIA LIMITED
137 Euston Road
London
NW1 2AA

870 Market Street, Ste 720
San Francisco
CA 94109

ISBN 1 900 151 76 6

First published 2001

A catalogue record for this book is available from the British Library.

Visit our website at:
www.greenwich-medical.co.uk

Distributed worldwide by Plymbridge Distributors Ltd and in the USA by Jamco Distribution

Typeset by Phoenix Photosetting Ltd, Chatham, Kent
Printed by Grafos, Spain

Contents

Preface vii

1 Introduction to clinical cytopathology of head and neck 1
Introduction 3
Fine needle aspiration 3

2 Salivary glands 9
Introduction 11
Non-neoplastic and inflammatory conditions 15
Benign tumours of the salivary gland 30
Malignant tumours of the salivary glands 44
Miscellaneous tumours 66

3 Thyroid 79
Introduction 81
Non-neoplastic and inflammatory conditions 87
Neoplasms 97
Metastatic tumours in thyroid 112

4 Lymph nodes 119
Introduction 121
Non-neoplastic lymphoproliferative conditions 124
Hodgkin's lymphoma 145
Non Hodgkin's lymphoma 148
Metastatic carcinoma 170

5 Miscellaneous lesions of the head and neck 183
Introduction 185
Benign soft tissue lesions 185

Index 205

Preface

The past century has seen Cytopathology, as a discipline and Fine Needle Aspiration Cytology as a method of obtaining material, become established. From the pioneering work of Martin and Ellis, through the enthusiasm of Zajicek and his colleagues, to the perseverance of numerous cytopathologists throughout the world, this simple technique has become part of the routine diagnostic investigations.

To this end, this book summarizes recent experiences with the role Cytopathology is playing in current clinical practice, particularly in relation to Head and Neck. This work is based on the experience drawn from a large referral practice – from ear, nose and throat, maxillofacial and general surgeons, endocrinologists, oncologists and others. From skeptical beginnings the FNAC service has grown and developed, to the extent that it is now accepted as a routine investigation and cytopathologists are considered the best people to deliver this service. Mutual understanding and trust between clinical colleagues and cytopathologists has led to further development of skills and a desire for improvement in respective disciplines. Clinically oriented work is a valuable source for the education and training of laboratory and junior pathology staff. To a cytopathologist, who meets new patients daily, this work is enormously satisfying.

In the new millenium, our efforts should no longer be to prove the validity of FNAC. Instead, with the advances in new technologies, our aim should be the refinement of morphological diagnoses in order to match the existing or improve future treatment options.

My sincere thanks for producing this book go, firstly, to my parents who posed for the sometimes, unflattering photographs; to my medical and technical colleagues in the Cytopathology Laboratory, University College Hospital London, to eminent clinical colleagues for their advice and support and to Mr Paratian for processing the photographs. Lastly, I would like to thank Tony and Arabella for putting up with my absences during the long gestation of this book.

G Kocjan
London, May 2001

1

Introduction to clinical cytopathology of the head and neck

Introduction
Fine needle aspiration

INTRODUCTION

Very few areas in the body are so exposed to our scrutiny as the head and neck. Lumps and bumps in this area rarely go unnoticed; patients either notice changes themselves, or are alerted to them by others. Fine needle aspiration cytology (FNAC) is a valuable technique in investigation of nodules and masses arising within the head and neck. FNAC is particularly helpful because biopsy of this area should be avoided unless all other diagnostic modalities have failed to establish a diagnosis. As such, FNAC represents an accurate, inexpensive and rapid investigative technique of head and neck masses.[1–22]

The pattern of referral to FNAC is usually from the general practitioner, via the specialist to the pathologist. The referral pattern via the specialist reduces the need for FNAC in a majority of cases that are due to infection and have settled after the initial treatment. This particularly relates to the paediatric age group.

The majority of aspirates from cervical lymph nodes will disclose either reactive lymphadenopathy or metastatic squamous cell carcinoma. Occasional nodules will be due to lymphoma. While primary diagnosis of lymphoma by FNAC is generally not considered definitive, it is helpful in further management. Similarly, establishing the presence of carotid body tumours, branchial cleft cysts or epidermoid cysts excludes metastatic carcinoma and avoids the open biopsy as well as reassuring both clinician and patient. FNAC of lesions within the mouth, oropharynx, nasopharynx and nasal sinuses eliminates squamous cell carcinoma as its primary objective. FNAC can establish diagnosis of salivary gland tumours, which should not be biopsied prior to definitive treatment. It can diagnose the majority of thyroid enlargements and helps reduce the rate of surgery for thyroid lumps. In addition, FNAC can diagnose many specific conditions, both of local origin or a reflection of a more generalised disease. Each of these represents an important clinical entity with a specific therapy. Ancillary techniques, namely immunocytochemistry, flow cytometry and sometimes molecular techniques, can greatly broaden the diagnostic range and specificity of FNAC. They are particularly useful in the diagnosis of lymphoproliferative processes and in determining the precise nature of lesions as variable as rhabdomyosarcoma, olfactory neuroblastoma and granular cell tumour. The prudent use of these techniques can be cost-effective and avoid the need for more invasive diagnostic procedures. FNAC has a high degree of accuracy for the diagnosis of both primary and metastatic disease.[23]

FINE NEEDLE ASPIRATION

Clinical history

Clinical history forms an integral part of FNAC investigation. In our institution, the specialist refers patients to the FNAC clinic (Fig. 1.1). A pathologist (who examines patients, takes the samples and reports them) runs the FNAC clinic. Patients bring a request form or a letter from the referring physician stating a short clinical history and indication for FNAC. The pathologist confirms the patient's identity, takes the past and present clinical history, examines the patient and confirms the site of investigation (Fig. 1.2). The procedure is explained to the patient. In cases where a need for multiple passes is anticipated, a local anaesthetic is applied. As a result, most patients do not experience any significant degree of pain. Clinical history and physical properties of the lesion (anatomy, consistency, mobility, pain) are very useful information helping to reach a correct diagnosis.

Physical examination

The pathologist examines the patient, focusing on the area indicated by the referring specialist but also any other areas indicated by the patient or discovered by thorough scrutiny. This is a very important part of the consultation since

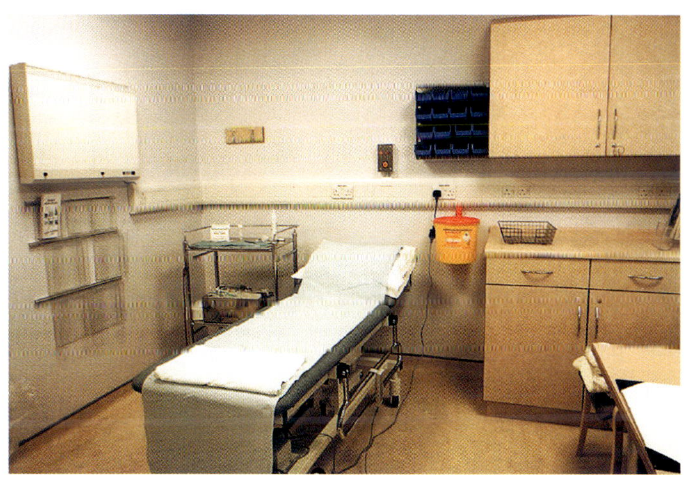

Figure 1.1 FNAC clinic room. Consulting room with an examination couch, work surface, waste disposal, sink, microscope and facility for rapid staining.

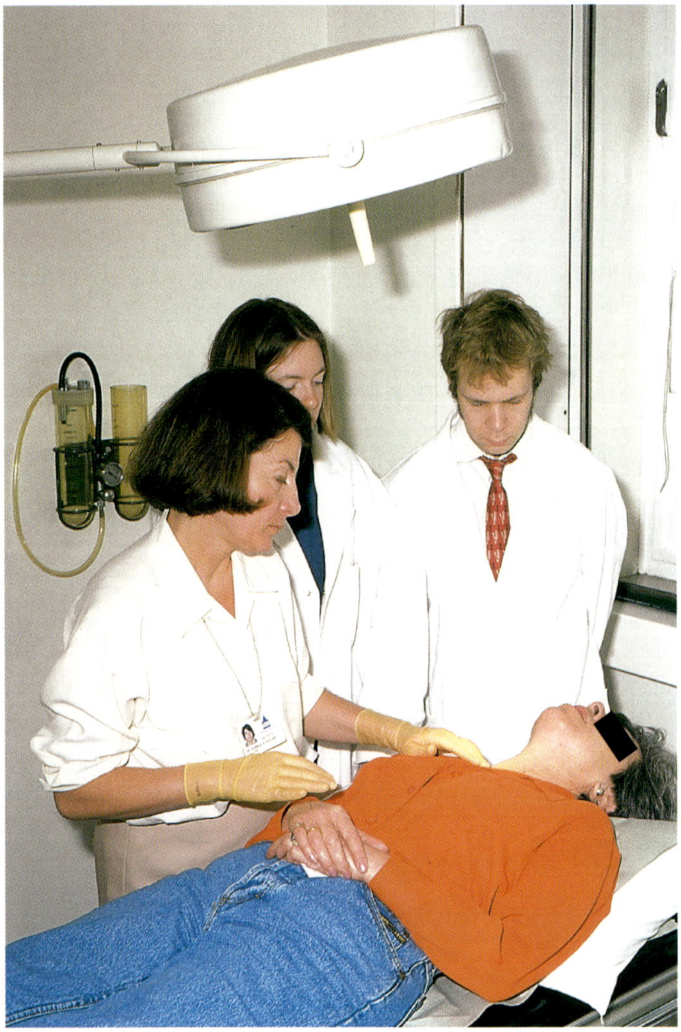

Figure 1.2 Clinical history and examination. Pathologist at the bedside examines the area referred to by the specialist. Patient is asked further relevant questions about the duration of the swelling, level of pain and any other associated systemic symptoms.

valuable data can be obtained about the anatomy and nature of the lesion as well as getting relevant clinical history, e.g. a patient with a submandibular swelling will readily describe that the swelling changes in size. Palpable lumps can be hard or soft, mobile in different directions or adherent to surrounding tissues and skin, painful, oval, round or irregular, or pulsating. On needling, they can feel soft, hard, gritty, fatty, can yield clear fluid, purulent fluid, keratinous viscous fluid, mucoid material and blood. All these signs are significant and are noted on the patient's request form.

FNAC procedure

With the FNAC procedure having been explained, the patient is put in a supine position. The choice of whether or not to apply anaesthetic largely depends on the patient, the site involved and the extent of FNAC sampling planned. Since the average FNAC does not involve more than one pass with a 22+G needle, most patients do not require local anaesthetic. However, if the patient is a child or a needle-phobic, or if the site is particularly tender (e.g. lip, nose, areola), or if it is expected that several passes will be necessary, a local anaesthetic is applied in the form of subcutaneous injection of 0.5 ml of 2% lignocaine. More recently we have been using a needle-free syringe where pressurised air expels the anaesthetic, penetrating the skin, without a needle (Fig. 1.3).[24] The anaesthetic forms a small white ring through which the subsequent test needle is applied, once or more (Fig. 1.4). Patients do not experience any pain on application of the anaesthetic and experience no or minimal pain at FNAC.

The palpable area in question is cleaned with an antiseptic agent and fixed between the two fingers of the non-dominant hand. A 22G, 23G or smaller needle is then passed into the lump. Usually, a syringe and a syringe holder are attached to the needle to help aspiration (Fig. 1.5). More recently we have been using a non-aspiration technique (capillary sampling) with the aid of a needle only (without the syringe attachment) (Fig. 1.6).[23,25–29] The needle is passed round several times in the cases of non-thyroid lumps. In the case of thyroid, several vertical movements in the same direction are usually sufficient to gain representa-

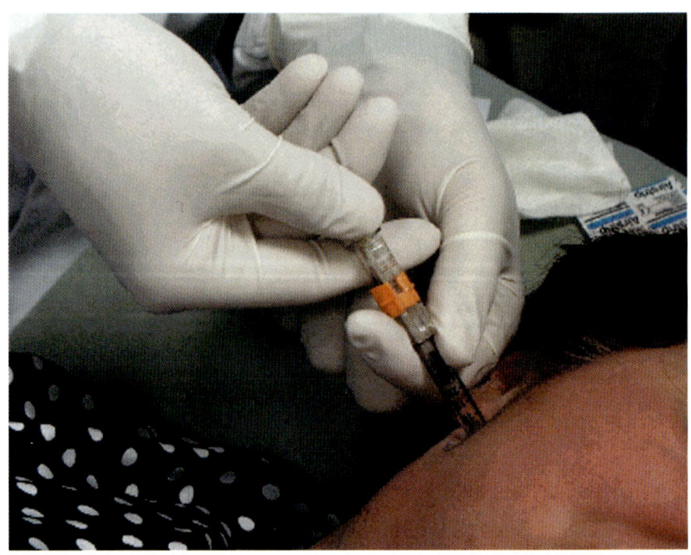

Figure 1.3 Needle-free anaesthetic system. Initially designed for patients who need daily injections (e.g. insulin), but applicable to local anaesthesia. This is particularly useful in children, in needle-phobic patients, in sensitive skins and where multiple needle passes are anticipated.

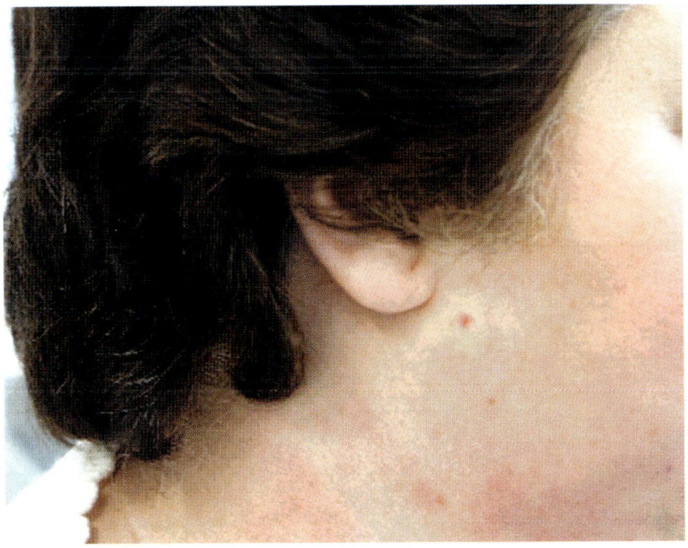

Figure 1.4 Needle-free anaesthetic system. A pale ring indicates the area of subdermal infiltration. The test needle should be passed through this area.

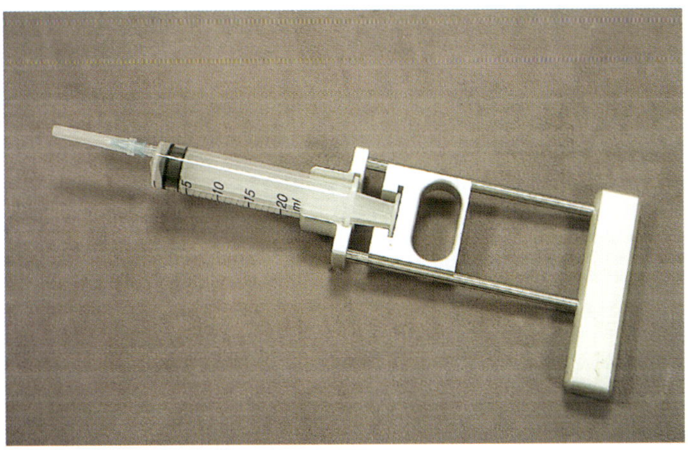

Figure 1.5 Standard FNAC procedure. A 20 ml syringe attached to a CAMECO syringe holder. A 23G needle is used.

tive material. Whilst using a syringe attachment, it is important to release the negative pressure before exiting the lump, otherwise the material is aspirated into the syringe and can only be retrieved with the aid of a needle wash.

FNAC MATERIAL PREPARATION

FNAC material obtained with the needle is expelled onto glass slides or into a solution (Fig. 1.7). Material on the slides is smeared by sliding another glass slide over it gently (Fig. 1.8), resulting in an evenly spread thin smear with the

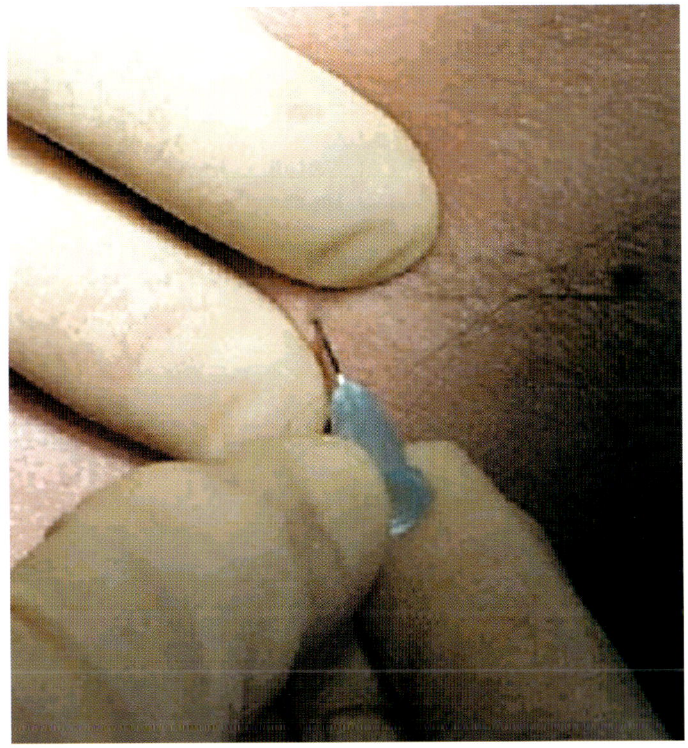

Figure 1.6 Free needle FNAC procedure. In recent years, a free needle technique of aspiration has been used. This is particularly useful in very small, mobile lesions (e.g. lymph nodes). The aspirator has a much better feel of the tip of the needle and better control of the area sampled. It is not the method of choice for cystic or very sclerosed lesions.

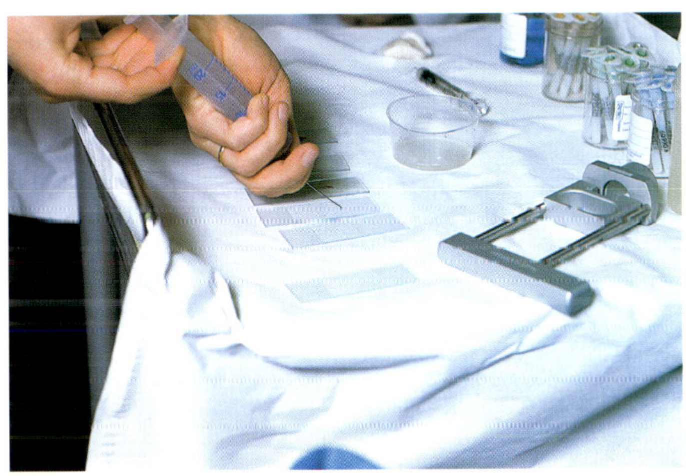

Figure 1.7 FNAC procedure. After the needle is withdrawn from the patient, a 20 ml syringe is attached to the needle with the air having been already drawn prior to attachment. The material is expelled from the needle onto the centre of a glass slide. The process is repeated, each time making sure that the needle is removed from the syringe when the air is drawn. Excess material expelled may be imprinted onto another slide thus multiplying the slides obtained.

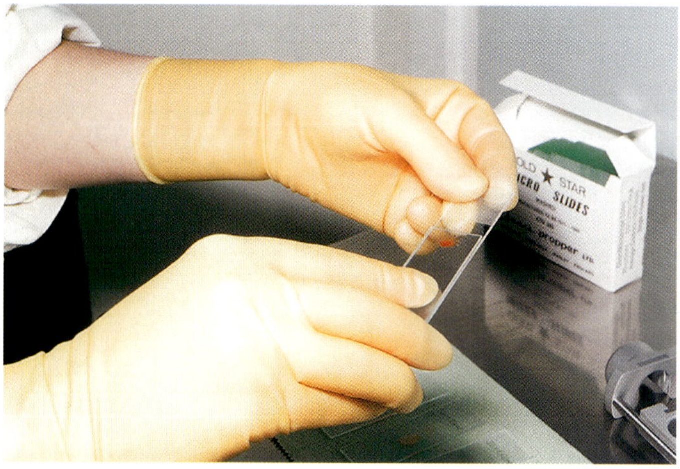

Figure 1.8 FNAC smearing procedure. Although there are various ways of spreading material onto the slide, we find that the most uniformly spread material is obtained when two glass slides are pulled over each other parallel. The top slide should not be at an angle but flat on top of the bottom slide. Otherwise it creates uneven thickness of the smear and ridges with accumulation of cells and various fixation artefacts.

majority of material in the centre of the slide (Fig. 1.9). This enables easier stain penetration and clearer microscopic image. Excess of blood is undesirable since this dilutes cellular material. Fibrin clots tend to aggregate cellular material and make them uninterpretable (Fig. 10). The solution is spun in the laboratory with the aid of a cytocentrifuge. Material on the slides, either smeared directly or spun, is either air dried or immediately fixed in 95% alcohol. Air dried smears are stained with May Grunweld Giemsa (MGG) (Romanowski). Alcohol fixed preparations are stained with Papanicolaou (PAP) stain. In the outpatient clinics, a rapid staining method is used to obtain an immediate microscopic image (Fig. 1.10). In our practice, we use mostly air dried smears since they are amenable to rapid staining techniques and immunocytochemistry. When deciding which method of cell preparation and fixation to use, the aspirator is guided by the clinical and pathological findings at the time of FNAC.

Some of the material at the time of aspiration may be sent for bacterial culture or washed in saline for molecular techniques.

WHO SHOULD BE PERFORMING FNAC?

It is our experience and that of others, that a good sampling technique is essential for the successful interpretation of

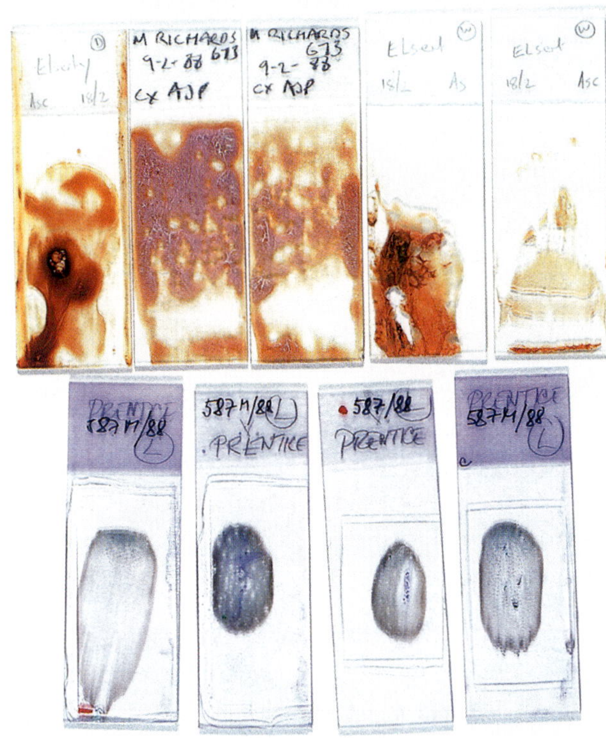

Figure 1.9 FNAC spreading. Material spread on the slides should be placed centrally and spread evenly so that the staining is even and screening easier (see bottom row of slides). Bloodstained smears (see top row) are unevenly spread, contain many blood clots and empty areas. When stained, much of the material may be washed off (see Fig. 1.10).

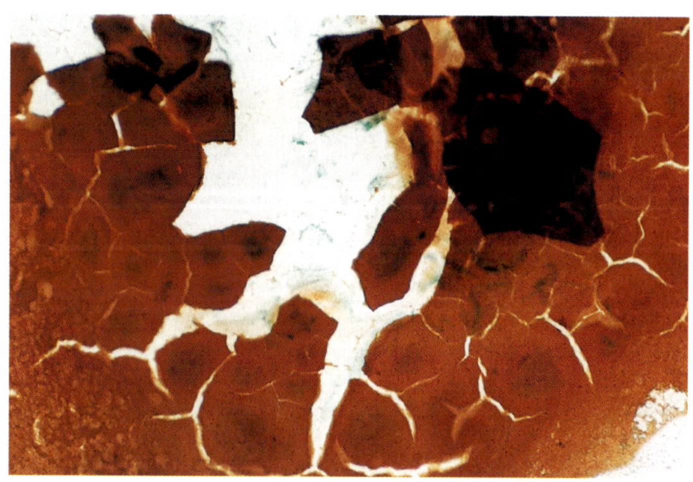

Figure 1.10 FNAC artefacts. Poorly spread bloodstained smears, as seen in Fig. 1.9 (top row), result in thick material, in which cells are trapped in the strands of fibrin or detached in the staining process as in this case. Material obtained in this way is unusuable.

FNAC. Comparing the material obtained in the FNAC clinic by the cytopathologist with the material sent from various aspirators, we found that the rate of material unsuitable for diagnosis was 9% and 46% respectively.[30] It is this that has prompted us to centralise the FNAC service where a cytopathologist performs aspiration. Similar experience was described by Cajulis et al, where the cytopathologist performed 59% of FNAC and clinicians performed 49%, achieving 100% and 77% diagnostic accuracy respectively.[31] The greater the experience of the operator the more improved the accuracy rate.[32]

The FNAC clinic, where the pathologist takes and reports optimally prepared and stained specimens, provides a high-quality and accurate service on which clinicians can confidently base clinical management decisions (Figs 1.11–1.13). Unnecessary investigations and operations are avoided, allowing resources to be released for other procedures.[33]

The triad of physical examination/clinical history, appropriate cell preparation and subsequent interpretation is essential for a successful FNAC service and is in our view best performed by fewer persons. Like others, we have experienced difficulties when different people have undertaken one or more components of this triad. Lack of skill, clinical information and communication has on occasions been detrimental to the result. The success rate of FNAC

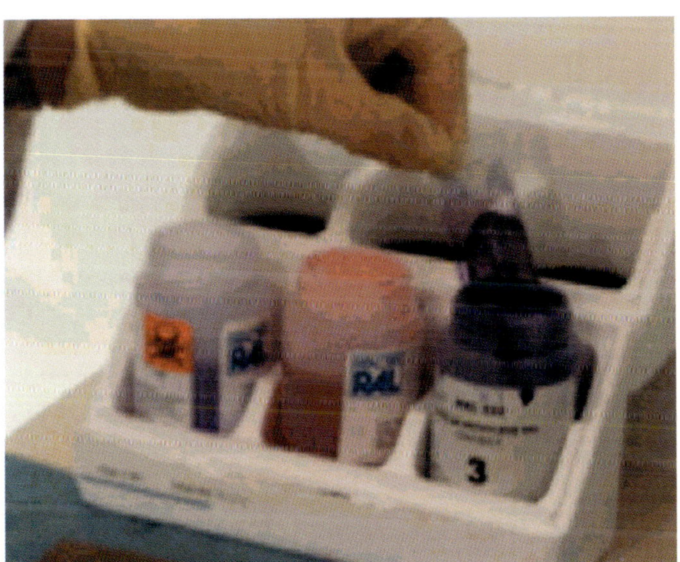

Figure 1.11 Rapid staining and examination. Slides are stained with one of the rapid stains and examined under the microscope for cellularity. This gives a good indication of whether further material is needed or if a different cell preparation technique should be applied.

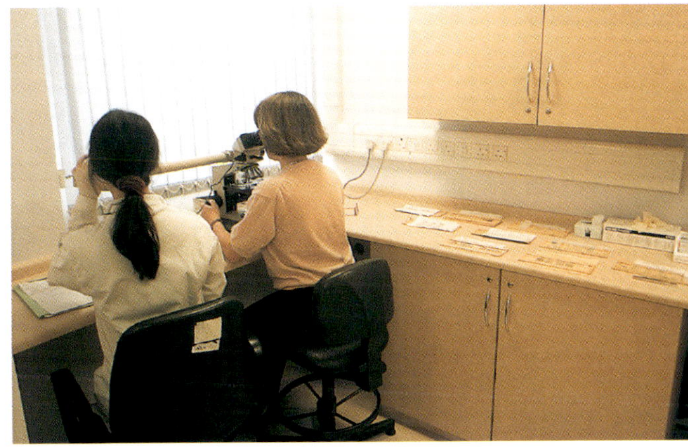

Figure 1.12 Examination of the slides in the clinic. This gives orientation of cellularity and indicates whether further samples need to be taken for special techniques and/or microbiology cultures.

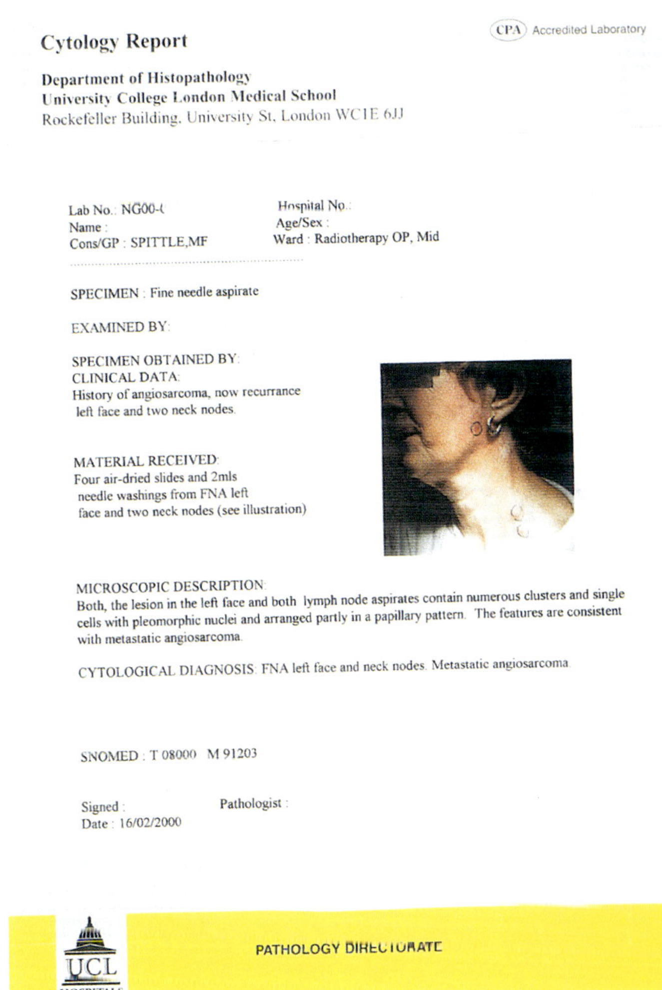

Cytology Report

CPA Accredited Laboratory

Department of Histopathology
University College London Medical School
Rockefeller Building, University St, London WC1E 6JJ

Lab No.: NG00-
Name :
Cons/GP : SPITTLE,MF

Hospital No.:
Age/Sex :
Ward : Radiotherapy OP, Mid

SPECIMEN : Fine needle aspirate

EXAMINED BY:

SPECIMEN OBTAINED BY:
CLINICAL DATA:
History of angiosarcoma, now recurrance left face and two neck nodes.

MATERIAL RECEIVED:
Four air-dried slides and 2mls needle washings from FNA left face and two neck nodes (see illustration)

MICROSCOPIC DESCRIPTION:
Both, the lesion in the left face and both lymph node aspirates contain numerous clusters and single cells with pleomorphic nuclei and arranged partly in a papillary pattern. The features are consistent with metastatic angiosarcoma.

CYTOLOGICAL DIAGNOSIS: FNA left face and neck nodes. Metastatic angiosarcoma

SNOMED : T 08000 M 91203

Signed :
Date : 16/02/2000

Pathologist :

UCL HOSPITALS

PATHOLOGY DIRECTORATE

Figure 1.13 Cytopathology report. The report should contain the patient's details and clinical history and the number and position of the site(s) sampled (preferably illustrated by photograph or diagram), as well as indicating the name of the aspirator, the date of the sample, the number of slides made and/or other material obtained, the microscopic description, the cytological diagnosis, the diagnostic code and the pathologist's signature and date.

diagnosis in material obtained by an experienced cytopathologist is far in excess of that where specimens are taken and sent to a laboratory for interpretation.[34]

References

1. Gertner R, Malberger E, Podoshin L, Fradis M, Lemberg S. [Fine needle aspiration in the cytologic diagnosis of head and neck lesions]. *Harefuah* 1978; 95(7): 203–5.
2. Murthy P, Laing MR, Palmer TJ. Fine needle aspiration cytology of head and neck lesions: an early experience. *J R Coll Surg Edinb* 1997; 42(5): 341–6.
3. Stevenson DS, Allison RS, Robertson MS, Hamer JW. Aspiration cytology in the diagnosis of head and neck masses: the early Christchurch experience. *N Z Med J* 1989; 102(881): 639–41.
4. Oyafuso MS, Longatto Filho A, Ikeda MK. The role of fine needle aspiration cytology in the diagnosis of lesions of the head and neck excluding the thyroid and salivary glands. *Tumori* 1992; 78(2): 134–6.
5. Ono T, Kawai F, Nakamura M, Taniguchi N, Itoh K. [Ultrasound-guided fine-needle aspiration cytology for neck lesions]. *Rinsho Byori* 1999; 47(12): 1173–6.
6. Guyot JP, Obradovic D, Krayenbuhl M, Zbaeren P, Lehmann W. Fine-needle aspiration in the diagnosis of head and neck growths: is it necessary? *Otolaryngol Head Neck Surg* 1990; 103(5 pt 1): 697–701.
7. Pradhan KC, Padhi NC, Dandapat MC. Evaluation of fine needle aspiration cytology in the diagnosis of head and neck masses. *J Indian Med Assoc* 1988; 86(4): 96–8.
8. Schelkun PM, Grundy WG. Fine-needle aspiration biopsy of head and neck lesions. *J Oral Maxillofac Surg* 1991; 49(3): 262–7.
9. Patt BS, Schaefer SD, Vuitch F. Role of fine-needle aspiration in the evaluation of neck masses. *Med Clin North Am* 1993; 77(3): 611–23.
10. Wilson JA, McIntyre MA, Tan J, Maran AG. The diagnostic value of fine needle aspiration cytology in the head and neck. *J R Coll Surg Edinb* 1985; 30(6): 375–9.
11. van den Brekel MW, Castelijns JA, Stel HV et al. Occult metastatic neck disease: detection with US and US-guided fine-needle aspiration cytology. *Radiology* 1991; 180(2): 457–61. (Published erratum appears in *Radiology* 1992; 182(1): 288.)
12. Lin CK. Fine needle aspiration biopsy cytology of head and neck masses: a personal experience in Republic of China. *Chung Hua I Hsueh Tsa Chih* 1988; 42(4): 255–60.
13. Oyafuso MS, Ikeda MK, Longatto Filho A. [Fine needle aspiration cytology in the diagnosis of head and neck tumors]. *Rev Paul Med* 1990; 108(4): 162–4. (Published erratum appears in *Rev Paul Med* 1991; 109(3): 140).
14. Fulciniti F, Califano L, Zupi A, Vetrani A. Accuracy of fine needle aspiration biopsy in head and neck tumors. *J Oral Maxillofac Surg* 1997; 55(10): 1094–7.
15. Slack RW, Croft CB, Crome LP. Fine needle aspiration cytology in the management of head and neck masses. *Clin Otolaryngol* 1985; 10(2): 93–6.
16. Carroll CM, Nazeer U, Timon CI. The accuracy of fine-needle aspiration biopsy in the diagnosis of head and neck masses. *Ir J Med Sci* 1998; 167(3): 149–51.
17. Makowska W, Bogacka-Zatorska E, Waloryszak B. [Fine needle aspiration biopsy in the diagnosis of head and neck tumors]. *Otolaryngol Pol* 1992; 46(3): 268-72.
18. McLean NR, Harrop-Griffiths K, Shaw HJ, Trott PA. Fine needle aspiration cytology in the head and neck region. *Br J Plast Surg* 1989; 42(4): 447–51.
19. Donahue BJ, Cruickshank JC, Bishop JW. The diagnostic value of fine needle aspiration biopsy of head and neck masses. *Ear Nose Throat J* 1995; 74(7): 483–6.
20. Flynn MB, Wolfson SE, Thomas S, Kuhns JG. Fine needle aspiration biopsy in clinical management of head and neck tumors. *J Surg Oncol* 1990; 44(4): 214–7.
21. Raju G, Kakar PK, Das DK, Dhingra PL, Bhambhani S. Role of fine needle aspiration biopsy in head and neck tumours. *J Laryngol Otol* 1988; 102(3): 248–51.
22. Mondal A, Gupta S. The role of peroral fine needle aspiration cytology (FNAC) in the diagnosis of parapharyngeal lesions – a study of 51 cases. *Indian J Pathol Microbiol* 1993; 36(3): 253–9.
23. Layfield LJ. Fine-needle aspiration of the head and neck. *Pathology (Phila)* 1996; 4(2): 409–38.
24. Keshtgar MR, Barker SG, Ell PJ. Needle-free vehicle for administration of radionuclide for sentinel-node biopsy [letter]. *Lancet* 1999; 353(9162): 1410–1.
25. Dey P, Ray R. Comparison of fine needle sampling by capillary action and fine needle aspiration. *Cytopathology* 1993; 4(5): 299–303.
26. Hamaker RA, Moriarty AT, Hamaker RC. Fine-needle biopsy techniques of aspiration versus capillary in head and neck masses. *Laryngoscope* 1995; 105(12 pt 1): 1311–4.
27. Kate MS, Kamal MM, Bobhate SK, Kher AV. Evaluation of fine needle capillary sampling in superficial and deep-seated lesions. An analysis of 670 cases. *Acta Cytol* 1998; 42(3): 679–84.
28. Mair S, Dunbar F, Becker PJ, Du Plessis W. Fine needle cytology – is aspiration suction necessary? A study of 100 masses in various sites [see comments]. *Acta Cytol* 1989; 33(6): 809–13.
29. Yue XH, Zheng SF. Cytologic diagnosis by transthoracic fine needle sampling without aspiration. *Acta Cytol* 1989; 33(6): 805–8.
30. Kocjan G. Evaluation of the cost effectiveness of establishing a fine needle aspiration cytology clinic in a hospital out-patient department. *Cytopathology* 1991; 2(1): 13–8.
31. Cajulis RS, Gokaslan ST, Yu GH, Frias-Hidvegi D. Fine needle aspiration biopsy of the salivary glands. A five-year experience with emphasis on diagnostic pitfalls. *Acta Cytol* 1997; 41(5): 1412–20.
32. Jandu M, Webster K. The role of operator experience in fine needle aspiration cytology of head and neck masses. *Int J Oral Maxillofac Surg* 1999; 28(6): 441–4.
33. Yu X, Zhang C, Huang S. [Study on measures to increase diagnostic accuracy of FNAC of breast masses]. *Chung Hua Ping Li Hsueh Tsa Chih* 1997; 26(6): 334–6.
34. Morton KD. Fine needle aspiration cytology of lesions of the head and neck and factors affecting outcome. *Scott Med J* 1989; 34(5): 523–5.

2

Salivary glands

Introduction
Non-neoplastic and inflammatory conditions
Benign tumours of the salivary gland
Malignant tumours of the salivary glands
Miscellaneous tumours

INTRODUCTION

Cytological diagnosis of salivary gland lesions is becoming one of the most sought after requests in the preoperative clinical management of patients. Therefore, cytopathologists have to be familiar with the main principles necessary for safe practice. First, the anatomical site of the material is important. If it is within the area of major and minor salivary glands, it is important to establish if the lesion involves salivary gland or has arisen in adjacent tissues such as lymph nodes or skin (Fig. 2.1). Second, it is important to decide whether or not the lesion is neoplastic. In many series, non-neoplastic lesions make for over 50% of fine needle aspiration cytology (FNAC) requests and fewer than 10% of these had subsequent surgery.[1] Third, if the lesion is neoplastic, the cytopathologist has to decide whether it is benign or malignant (low or high grade). The distinction is desirable since benign tumours may not require surgery and highly malignant tumours may require the planning of a more radical surgical procedure. Cytological diagnosis of malignancy is based on well-established cytological criteria: nuclear enlargement, pleomorphism, chromatin pattern, nucleoli, cytoplasmic differentiation, cell cohesiveness and arrangement and presence of background stromal material, as well as on the clinical history and presentation.[2] From a practical point of view, cytological subtyping of malignant salivary gland tumours is unnecessary since it rarely influences management. Although diagnosis of some common tumours is not difficult in most cases, sampling error may cause difficulties in interpretation.

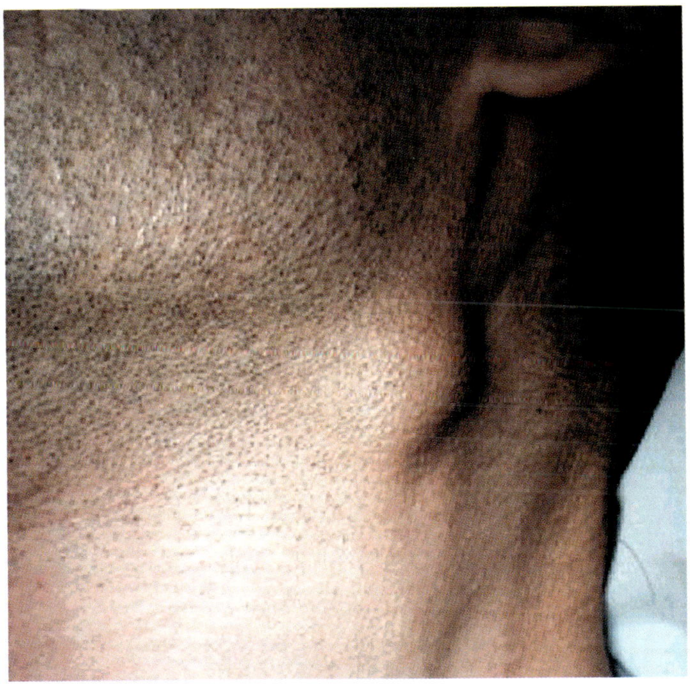

Figure 2.1 A patient presented with a swelling at the upper neck of 4 weeks duration. Clinically it was thought to be a Warthin's tumour. FNAC was requested to establish the anatomy and nature of the lesion. The patient was found to have a granulomatous lymphadenitis consistent with tuberculosis. The material obtained was sent for mycobacterial culture and the patient was treated appropriately.

Diagnostic accuracy

Cytopathologists interpreting FNAC of the salivary gland should be aware of the diagnostic features of common conditions. However, as large series have shown, even in the best hands, cytological interpretation of salivary gland cytology does not have a 100% sensitivity and specificity (Table 2.1).[3–13] False-negative and false-positive diagnoses are described in most series. However, if type-specific diag-

Table 2.1 Sensitivity and specificity of salivary gland FNAC in some of the series carried out between 1990 and 2000

Author (year)	No. of cases	Sensitivity	Specificity
Orell (1995)[1]	325	85.5	99.5
Candel et al (1993)[6]	1022	95.7	100
Frable & Frable (1991)[8]	552	93.3	99
Cajulis et al (1997)[7]	151	91	96
Kocjan et al (1990)[9]	45	89	94
Young et al (1990)[13]	79	84	98.4
Jayaram (1994)[13a]	195	87.8	98.0
Stewart et al (2000)[10]	341	92	100
Goh (1998)[10a]	93	94.7	100
Cristallini et al (1997)[5]	153	97.6	98.4
Al-Khafaji et al (1998)[4]	154	82	86
Shintani et al (1997)[11]	43	88.9	94.1
Chan et al (1992)[3]	112	86	99
Murthy et al (1997)[12]	91	77.7	93.3

noses are made only when all diagnostic criteria are present and any uncertainty clearly conveyed to the clinician, FNAC is a safe and accurate tool in the investigation of salivary gland lesions.[1] The pitfalls in cytological interpretation can be avoided with increased practice. Special training is required to become proficient in both obtaining and interpreting aspirated material. It is not sufficient for pathologists to apply personal experience from tissue pathology to the diagnosis of cytological specimens.

Role of FNAC in management of salivary gland lesions

Although it is accepted that clinical and radiological assessment (including two-phase helical CT) of parotid masses cannot distinguish reliably between benign and malignant lesions,[14] the value of FNAC in the evaluation and management of salivary gland pathology has been controversial for a long time. The major reasons for this controversy are the difficulty in cytological evaluation and the fact that the extent of surgery can be easily defined based on clinical judgement, particularly at a cancer referral centre (where clinicians may be experienced at diagnosing parotid gland malignancies).[4] However, a preoperative diagnosis is helpful in discussions with patients regarding the extent and type of surgery necessary. Most centres using salivary gland FNAC do so selectively, in an attempt to obtain a preoperative diagnosis in order to distinguish between neoplasms and non-neoplastic conditions and thus avoid surgery in conditions that clinically mimic neoplasm. A combination of MRI findings and cytology results is optimal for diagnosing malignancies of the parotid lesions.[15]

Apart from the fact that FNAC can distinguish benign from malignant conditions, it is also very useful in distinguishing between salivary and other non-salivary pathology. Preoperative diagnosis of Warthin's tumour, lymphoma or benign lymphoepithelial disease is essential to the correct management of these patients.[16] With FNAC, surgical excision is often unnecessary.

When assessing the impact of FNAC of salivary gland masses in clinical decision making, Heller et al[17] compared the clinician's initial clinical impression with the FNAC diagnosis and the final diagnosis in each case. Overall, FNAC resulted in a change in the clinical approach to 35% of the patients. As a result, they recommend the performance of FNAC in almost all patients with salivary masses.[17] FNAC provides accurate diagnosis of most salivary gland lesions and contributes to conservative management in many patients with non-neoplastic conditions.[10] By using FNAC, an operation was avoided in 70% and 79% of patients with a non-neoplastic lesion and a metastasis respectively.[18] FNAC plays an important role in the preoperative and postoperative assessment of parotid masses by aiding in the evaluation of tumours in poor surgical candidates and unresectable tumours, and by identifying metastases from other sites. Although definitive subclassification of some lesion types remains poor, FNAC is invaluable in patient triage.

Diagnostic difficulties

The wide spectrum of benign and malignant tumours as well as the heterogeneity of many tumours poses a formidable task for any cytopathologist with an ambition for a good histological correlation of his or her findings. The original series of salivary gland tumours described by Zajicek and co-workers at the Karolinska hospital in the 1960s and 1970s described the tumour types known at the time.[19] Since that time, many new entities have been described. The newest World Health Organization classification of salivary gland tumours now includes 9 benign tumours (adenomas) and 18 malignant tumours (carcinomas), with the addition of non-epithelial tumours, malignant lymphoma, tumour-like lesions and metastatic tumours (Box 2.1).[20] There is sometimes overlap between different conditions showing similar appearances.

Problem areas in FNAC of salivary gland lesions are: cystic lesions (neoplastic and non-neoplastic); atypical cells in pleomorphic adenoma; cellular smears with epithelial cells and no stroma; squamous or 'squamoid differentiation', tumours with a 'clear cell' pattern, hyaline stromal globules and prominent lymphoid component in some lesions.[21–25] These present potential pitfalls, of which the cytopathologist needs to be aware and, if necessary, include differential diagnosis as part of the final report. The clinician will thus plan further management and decide about the need for surgery on clinical grounds, knowing that only the final histology will give the full answer.

Salivary gland tumours are composed of epithelial cells, myoepithelial cells and stroma in various proportions. Cytological smears lack the architecture that is particularly important in differentiating some of the tumours. Some

Box 2.1 Revised World Health Organization classification of salivary gland tumours and tumour-like conditions[20]

1. Adenomas
1.1 Pleomorphic adenoma
1.2 Myoepithelioma (myoepithelial adenoma)
1.3 Basal cell adenoma
1.4 Warthin's tumour (adenolymphoma)
1.5 Oncocytoma (oncocytic adenoma)
1.6 Canalicular adenoma
1.7 Sebaceous adenoma
1.8 Ductal papilloma
1.8.1 Inverted ductal papilloma
1.8.2 Intraductal papilloma
1.8.3 Sialadenoma papilliferum
1.9 Cystadenoma
1.9.1 Papillary cystadenoma
1.9.2 Mucinous cystadenoma

2. Carcinomas
2.1 Acinic cell carcinoma
2.2 Mucoepidermoid carcinoma
2.3 Adenoid cystic carcinoma
2.4 Polymorphous low-grade adenocarcinoma (terminal duct adenocarcinoma)
2.5 Epithelial-myoepithelial carcinoma
2.6 Basal cell adenocarcinoma
2.7 Sebaceous carcinoma
2.8 Papillary cystadenocarcinoma
2.9 Mucinous adenocarcinoma
2.10 Oncocytic carcinoma
2.11 Salivary duct carcinoma
2.12 Adenocarcinoma (not otherwise specified)
2.13 Malignant myoepithelioma (myoepithelial carcinoma)
2.14 Carcinoma in pleomorphic adenoma
2.15 Squamous cell carcinoma
2.16 Small cell carcinoma
2.17 Undifferentiated carcinoma
2.18 Other carcinomas

3. Non-epithelial tumours

4. Malignant lymphomas

5. Secondary tumours

6. Unclassified tumours

7. Tumour-like lesions
7.1 Sialadenosis
7.2 Oncocytosis
7.3 Necrotizing sialometaplasia (salivary gland infarction)
7.4 Benign lymphoepithelial lesion
7.5 Salivary gland cysts
7.6 Chronic selerosing sialadenitis of submandibular gland (Kuttner's tumour)
7.7 Cystic lymphoid hyperplasia in AIDS

tumours are so rare that a practising cytopathologist may not have come across the entity before, either during training or in practice. The lesions most frequently misdiagnosed are pleomorphic adenoma, mucoepidermoid carcinoma, chronic sialadenitis and malignant lymphoma. Problems may also be encountered in differentiating hematopoietic from non-hematopoietic lesions and with the interpretation of spindle cell neoplasms, acinic cell carcinoma, adenoid cystic carcinoma, lymphoproliferative disorders and post-irradiation changes.[7]

In a series reported by MacLeod & Frable, diagnostic pitfalls present only a minority (21 out of 582 in 17 years) and therefore should not distract from the fact that most salivary gland lesions can be diagnosed with confidence as benign or malignant from cytological material.[26]

Despite the relative rarity of salivary gland tumours, if established diagnostic criteria are present and strictly observed, the great majority of the common variants of the non-neoplastic and both benign and malignant salivary gland tumours can be diagnosed with a high level of accuracy.[27]

FNAC versus frozen section diagnosis histology

The minimal recommended surgical approach to parotid tumours is partial parotidectomy with resection of the superficial lobe of the gland. Histological diagnosis prior to surgery is not possible, as incisional biopsies are contraindicated due to the possibility of facial nerve injury or incomplete tumour resection. Thus, if performed at all, the biopsies tend to be perioperative.[28] When comparing the outcomes of 171 salivary gland FNACs with subsequent histology, Layfield et al[29] found that the false-positive rate of fine needle aspiration in this series was 3.5% and false-negative 4.7%. Corresponding frozen sections in 38 cases showed an exact histological correlation in 58% of cases, with no false positives but with 11% false negatives.[29] A comparison of the cytological diagnosis and frozen section made by Chan et al[3] showed that the overall diagnostic accuracy of FNAC for diagnosis of malignant and benign salivary gland tumours was 95% and for frozen section, 91%.[3] The accuracy in diagnosing the exact category of neoplastic disease was 70% and 77% respectively. The diagnostic sensitivity for malignant disease was 86% and 70%, and specificity 99% and 100% respectively. Frozen section, however, did supplement the FNAC diagnosis in some cases. Carvalho et al[28] found that sensitivity of the frozen sections for malignancy was 61.5% (95% CI 54–69%) and specificity was 98% (95% CI 94–100%).[28]

Cost-effectiveness

FNAC is a quick, safe and inexpensive method for obtaining material for pathological diagnosis. It is most useful in the diagnosis of a malignant tumour but it is probably most cost-effective in avoiding surgery. Current indications are that the FNAC will be used with increasing frequency for reasons involving both clinical practice and cost containment.[30,31]

Rapid cytology reporting of salivary gland FNAC

The speed with which FNAC can provide a diagnosis has so far been utilised mostly in the so-called 'one-stop breast clinic'. However, there are reports on the application of rapid reporting of FNAC in patients with salivary gland lesions in a head and neck surgery clinic.[32] The aspirates are reported immediately by a cytopathologist and the reports conveyed to the surgeon during the same clinic visit. FNAC results are then compared with histology in those patients who undergo surgery or with the clinical course of the disease at subsequent clinic visits for patients in whom surgery was not performed. In a series of 92 patients, Roland et al[32] found that the cytological diagnosis was incorrect in 5 cases, 1 of which was a false-negative result. There were no false-positive results. The sensitivity was 90.9% and the specificity 100%. This rapid report system of FNAC has been found to be safe, free of complications and helpful in the planning of treatment.[32]

FNAC procedure and potential complications

In most instances, FNAC is performed in a standard manner with the aid of a Cameco syringe or according to a non-aspiration technique (Figs 2.2 and 2.3).[19,33–38] In both instances, a 22G or thinner needle is applied. A local anaesthetic is usually not given except in cases where the patient is needle-phobic or the area is tender. One or two passes with a needle usually produces sufficient material. The material is spread onto a slide as a direct smear and needle

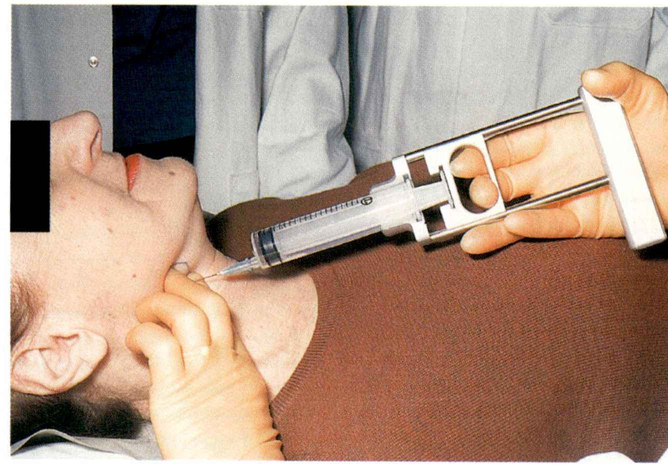

Figure 2.2 FNAC of a submandibular swelling is performed with the aid of a syringe holder, using a 23G needle.

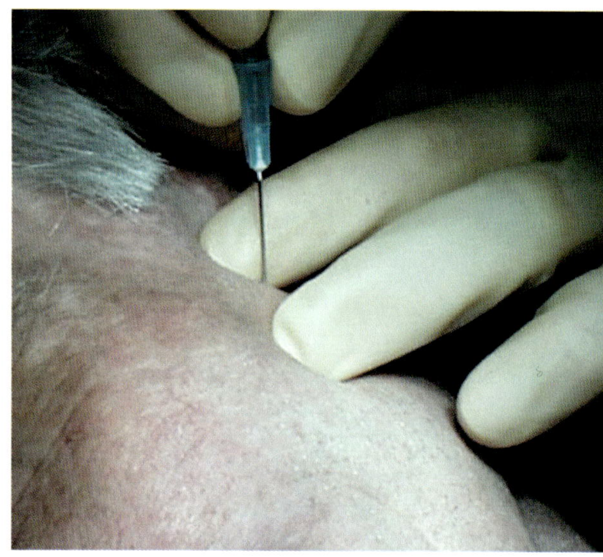

Figure 2.3 Capillary FNAC is used in most cases of head and neck swellings. A 3G or thinner needle can be used and rapid movements of the needle within the swelling provide sufficient cells.

washings are taken for special stains where appropriate. Slides are either air dried or alcohol fixed. Rapid staining in the clinic usually establishes the cellularity and gives an indication of the type of the lesion so that extra material can be obtained if necessary.

FNAC of the salivary gland is a safe procedure with no sinister complications, although patients often experience discomfort, particularly with FNAC of non-neoplastic conditions. However, the main concern is obviously whether the needle interference with the lesion will eventually lead to a higher recurrence rate in some tumours. Provided the standard FNAC technique is applied and a standard-calibre needle (<21G, preferably 23 or 25G) is used, there is no evidence in many long-term follow-up studies of patients who have had preoperative FNAC, that it influences recurrence of tumours. Occasionally, haemorrhage is encountered. In the case of the submandibular glands, this sometimes results in the mouth bleeding through the salivary gland ducts. Although the immediate effect of FNAC procedure is dramatic, the bleeding is at the same time reassuring in terms of patency of the salivary gland duct.

Recent reports[39,40] suggest certain histological changes associated with preoperative FNAC of benign parotid lesions and point to the features that distinguish these changes from malignant neoplasms. A spectrum of histological alterations was observed, including squamous cell metaplasia, infarction and necrosis, subepithelial stromal hyalinisation, acute and chronic haemorrhage and inflammation with multinucleated giant cells, granulation tissue with subsequent fibrosis, cholesterol cleft formation, pseudoxanthomatous reaction, pseudocapsular invasion and microcystic degeneration. In cases with exuberant squamous metaplasia, necrosis or subepithelial stromal hyalinisation, a diagnosis of squamous cell carcinoma or low-grade mucoepidermoid carcinoma may be seriously considered. The knowledge of a previous FNAC procedure and awareness of its effects on histology of the subsequent parotidectomy specimens are necessary to avoid potential misdiagnosis.[39,40]

Incidence of salivary gland tumours

Salivary gland tumours are uncommon. Most swellings are due to inflammation or non-neoplastic disease. Fewer than 3% of tumours of the head and neck arise in the salivary glands. Most tumours are seen in the parotid gland; the ratio is approximately 100 parotid tumours to 10 submandibular tumours to 10 minor salivary gland tumours to 1 sublingual gland tumour.[41] Approximately 1 in 6 parotid tumours is malignant, 1 in 3 submandibular tumours is malignant and 3 in 4 tumours in minor salivary glands are malignant. The average annual age-adjusted incidence rate per 100 000 is 4.7 for benign tumours and 0.9 for malignant tumours. Incidence rates for both benign and malignant tumours increase with age until age 65–74 years and then decline. Benign mixed tumours occur more frequently in female patients, whereas Warthin's tumours and malignant tumours occur more frequently in male patients ($P < 0.05$). Warthin's tumour is rare in black patients. Salivary gland tumours are an uncommon but epidemiologically diverse group of tumours.

The value of ancillary techniques in evaluating salivary gland lesions

The immunohistochemical evaluation of diagnostic and prognostic value of the proliferating cell nuclear antigen (PCNA) and Ki-67 showed that the values of MIB-1 parameters increased progressively in benign lesions in comparison with the normal and in malignant neoplasms in comparison with non-neoplastic and benign lesions. PCNA and MIB-1 indices may be one of the markers for discriminating between benign and malignant tumours of the parotid gland (see page 44).

NON-NEOPLASTIC AND INFLAMMATORY CONDITIONS

Normal salivary gland cytology

FNAC samples from normal salivary glands are usually performed when there is an anatomical dilemma as to the nature of the swelling (lymph node, salivary gland, other?). The procedure is usually unduly painful and the material aspirated is poorly cellular. Smears consist of acinar cells, occasional ductal cells and fat cells (Fig. 2.4). Acinar cells are usually present in cohesive, branching aggregates with rounded edges. Serous acinar cells have eccentric, small, round nuclei with inconspicuous nucleoli and abundant vacuolated cytoplasm. Mucinous acinar cells, which are present abundantly in the submandibular gland, have intracytoplasmic mucin. Ductal cells are usually closely associated with acinar cells but may lie separately. They are arranged in flat, honeycomb sheets of small, cuboidal, tightly cohesive cells with centrally placed, relatively large nuclei and inconspicuous nucleoli (Fig. 2.5).

Normal salivary gland cells may show degenerative and regenerative changes due to inflammation, cyst formation, radiotherapy and chemotherapy. Acinar cell nuclei may present as bare nuclei surrounding the aggregates, sometimes in large numbers. They should not be mistaken for lymphocytes. The latter have a well-defined rim of cytoplasm and, apart from having a different chromatin pattern, are usually oval rather than round. Ductal cells may undergo squamous metaplasia.

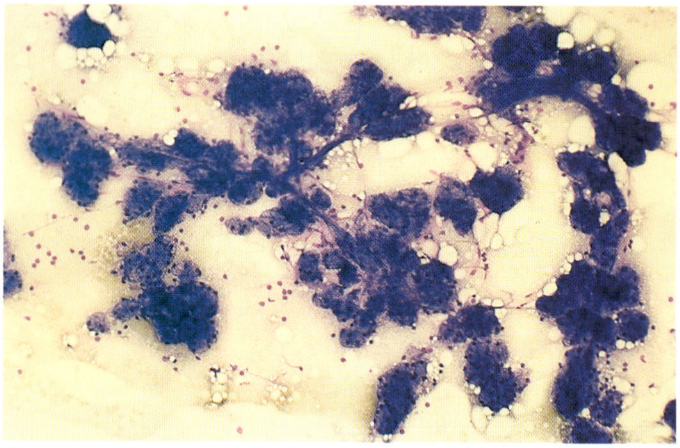

A

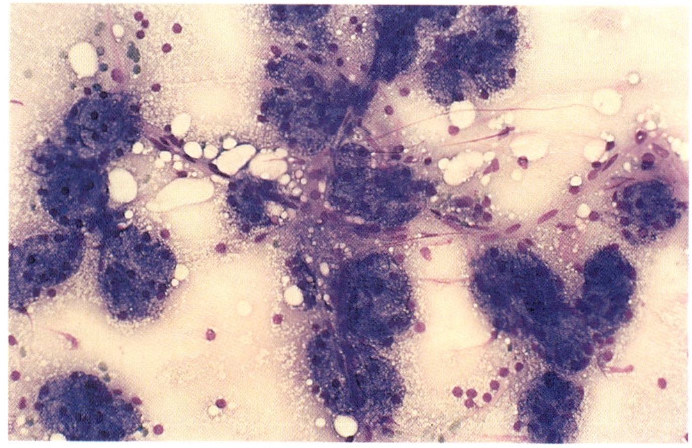

B

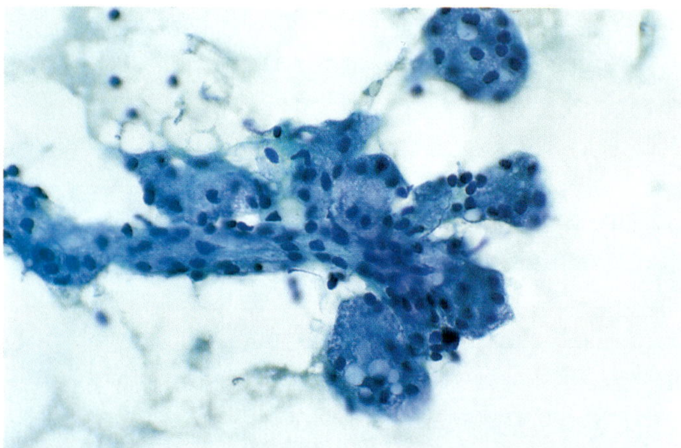

C

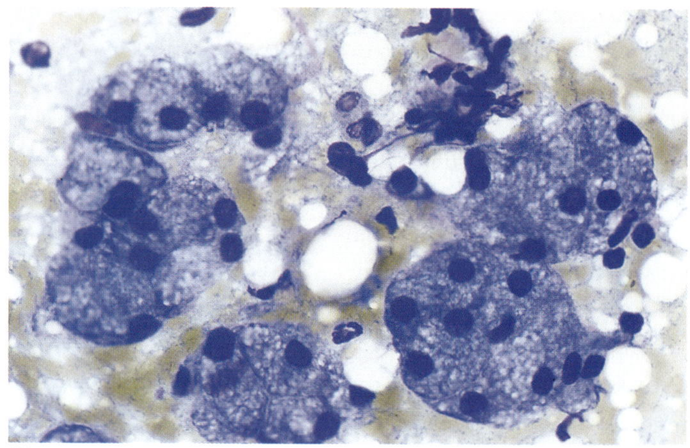

D

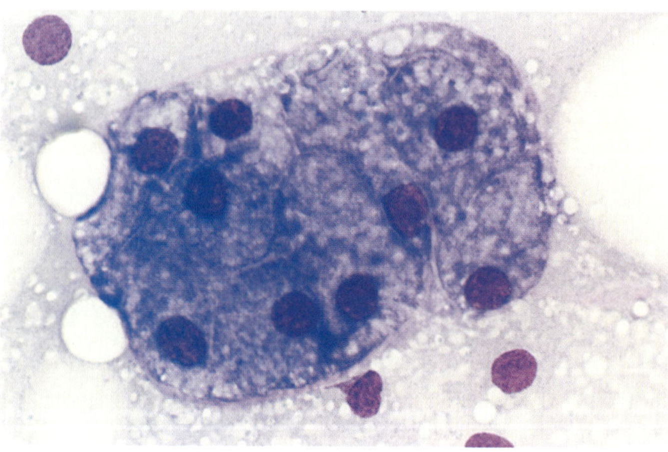

E

Figure 2.4 Normal salivary gland cytology. **A.** A low-power view reveals numerous tightly cohesive round aggregates held together like a bunch of grapes by capillaries and ducts (MGG ×100). **B.** Same case, higher power acinar cells in aggregates, only a few naked nuclei in the background. Capillaries and small fat vacuoles are frequently seen (MGG ×200). **C.** Similar features are shown on this alcohol-fixed smear. Well-outlined acini, ducts and fat cells (Papanicolaou ×200). **D.** Ducts and acini are often in close proximity (MGG ×600, oil immersion). **E.** Acinar cells have eccentric, relatively small nuclei and inconspicuous nucleoli. Cytoplasm is vacuolated, abundant and well outlined in well-preserved cells. There are, however, often bare nuclei of acinar cells in the background. These should not be confused with lymphocytes.

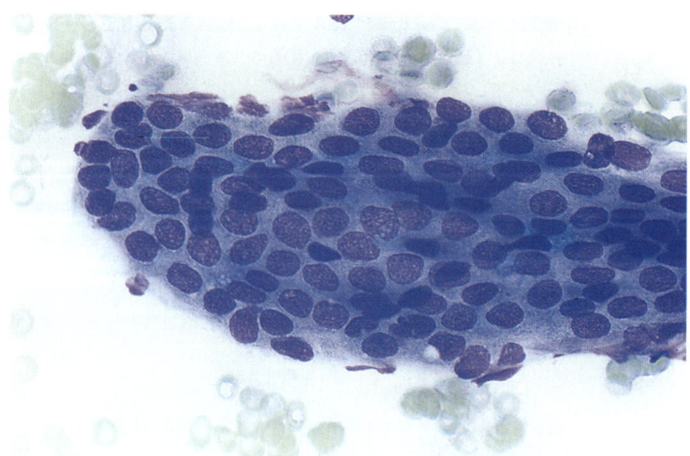

Figure 2.5 Ductal cells. Ductal epithelium of the normal salivary gland is usually closely associated with acinar cells but may lie separately. It is arranged in flat, honeycomb sheets of small cuboidal cells (MGG ×600).

Sialadenosis

Sialadenosis refers to a non-inflammatory, painless, non-neoplastic, often recurrent enlargement of the salivary glands, usually associated with an underlying systemic disorder. Bilateral and symmetric, it usually affects parotid and occasionally submandibular or minor salivary glands.[42] It is seen in alcoholism, malnutrition, diabetes, anorexia nervosa, bulimia and some other disorders. There is no sex predilection, and the peak age incidence is between 30 and 70 years. The common underlying pathogenesis for this seemingly disparate group of patients is a peripheral autonomic neuropathy, seen as a demyelinating polyneuropathy. This seems to be responsible for disordered metabolism and secretion, resulting in acinar enlargement.[43,44] Histologically, salivary glands show enlargement of the acini and increased granulation of serous cells; in chronic disease there is acinar atrophy and fatty replacement of the salivary gland.

Fine needle aspiration is performed on painless, diffuse parotid swellings (Fig. 2.6). FNAC smears reveal relatively cellular aspirates containing clusters of enlarged acini and numerous naked nuclei of acinar origin in the background (Fig. 2.7A, B). There is an absence of inflammatory cells. In the chronic phase, degeneration of acini and replacement of epithelium with fat cells is seen (Fig. 2.7C, D). Gupta et al[47] performed morphometric measurements, which showed a significant increase in mean acinar diameter in a sialadenotic gland as compared to a normal gland (76.03 μ vs. 53.79 μ). Cytomorphological features of sialadenosis are distinctive enough to enable a diagnosis 'consistent with sialadenosis'.[45]

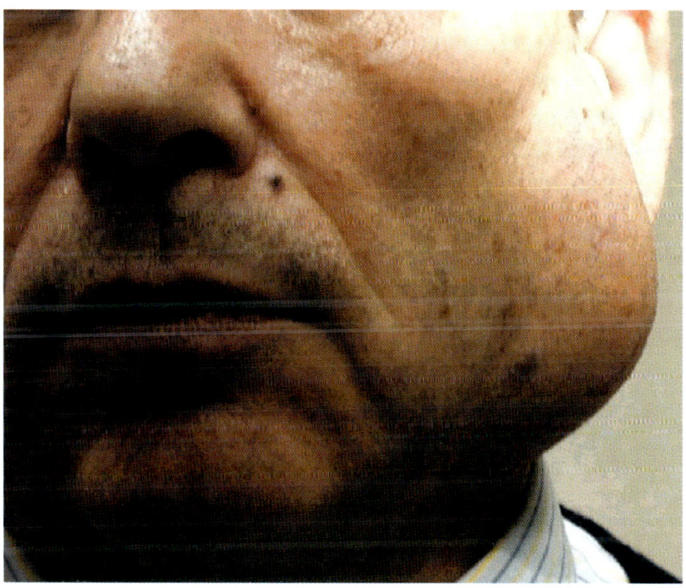

Figure 2.6 Sialadenosis. Patients present with a longstanding history of diffuse painless swelling. The lesion is soft, not clearly demarcated but mobile. FNAC produces fatty material.

Recognising sialadenosis is important because it may point to the unsuspected presence of underlying systemic disease.[46] It also excludes other causes of diffuse, painless enlargement of the salivary gland, e.g. lymphoepithelial lesions. It is important to be aware of this entity, as most cases do not require surgical intervention.[47] Management of sialadenosis depends upon identification of the underlying cause, which must then be corrected. In bulimic patients, the swellings may be refractory to standard treatment modalities, and parotidectomy may be considered as a last resort to improve unacceptable aesthetics.

Salivary gland cysts

Mucocele

Mucocele is a painless, soft, diffuse swelling of the salivary gland due to extravasation of saliva/mucus. It is rare in submandibular glands. Clinically it may be mistaken for tumour (Fig. 2.8). It may occur as a sequel of surgery for benign tumours. Cytologically, there is dense mucinous background (PAS-D positive) with foamy macrophages (Fig. 2.9). Absence of inflammation or epithelium is significant in excluding other pathology. Treatment is surgical excision (Box 2.2).

Box 2.2 Cystic lesions of the salivary glands

Non-neoplastic
Lymphoepithelial cyst
Retention cyst
Mucocele
Branchial cleft cyst
Dermoid cyst
Epidermoid cyst

Neoplastic

Benign
Warthin's tumour
Pleomorphic adenoma
Cystadenoma

Malignant
Mucoepidermoid carcinoma
Acinic cell carcinoma

Modified from Orell[1]

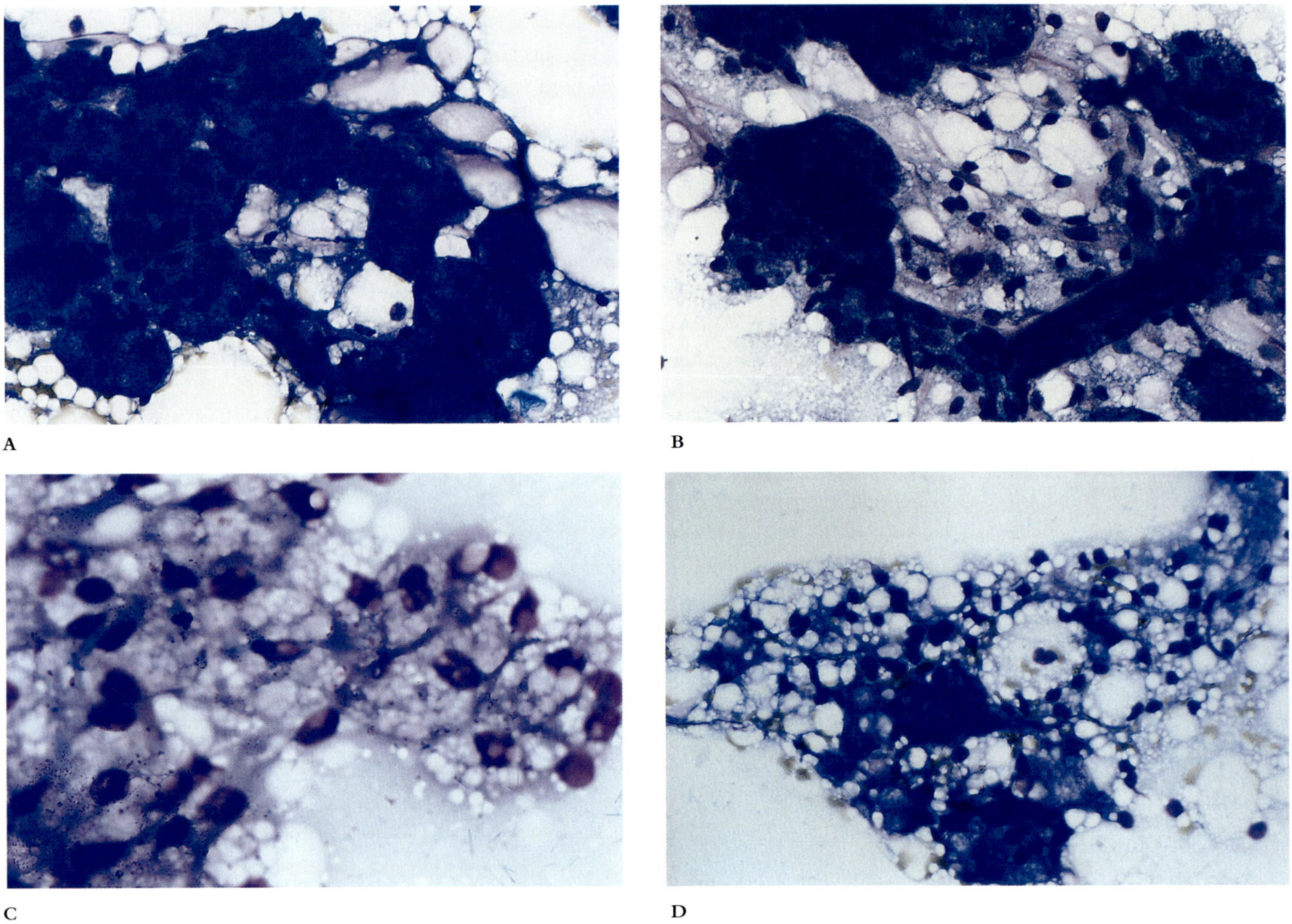

Fig. 2.7 FNAC of sialadenosis. **A.** Smears contain enlarged acini interspersed with fat cells. **B.** High-power view, same case (MGG ×400). **C.** Increased granulation of cells reflecting the acinar atrophy and fatty replacement of the salivary gland (MGG ×600). **D.** Epithelium is gradually bring replaced by fat (MGG ×400).

Retention cyst

Retention cyst is a salivary gland swelling due to obstruction. The content of the cyst is usually turbid fluid. Microscopy reveals dense proteinaceous background, debris, macrophages, some epithelial cells (columnar or squamous) and variable degrees of inflammation (Fig. 2.10). Differential diagnosis of squamous cells in FNAC of salivary gland lesions includes chronic sialadenitis, lymphoepithelial cyst, branchial cleft cyst (Fig. 2.10C), pleomorphic adenoma (Fig. 2.32C), Warthin's tumour (Fig. 2.36), mucoepidermoid carcinoma (Fig. 2.42) and squamous cell carcinoma (Fig. 2.60). The squamous cells may be a defining feature of the lesion, or an occasional and thus unexpected finding, with a consequent potential for misdiagnosis (Table 2.3).[48,49]

Lymphoepithelial cyst

Lymphoepithelial cyst of the salivary gland has been known about for nearly 100 years but was uncommon until the 1990s. Since then it has been seen more frequently in association with HIV infection. The equivalent proliferation fraction of the epithelial compartment in both lymphoepithelial cysts (HIV related) and salivary retention cysts (HIV non-related) are consistent with the hypothesis that cyst formation is secondary to the obstruction of salivary ducts by exuberant lymphoid infiltration (Box 2.2).[50]

FNAC is an appropriate tool for diagnosing these lesions and may sometimes be the first indication of an underlying retroviral infection. Histologically, cysts are lined by

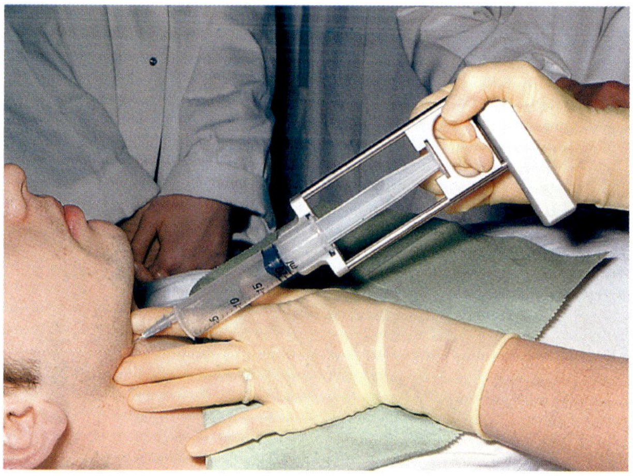

Figure 2.8. Submandibular swelling in this 13-year-old boy provoked alarm since it did not subside after treatment with antibiotics or reduce in size with time. He was sent to us for investigation of a possible Hodgkin's lymphoma. FNAC yielded tenacious mucoid transparent material.

stratified squamous epithelium, have cystic areas and lymphoid cells including lymphoid follicles with germinal centres.

Patients present with non-tender, diffuse swellings in either or both of the parotid glands, gradually increasing in size over 6 months (Fig. 2.11). FNAC yields 2-5 ml of yellow to brown, non-viscous fluid. Smears show a dense proteinaceous background with small and large lymphocytes and occasional lymphoid aggregates (residual follicle centre cell fragments) (Fig. 2.12). Small and polygonal non-keratinised squamous cells are dispersed in this material and are, in our experience, invariably sparse and show degenerate changes. Macrophages, siderophages and multinucleate giant cells are also seen.[51] These show p24 (HIV-1) protein positivity, which can be a useful diagnostic marker, particularly in cases that lack epithelial component. Amylase crystalloids, described in sialadenitis, may also be present.[52]

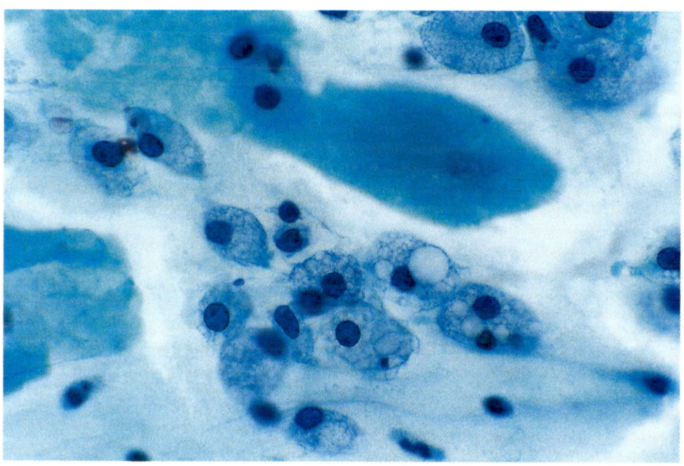

A

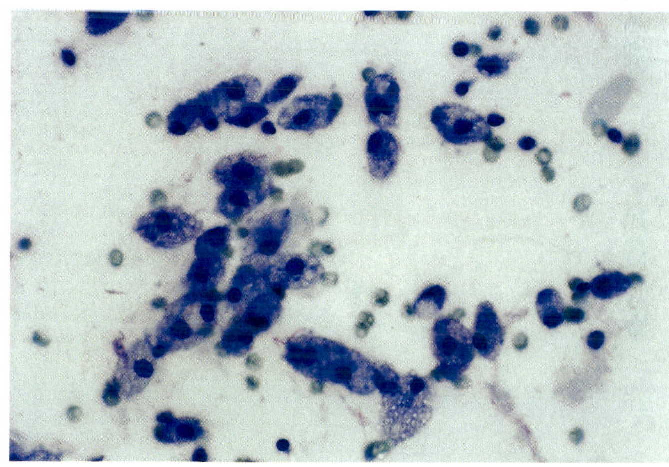

B

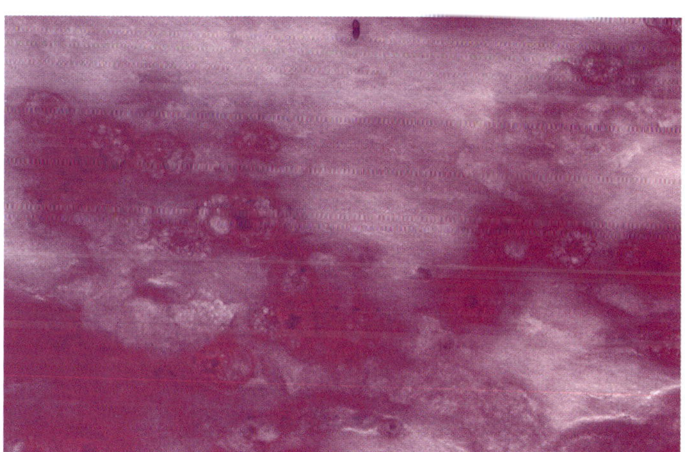

C

Fig. 2.9 Mucocele. Same patient as in 2.8. **A.** Mucocele FNAC smears contain macrophages against a mucinous background (PAP ×600 oil). **B.** MGG shows macrophages (×400). **C.** PAS diastase shows background mucin (PAS-D ×400).

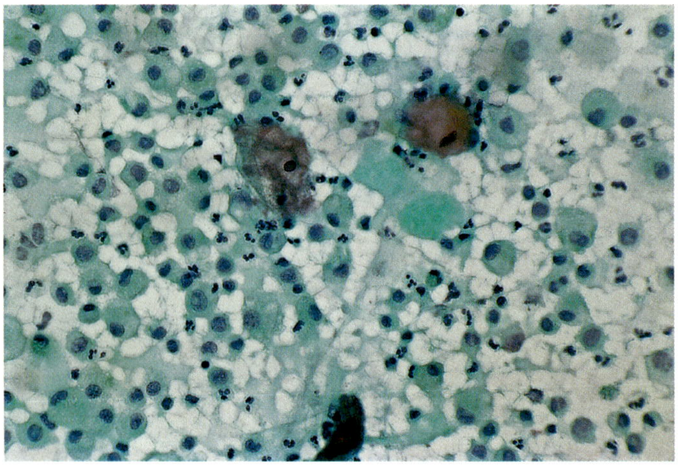

A

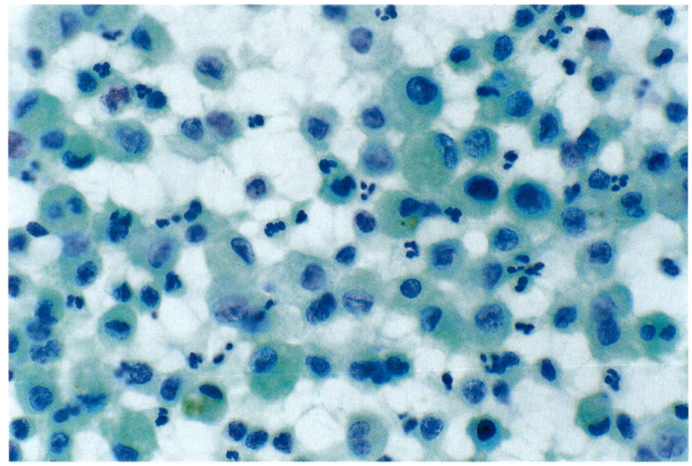

B

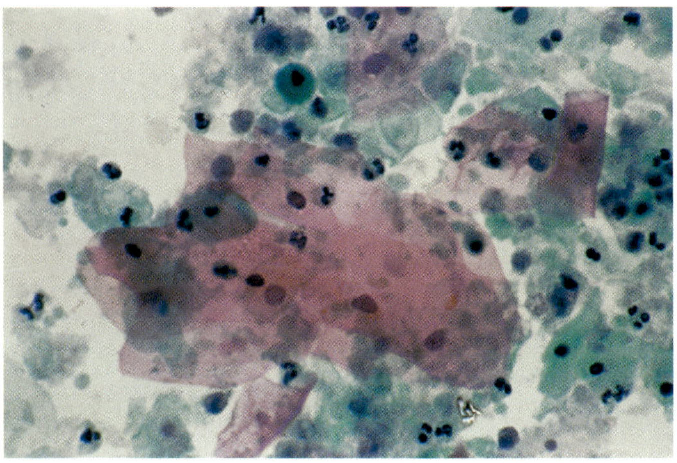

C

Figure 2.10 Retention cyst and branchial cleft cyst. Low-power view reveals many inflammatory cells, macrophages, debris and degenerate epithelial cells (PAP ×200). **B.** Same case. Secondary infection in a retention cyst, usually caused by sialolithiasis, is reflected by numerous polymorphs in addition to macrophages and degenerate epithelium (PAP ×400). **C.** Branchial cleft cyst. This contains many mature squamous cells, anucleate squamous cells and inflammatory cells. Macrophages are comparatively sparse (PAP ×400).

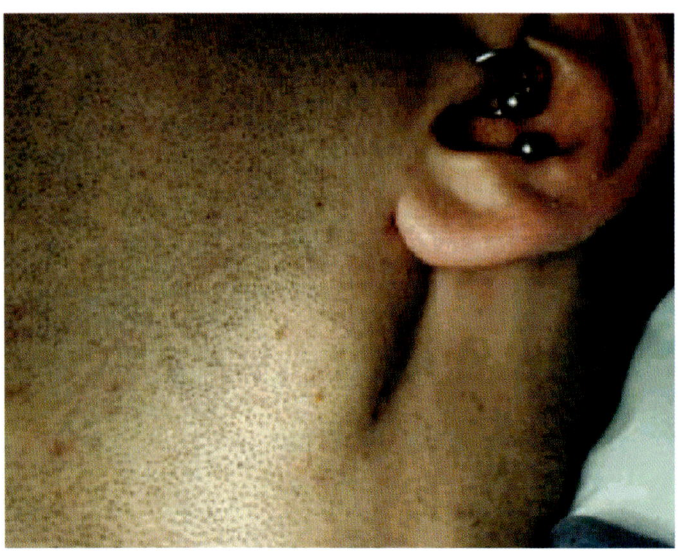

Figure 2.11 Lymphoepithelial cyst. 34-year-old HIV-positive patient presented with a 6-month history of painless, diffuse soft swelling at the angle of mandible. FNAC yielded bloodstained fluid.

Differential diagnosis, cytologically, includes epidermoid cyst, dermoid cyst, low-grade mucoepidermoid carcinoma, Warthin's tumour, cystic benign lymphoepithelial lesion and non-Hodgkin's lymphoma (Box 2.2). In epidermoid and dermoid cysts, there is an absence of lymphoid cells. Cystic low-grade mucoepidermoid carcinoma may produce mucin with a few lymphocytes, mucin-producing cells and a few squamous cells with minimal nuclear atypia. Mucoepidermoid carcinoma lacks the polymorphic population of lymphoid cells.[53] Warthin's tumour showing squamous metaplasia and secondary inflammation is also a potential source of error. Oncocytes and mast cells need to be present for a confident diagnosis of Warthin's tumour. Lymphoid cells from a lymphoepithelial cyst, particularly in HIV-positive patients, may come from hyperplastic germinal centres, which is reflected in a large number of centroblasts in the FNAC material. These may give the impression

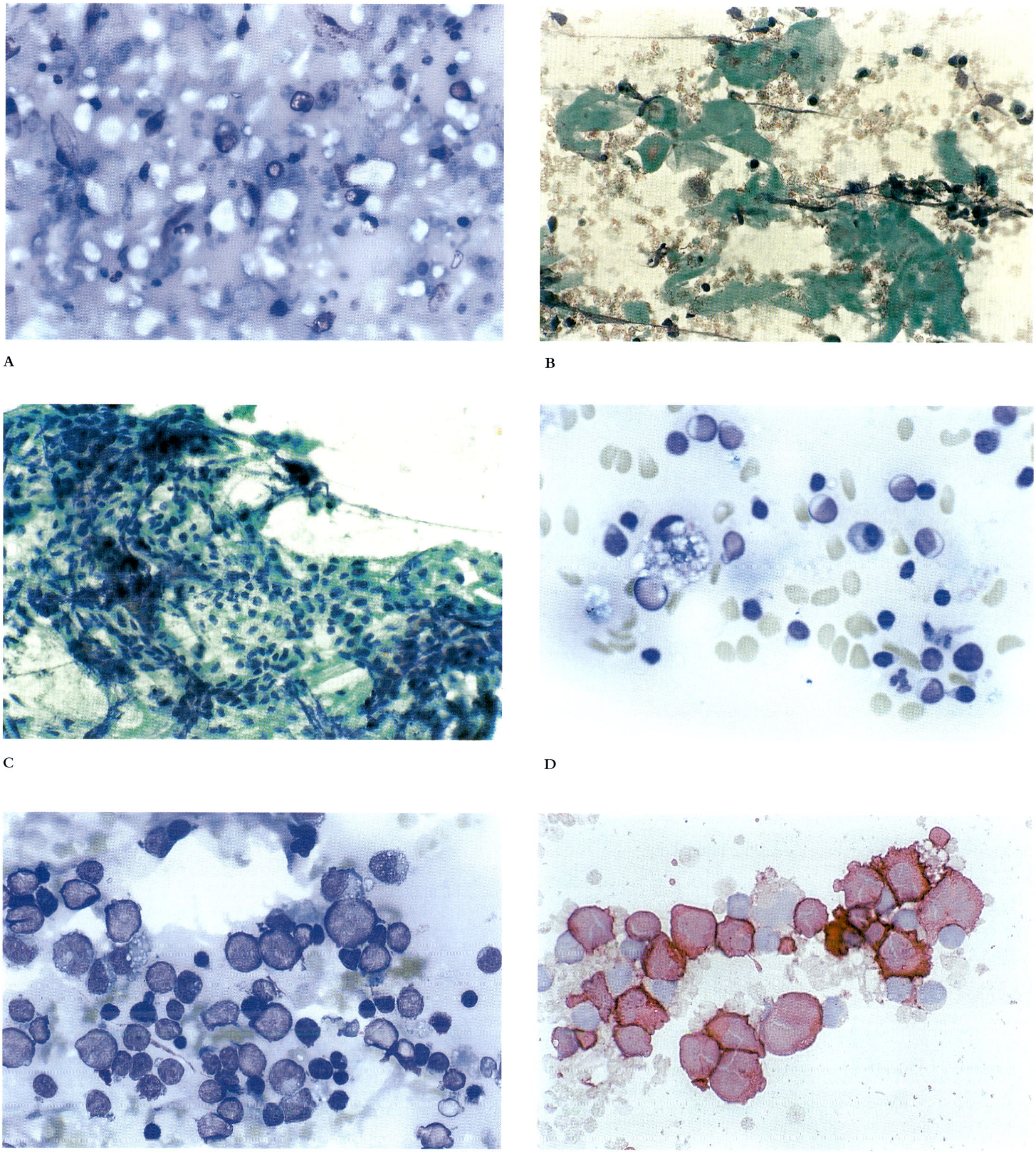

Figure 2.12 Lymphoepithelial cyst. **A.** Dense proteinaceous background with lymphoid cells and macrophages (MGG ×400). **B.** Same case. PAP stain (×400) reveals anucleate squamous cells and background debris. **C.** Only rarely are large epithelial fragments seen (PAP ×200). **D.** Lymphoid cells include a variety of follicle centre cells (MGG ×600 oil). **E.** Sometimes centroblasts are numerous and may mislead diagnosis (MGG ×600). **F.** CD20 positivity in the majority of blasts may be assumed incorrectly to be a lymphoma. ***(continued overleaf)***

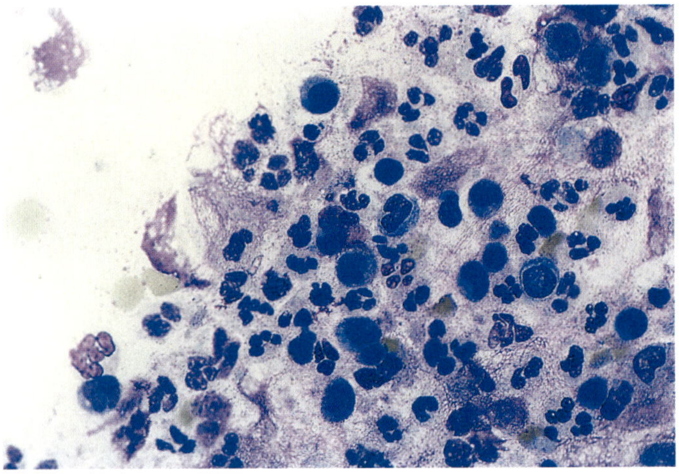

G

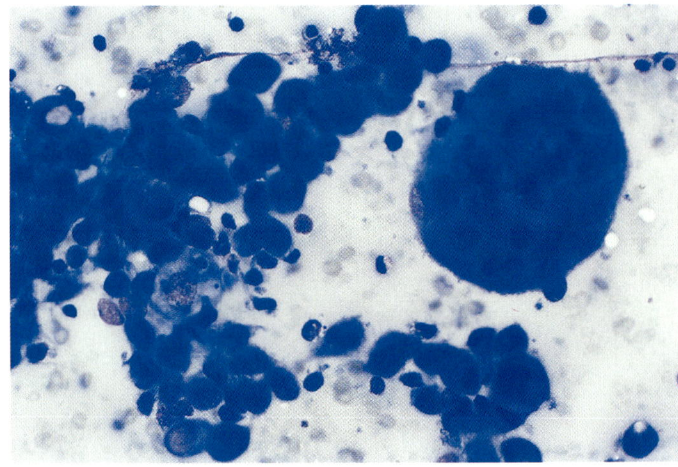

H

Figure 2.12 ***(continued)*** Lymphoepithelial cyst. **G.** Secondary infection may cause a mixed inflammatory exudate (MGG ×400). **H.** HIV sialadenitis with mulinucleate giant cells (MGG ×400).

of non-Hodgkin's lymphoma. The presence of epithelium and the polymorphous nature of lymphoid cells may be helpful.

The salivary gland is a frequent site of pathology in HIV-positive patients. Although lymphoepithelial lesions are the most common (74.8%), inflammatory processes (13.6%) and neoplasms (5.8%) may also be seen. The latter includes malignant lymphomas and metastatic carcinoma.[54] Malignancies are rare and since FNAC is reliable, most benign lesions can be managed conservatively.

Rare cysts

Odontogenic keratocysts, dermoid cysts and multiple oncocytic cysts have been described as occurring in the salivary gland.[55–57]

Sialadenitis

Inflammation of the salivary gland is most commonly caused by obstruction. Patients present with a short history of a painful swelling which may fluctuate in size and may be associated with eating or production of saliva (Fig. 2.13). Most commonly, obstruction is caused by sialolithiasis.

Acute sialadenitis

FNAC of acute sialadenitis shows many inflammatory cells with predominance of polymorphs, macrophages and occasional degenerate acinar and ductal cells (Fig. 2.14).

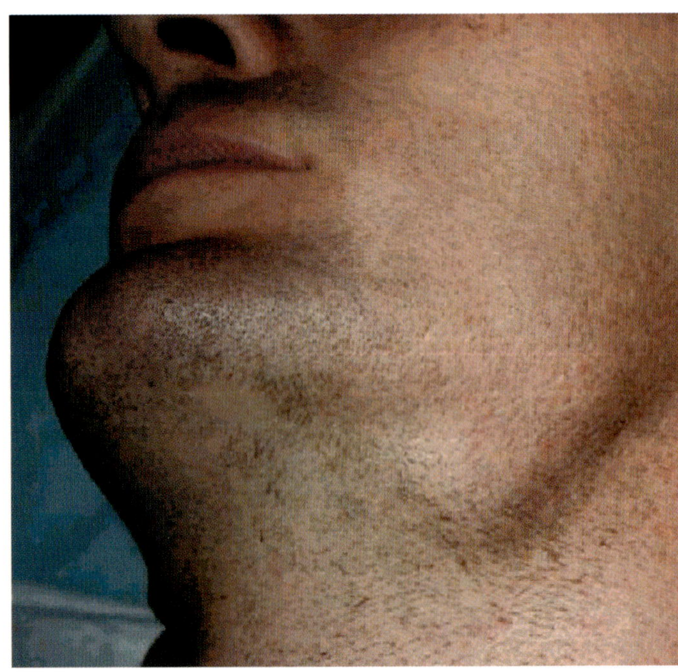

Figure 2.13 Acute sialadenitis. Patients present with a relatively recent onset of a firm, tender swelling, in this case, in the submandibular area.

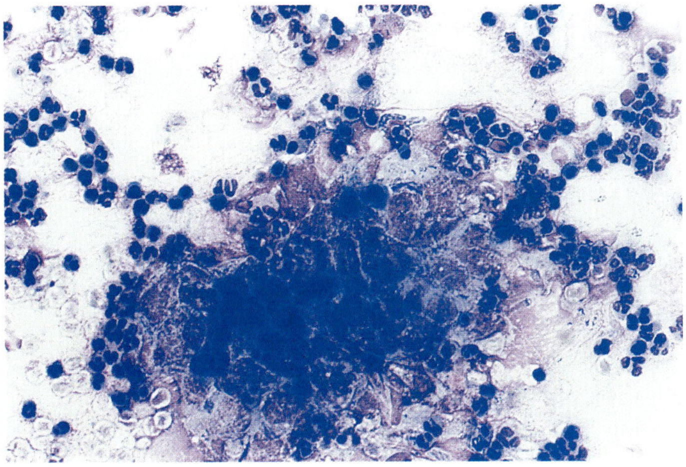

Figure 2.14 Acute sialadenitis. Numerous polymorphs surround degenerate salivary gland epithelium giving an impression of smearing artefact (MGG ×400).

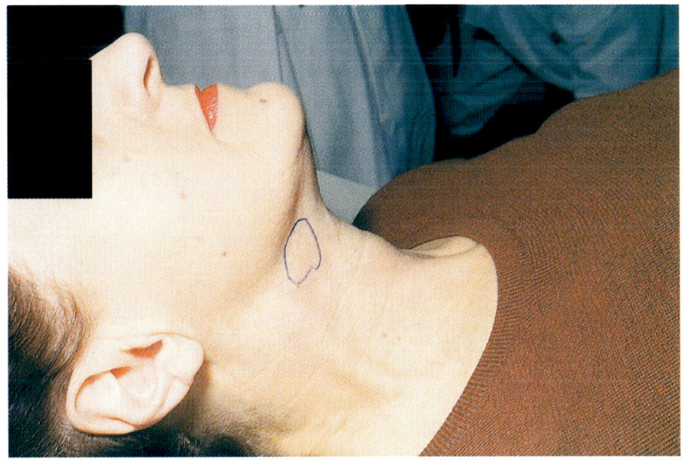

Figure 2.16 Chronic sialadenitis. Patients present with a firm, painless, mobile lump in the submandibular area that may clinically mimic tumour (Kuttner's tumour).

Chronic sialadenitis (Kuttner's tumour)

Chronic non-specific sialadenitis is an insidious inflammatory disorder, which is characterised by intermittent, often painful, swelling of the salivary glands (Fig. 2.15). The disease tends to progress and may lead to the formation of a fibrous mass, which may be clinically mistaken for a tumour (Fig. 2.16). Patients may have temporary facial nerve weakness and temporary paraesthesia of the cheek.[58] Sialography and scintigraphy may not always be helpful in diagnosing the lesion as benign, particularly when there are acute exacerbations of the condition. Histology shows marked atrophy of acinar epithelium, increased fibrous connective tissue and an intense lymphocytic infiltration.

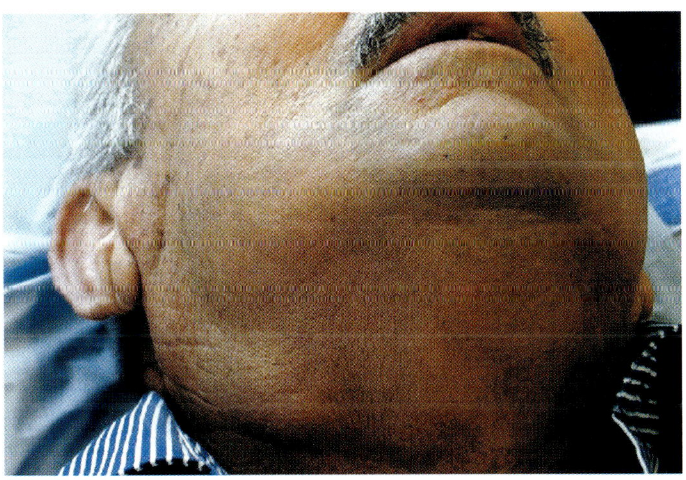

Figure 2.15 Sialadenitis. The patient presented with several months history of diffuse tender swelling with fluctuation in size.

Depending on the stage of the disease, FNAC contains variable amounts of inflammatory cells, but most frequently sparse duct epithelium and very few degenerate or no acinar cells (Fig. 2.17). Duct epithelium can sometimes show squamous metaplasia and may mimic squamous cell carcinoma (Fig. 2.17C, D, E). This is particularly the case with patients with history of neck irradiation for previous head and neck malignancy. These patients often present with a firm submandibular swelling which is clinically indistinguishable from lymph nodes and requires investigation prior to the possible radical neck dissection of lymph nodes.[9] Squamous metaplasia is known to occur in benign salivary gland lesions, such as pleomorphic adenoma and Warthin's tumours, as well as in salivary duct cysts and necrotising sialometaplasia.[49] A case of parotid duct carcinoma arising from chronic obstructive sialadenitis has been described.[59]

Sialadenitis with crystalloid formation

In some patients with sialadenitis, crystalloids of salivary alpha-amylase can be identified by May-Grunwald-Giemsa and Papanicolaou stains (Fig. 2.18).[60] These appear as numerous non-birefringent crystalloids of varying sizes and shapes: rectangles, needles, squares and rods mixed with neutrophils and rare multinucleated giant cells. No salivary gland components need be seen, and all special staining with alcian blue, mucicarmine, Von Kossa and congo red is negative.[61] In the salivary gland, several kinds of crystals or crystalloids can be found: cholesterol crystals, calcium oxalate crystals and tyro-

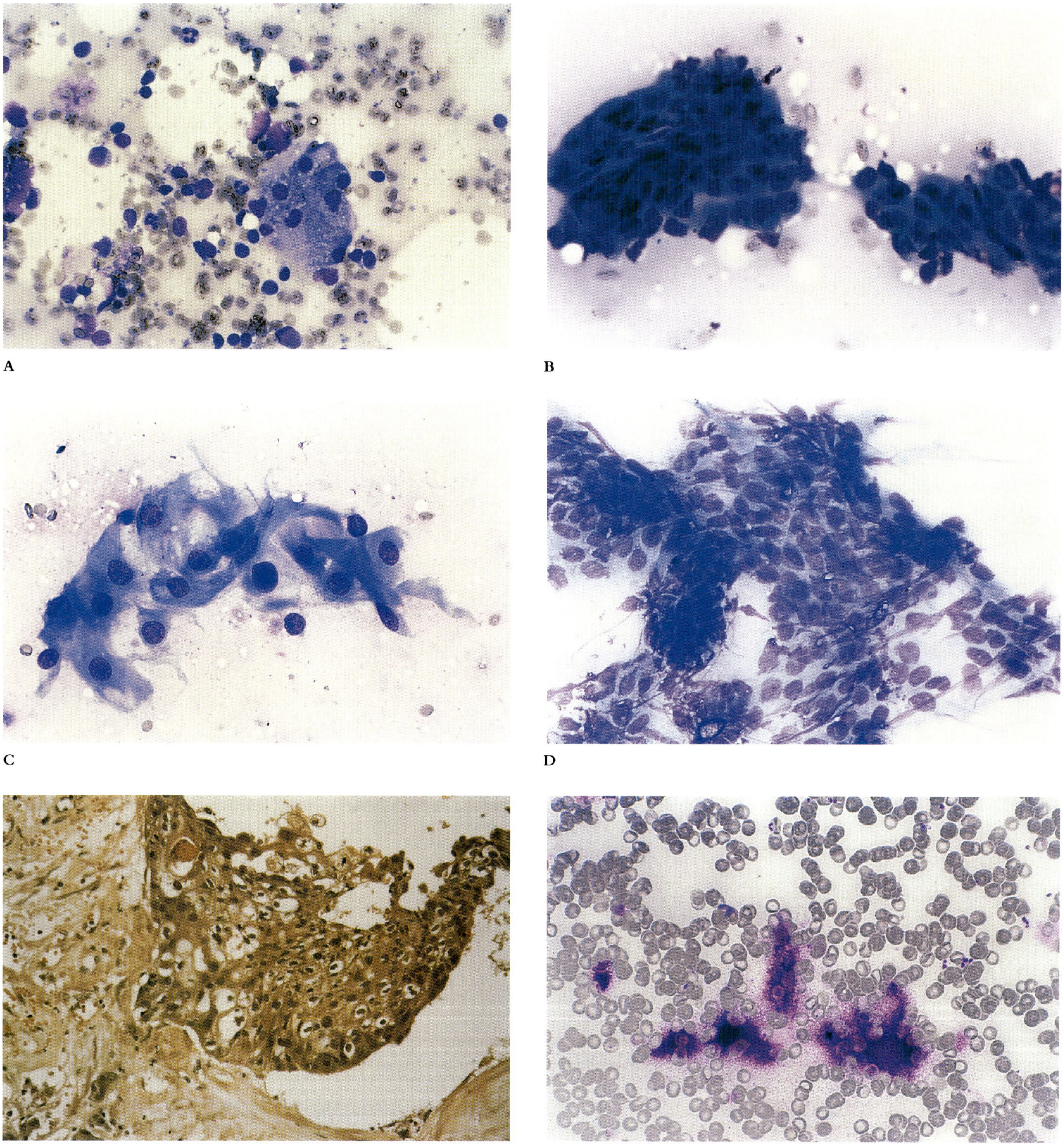

A B C D E F

Figure 2.17 Chronic sialadenitis. **A.** Sparse acini with occasional lymphocytes (MGG ×400). **B.** Tightly cohesive aggregates of ductal epithelial cells (MGG ×400). **C.** Ductal epithelium showing squamous metaplasia may be mistaken for squamous cell carcinoma (MGG ×600 oil). **E.** Same case as **D.** Squamous metaplasia may be mistaken for squamous metaplasia in chronic sialadenitis (H&E ×200). **F.** Specks of calcium shown as granular purple material in MGG stain are occasionally seen in chronic sialadenitis (MGG ×400).

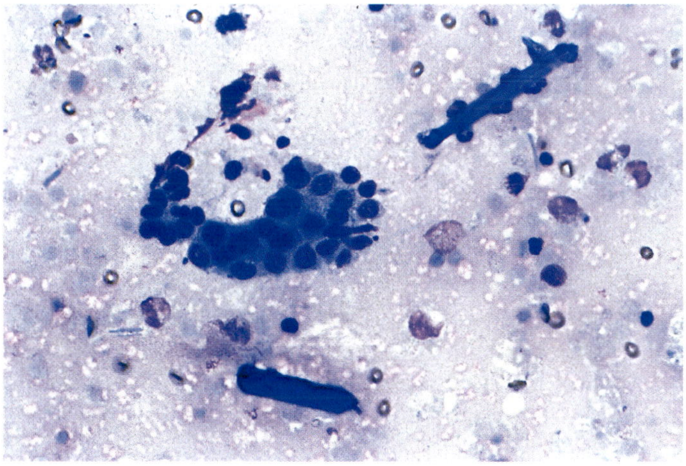

A

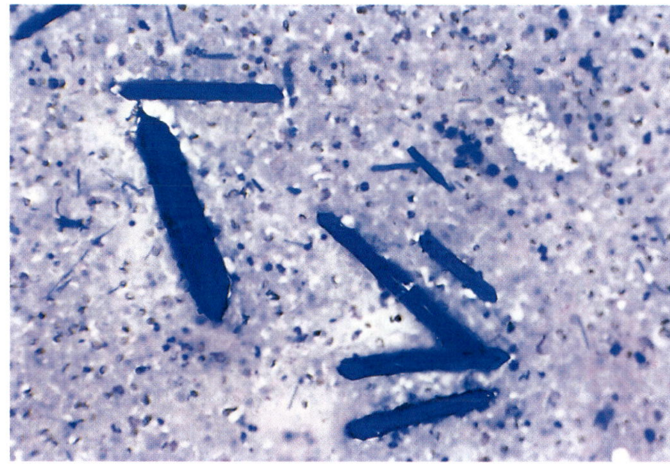

B

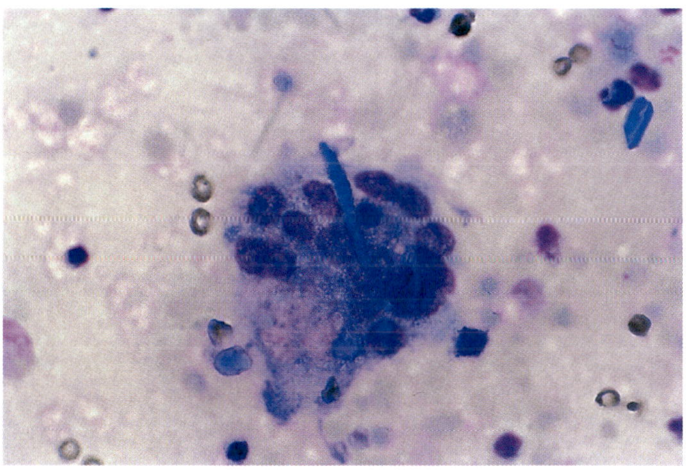

C

Figure 2.18 Sialadenitis with crystalloids. **A.** Salivary gland duct epithelium, sparse inflammatory cells and crystalloids (MGG ×400). **B.** Crystalloids are non-birefringent, of varying sizes and shapes; rectangles, needles, squares and rods mixed with neutrophils and occasional multinucleate giant cells (MGG ×400). **C.** Multinucleate giant cell in chronic sialadenitis with crystalloid (MGG ×600).

sine-rich crystalloids. Apart from sialolithiasis and sialadenitis, crystalline structures can be seen in neoplasms eg. Warthin's tumour, oncocytic papillary cystadenoma and pleomorphic adenoma. Tyrosine-rich crystalloids are rarely found in salivary gland tumours, but when present they support the diagnosis of pleomorphic adenoma. Non-tyrosine crystalloids are found in the highest concentrations in cystic spaces lined with oncocytic metaplastic cells and are possibly a product of oncocytic cell secretion.[62] For patients with parotid masses that contain non-tyrosine crystalloids, conservative management is indicated.[63]

Granulomatous sialadenitis

Granulomatous lesions of the salivary gland are rare. Granulomatous sialadenitis is most often a response to liberated ductal contents, particularly mucin, in various degrees of obstructive sialadenopathy, often a calculous duct obstruction.[64] Far less often, granulomatous sialadenitis is the result of specific infective granulomata or systemic granuloma-forming diseases. In these instances, the salivary parenchymal involvement is usually secondary to disease localisation in regional lymph nodes. Other causes of granulomatous sialadenitis are tuberculosis, sarcoidosis, carcinomatous duct obstruction and may be undetermined.[65] The tuberculous glands show caseation in the majority of cases but may consist predominantly of discrete granulomas with minimal necrosis. The sarcoid granulomata are typically non-caseating (Figs 2.19 and 2.20). The specific cytological features include histiocytes of both epithelioid and giant multinucleated types, without background necrosis.[66] Calculous and carcinomatous duct obstruction contains single to multiple small granulomata, which contain mucin and are related to ruptured ducts. It is suggested that the frequency of calculi and the mixture of serous and mucous acini in the submandibular gland account for the distribution of obstructive granulomata.

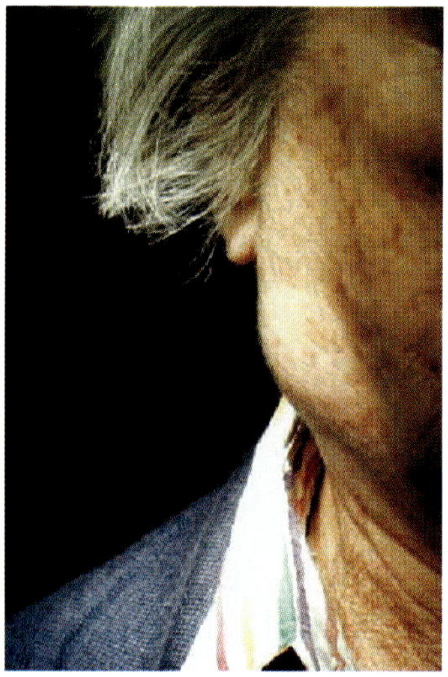

Figure 2.19 Sarcoid. Patients present with several months history of diffuse firm swelling clinically mimicking tumour.

Rare infections

In patients with immune deficiency, cytomegalovirus (CMV) sialadenitis can be diagnosed from FNAC. Characteristic viral intranuclear inclusions are best appreciated on a Papanicolaou stain.[67] The same applies to salivary gland mycoses. Histoplasmosis and *Candida* infections have been described and diagnosed on FNAC.[68] The incidence of HIV associated salivary gland disease is increasing as a result of the changing pattern of this disease in the era of protease inhibitor therapy[68a]. Serology should be a routine investigation when presented with a major salivary gland lump[68b].

Lymphoid proliferations of the salivary gland

Lymphoid proliferations of the salivary gland can be either reactive or neoplastic. The two are both clinically and

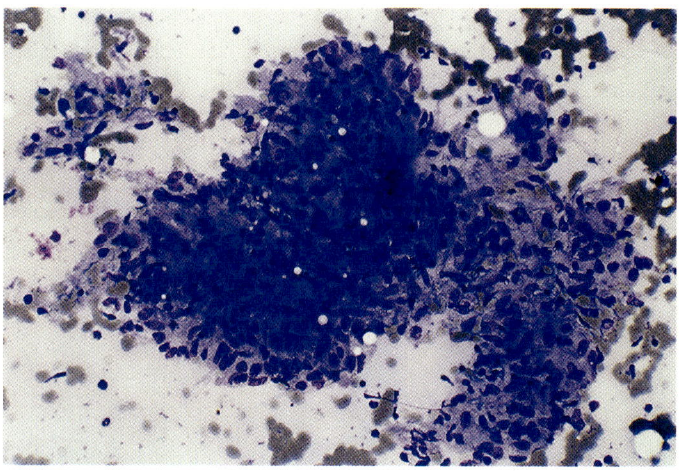

A

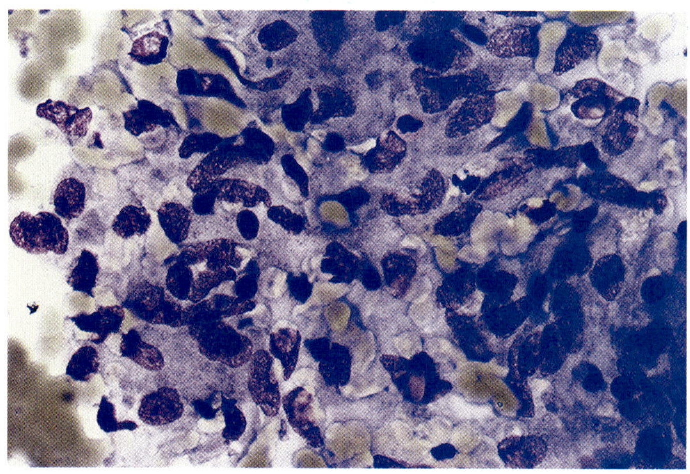

B

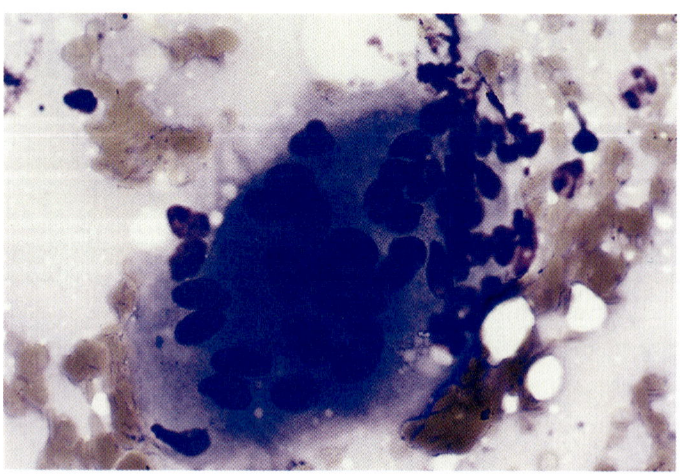

C

Figure 2.20 Granulomatous sialadenitis. **A.** Sarcoid affecting salivary gland. Numerous aggregates of epithelioid cells almost totally replacing salivary gland epithelium (MGG ×400). **B.** Epithelioid cells forming granulomata appear as 'shoal of fish', superimposed on each other without a clear cytoplasmic definition and typical twisted sausage-like appearance of the nucleus (MGG ×600). **C.** Multinucleate giant cell in the case of granulomatous sialadenitis due to sarcoid (MGG ×600 oil).

Box 2.3 Lymphoid-rich FNAC of parotid lesions

Salivary gland origin
Lymphoepithelial cyst
Myoepithelial sialadenitis (MESA)
Sjogren's syndrome
Chronic sialadenitis
Warthin's tumour
Malignant lymphoma
Mucoepidermoid carcinoma
Acinic cell carcinoma

Lymph node origin
Reactive lymph node hyperplasia
Malignant lymphoma of nodal origin

Modified from Young[2]

morphologically difficult to separate and are both included in this section for the purpose of closer comparison (Box 2.3). Further details on neoplastic lymphoid proliferations may be found in Chapter 4.

Reactive proliferations of lymphoid cells within the salivary gland include cystic lymphoid hyperplasia (a multicystic ductal proliferation with reactive germinal centres, seen most often in intravenous drug users infected with HIV) (see Figures 2.11 and 2.12) and the lymphoepithelial sialadenitis of Sjogren's syndrome (so-called benign lymphoepithelial lesion [BLEL] or myoepithelial sialadenitis [MESA]). In some cases it is preceded by a chronic sialectatic parotitis[69] or can be associated with hepatitis C liver disease.[70] The lymphoid proliferation involves infiltration of ductal epithelium by lymphocytes of marginal zone or monocytoid B-cell type, forming lymphoepithelial lesions (epimyoepithelial islands). There is a high prevalence of monoclonality in the lymphoepithelial lesions of the major salivary glands.[71] Patients with lymphoepithelial sialadenitis have a 44-fold increased risk of developing salivary gland or extrasalivary lymphoma, of which 80% are marginal zone/MALT type. These MALT lymphomas arise from sites normally devoid of lymphoid tissue but are preceded by chronic inflammatory, usually autoimmune, disorders that result in the accumulation of lymphoid tissue.[72–77] Like in MALT lymphoma of the stomach, there are reports of the possible association between the Helicobacter pylori infection and the development of the salivary gland MALT lymphoma[77a]. Broad strands of marginal zone or monocytoid B-cells around lymphoepithelial lesions and monotypic immunoglobulin detection by immunohistochemistry are considered diagnostic of MALT lymphoma.

'Nodal'-type B-cell lymphomas of the salivary glands are either follicular lymphoma (35%), which may arise in intrasalivary gland lymph nodes and behave similarly to follicular lymphoma in other sites, or diffuse large B-cell lymphoma (30%), which may arise de novo or secondary to either MALT or follicular lymphoma.[78] A simultaneous occurrence of both follicular and MALT lymphoma, phenotypically distinct but clonally identical, in a patient with Sjogren's syndrome has been described.[79]

The criteria for distinguishing benign lymphoepithelial lesions from low-grade B-cell lymphomas of MALT type in salivary glands and the significance of genotypically documented clonality in this setting are controversial. In addition, the clinical implications of a neoplastic diagnosis are unclear.[80] Patients have a history of long-lasting recurrent indolent swelling of one or both parotid glands (Fig. 2.21). Raised ESR, hypergammaglobulinaemia and persistent swelling despite immunosuppressive therapy clinically suggest lymphoma.[81]

Clinically, reactive intraparotid lymph nodes and lymphomas present as parotid enlargements that are indistinguishable from pleomorphic adenomas. FNAC is the only method of establishing a preoperative diagnosis of a

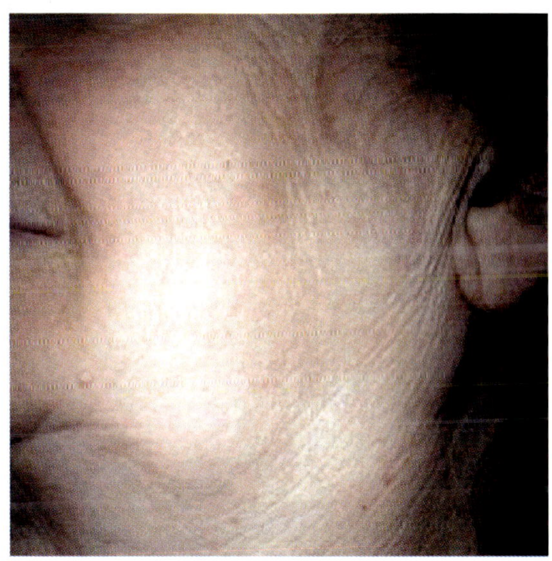

Figure 2.21 Lymphoid infiltrate in the parotid. This patient presented with 2-year history of a diffuse swelling at the angle of the mandible. The swelling did not change in size and was painless.

lymphoproliferative condition in these patients. Delineation of low-grade B-cell lymphoma from benign lymphoid lesions of MESA may be very difficult by means of cytomorphological criteria alone.[82] As in tissue material, monoclonal bands may be demonstrated on PCR (polymerase chain reaction) from FNAC material as means of differentiation between MESA and MALT. When evaluating the effectiveness of FNAC in the diagnosis of primary lymphoid processes of the salivary gland, MacCallum et al[83] reviewed 35 patients who underwent FNAC of the salivary gland and had a diagnosis of a primary lymphoid process. Most presented with palpable parotid (28 patients) or submandibular (4 patients) swellings. Sixteen cases of reactive hyperplasia and 9 cases of malignant lymphoma diagnosed by FNAC were confirmed by subsequent histopathological examination. Lymphoma was confirmed in 6 of 8 cases diagnosed as suspicious for lymphoma by FNAC. In all cases, the FNAC diagnosis of either a reactive or a malignant lymphoid process was unexpected and influenced the patient's further management. For a patient with a preoperative FNAC diagnosis of lymphoma, a more limited biopsy could be performed, thereby reducing the operative risk to the patient; also plans to process the tissue according to the institution's lymphoma protocol could be made.[83] Clinicians and pathologists should be aware of the possibility that MALT lesions including MALT lymphoma may be present in children who have AIDS.[84]

Cytological features of MESA or BLEL may be difficult to differentiate from lymphoma. In BLEL, a cellular aspirate is obtained. Smears should be examined on low to medium power for presence of epimyoepithelial islands. Lymphocytes, centrocytes, centroblasts, plasma cells, tingible body macrophages and occasional clusters of salivary gland cells are a common finding (Fig. 2.22). Clusters of myoepithelial cells may be present but they are not always identifiable on

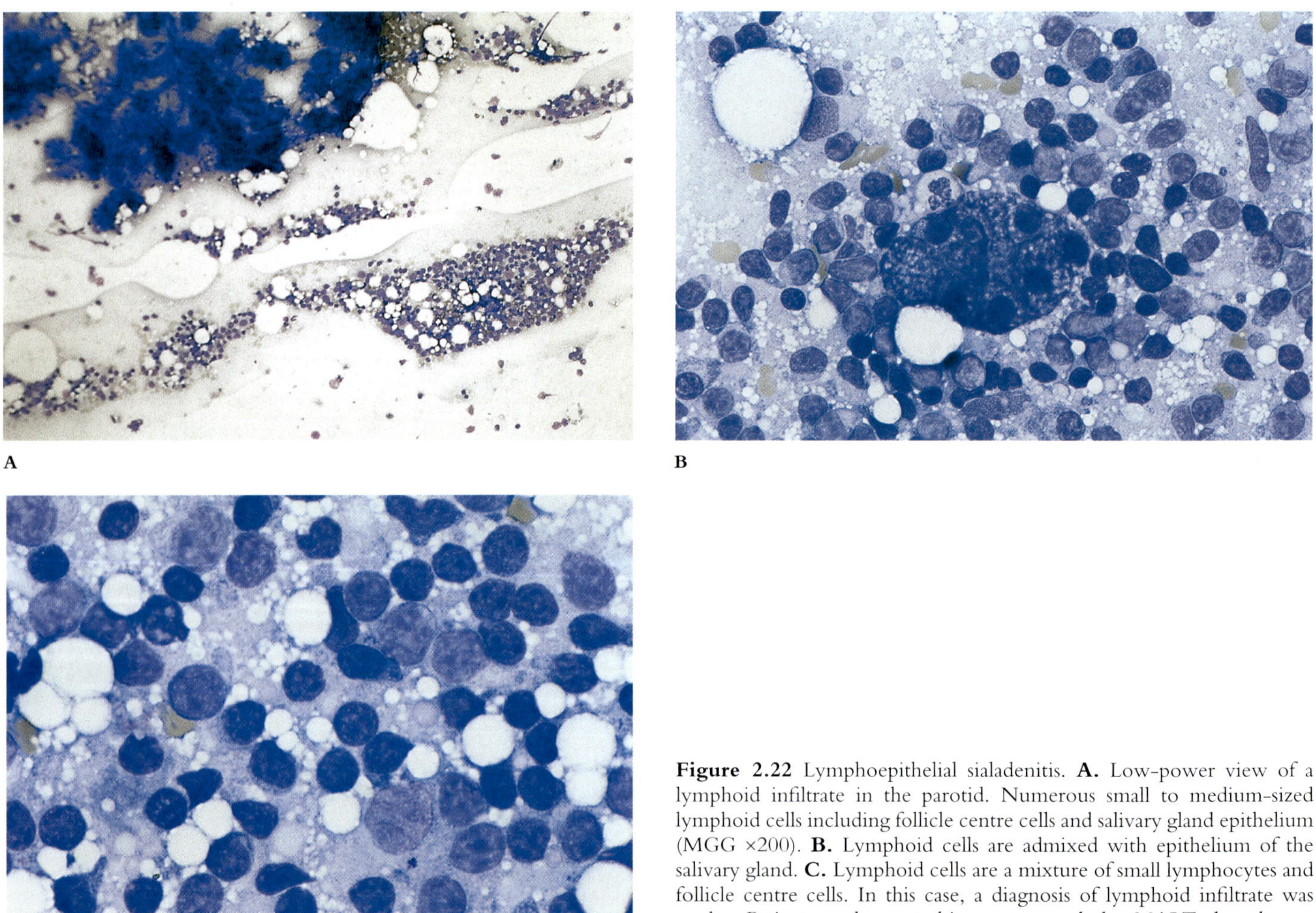

A

B

C

Figure 2.22 Lymphoepithelial sialadenitis. **A.** Low-power view of a lymphoid infiltrate in the parotid. Numerous small to medium-sized lymphoid cells including follicle centre cells and salivary gland epithelium (MGG ×200). **B.** Lymphoid cells are admixed with epithelium of the salivary gland. **C.** Lymphoid cells are a mixture of small lymphocytes and follicle centre cells. In this case, a diagnosis of lymphoid infiltrate was made. Patient underwent biopsy to exclude MALT lymphoma. Myoepithelial sialadenitis was diagnosed.

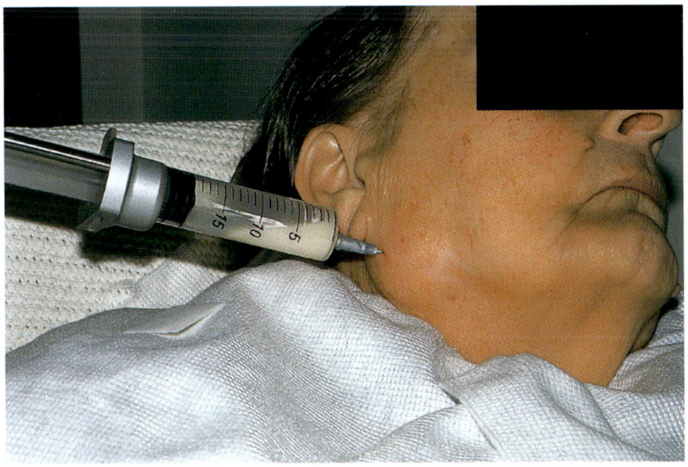

Figure 2.23 Lymphoid infiltrates in salivary gland. This 83-year-old patient presented with a parotid swelling. FNAC yielded white, milky fluid. Microscopy revealed numerous small lymphocytes in the absence of any other features. The lesion was considered benign, probably a lymphocele/lymphoepithelial cyst.

FNAC. Aspirates from intraparotid lymph nodes and some other salivary gland lesions may also result in 'lymphoid-rich' cytological preparations (Fig. 2.23; Box 2.1). Given the difficulty in distinguishing the condition from a MALT lymphoma, the possibility of lymphoma should be raised.

Cytological features of MALT lymphoma show intermediate-sized lymphocytes with a round to irregular nuclear outline and distinct pale cytoplasm intermixed with small mature lymphocytes (Fig. 2.24A–H). The chromatin is slightly paler and less clumped than in small, mature lymphocytes. A small, inconspicuous nucleolus is seen in most of the cells. These centrocyte-like cells may be seen to infiltrate epithelial island and form lymphoepithelial lesions (Fig. 2.24B–D). The persistent and often prominent follicle centre fragments in FNAC smears may create an impression

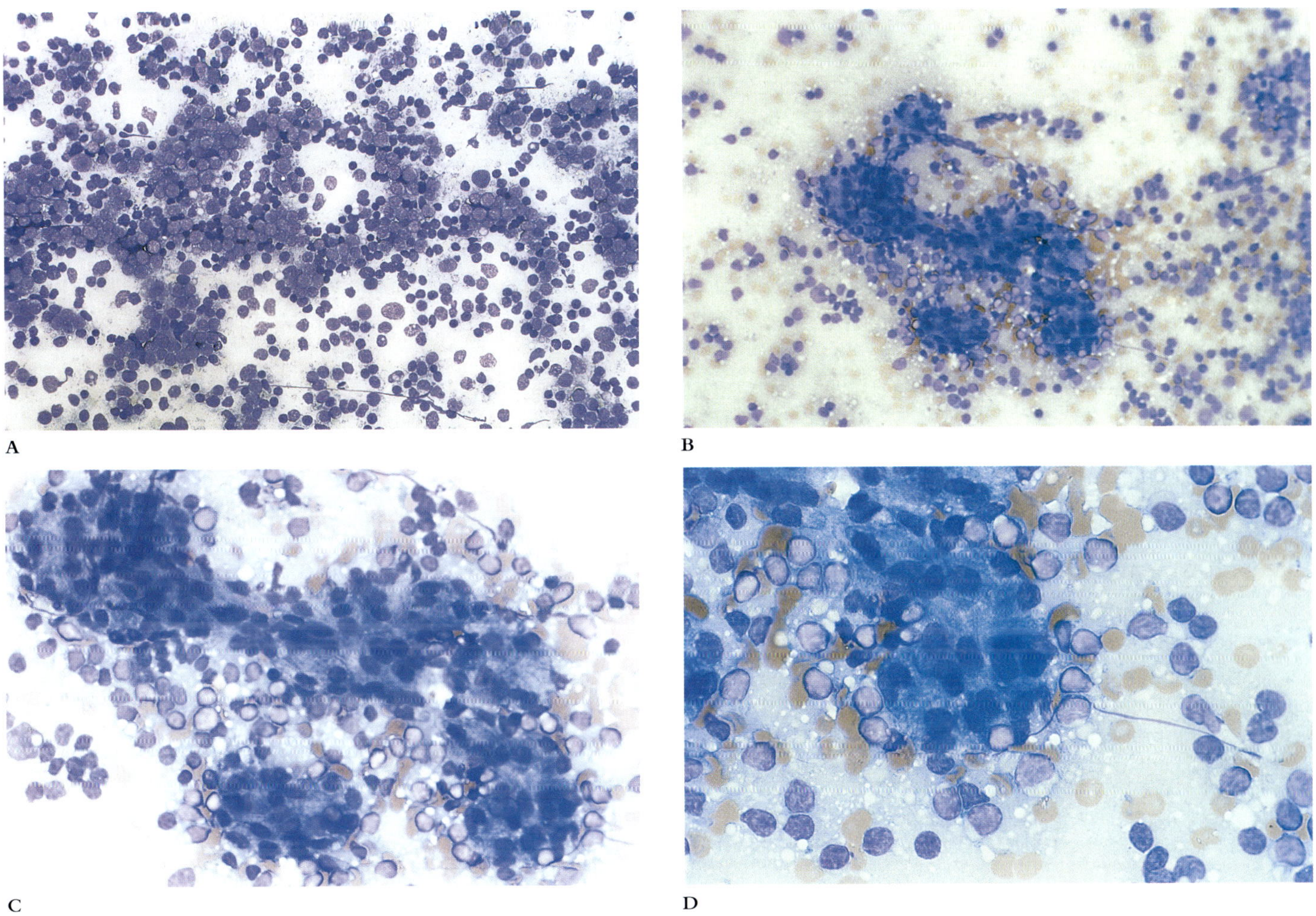

Figure 2.24 MALT lymphoma. **A.** Low-power view of the FNAC smear of a patient with MALT lymphoma. Hypercellular lymphoid infiltrate with monotonous pattern and no definite evidence of salivary gland epithelium (MGG ×100). **B.** When found, salivary gland epithelium appears surrounded by pale staining lymphocytes (MGG ×200). **C.** High-power view of the same duct which seems to be covered with lymphocytes (MGG ×600 oil). **D.** High-power view of the lymphoid cells infiltrating the epithelium (MGG ×1000 oil). ***(continued)***

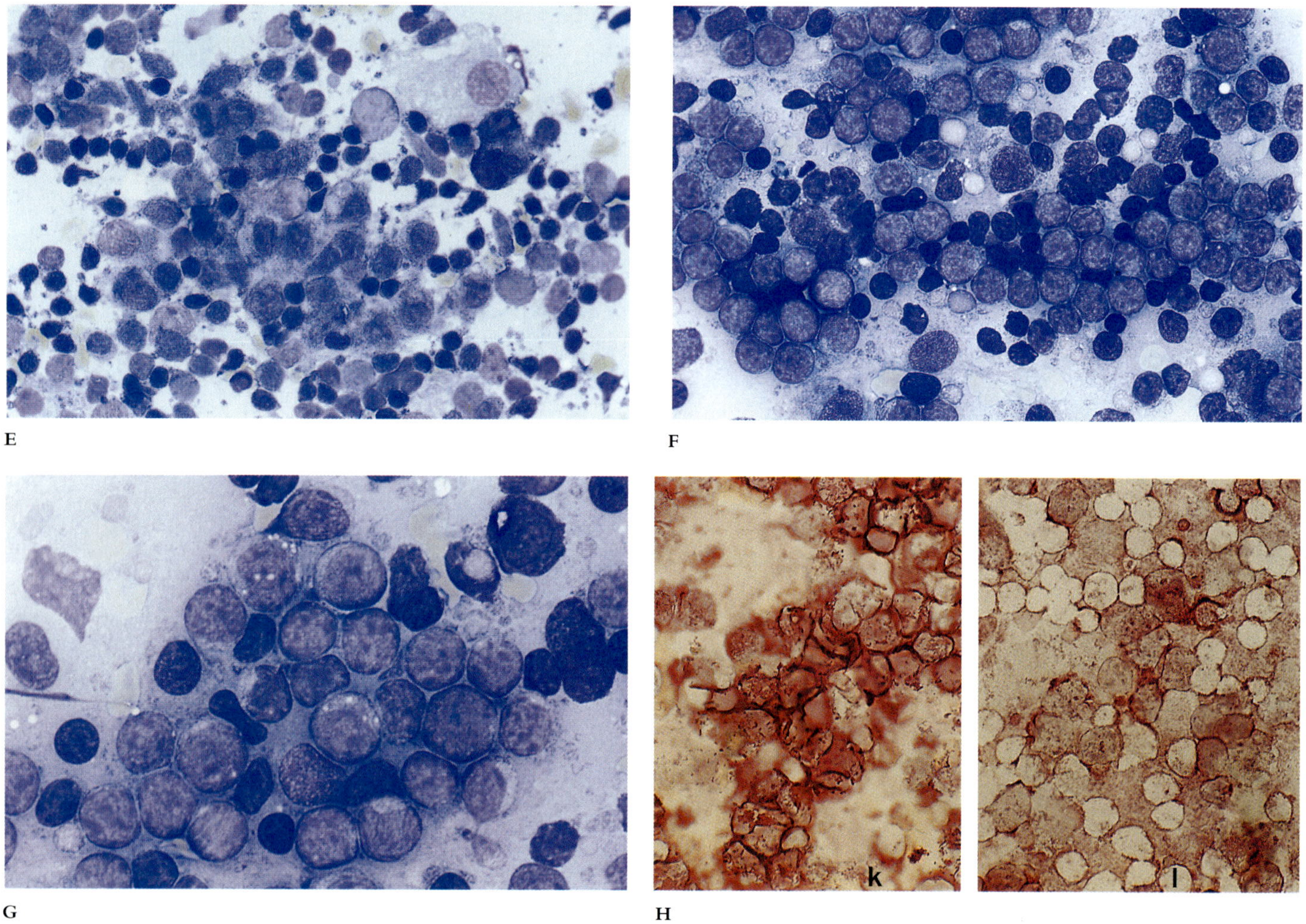

Figure 2.24 (***continued***) **E.** In other areas, it is more difficult to establish the presence of any epithelium, which has disappeared under the lymphoid infiltrate (MGG ×600, oil immersion). **F.** Lymphoid infiltrate is composed of centrocyte-like cells and small lymphocytes (MGG ×600). **G.** Centrocyte-like cells may be difficult to recognise as neoplastic (MGG ×1000). **H.** Tumour cells show light chain restriction for kappa chain.

of 'follicular' pattern and be mistaken for a follicular hyperplasia of an intraparotid node (Fig. 2.25). Flow cytometry immunophenotyping performed on the FNAC material shows a monoclonal population of B-cells usually with kappa light chain restriction (Fig. 2.24H). The cytomorphology coupled with the immunophenotyping study in this clinical context suggest the diagnosis of low-grade B-cell lymphoma of MALT.[85] Different MALT lymphomas show a tendency for diverse cytological expressions, such as: small lymphocytes in the lung, monocytoid cells in salivary glands and plasmacytic cells in the thyroid and skin.[86]

Given the difficulties with diagnosis of salivary gland lymphoid infiltrates and distinguishing between MESA, MALT and low-grade extranodal lymphomas, these lesions are best submitted for histological biopsy. (Figs 2.65 and 2.66).

BENIGN TUMOURS OF THE SALIVARY GLAND

Salivary gland tumours are very uncommon. The incidence of benign tumours of the salivary gland is 6.8 per 100 000 persons per year. The ratio of benign to malignant tumours is 4:1. Histological distribution shows a frequency of 54% pleomorphic adenomas, 28% adenolymphomas and 18% other tumours. The greatest number (85%) arise in the parotid. There is an average 3% recurrence rate, most frequently in pleomorphic adenoma.[87] The revised 1991 World Health Organization histological classification of benign tumours divides benign salivary gland tumours into 9 categories (Box 2.1).[20]

Cytologically, the most frequently diagnosed benign salivary gland tumours are pleomorphic adenoma and

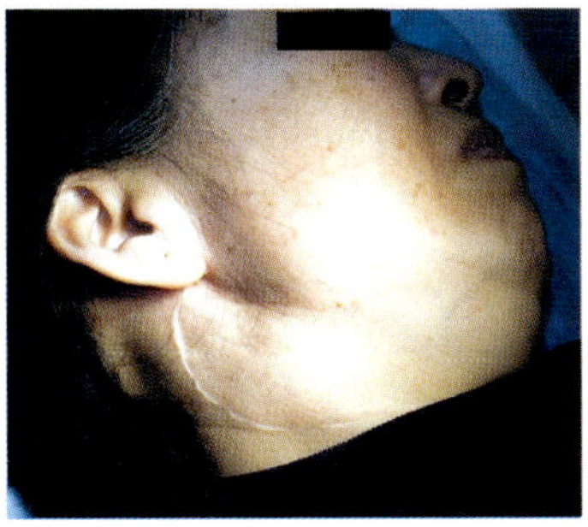

A

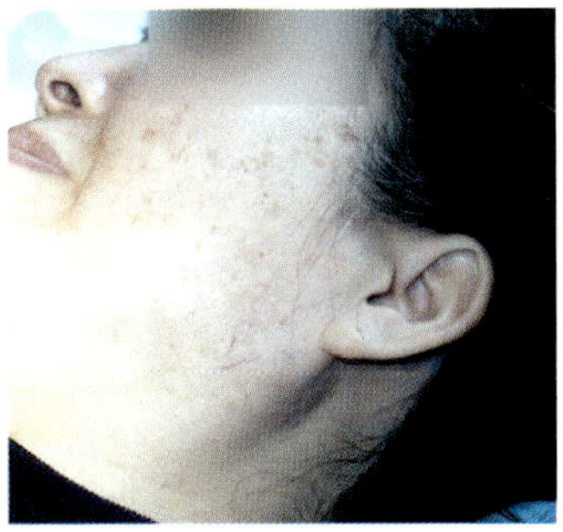

B

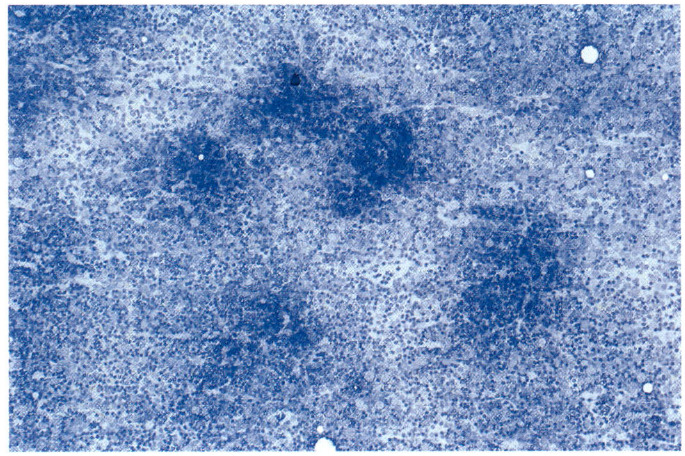

C

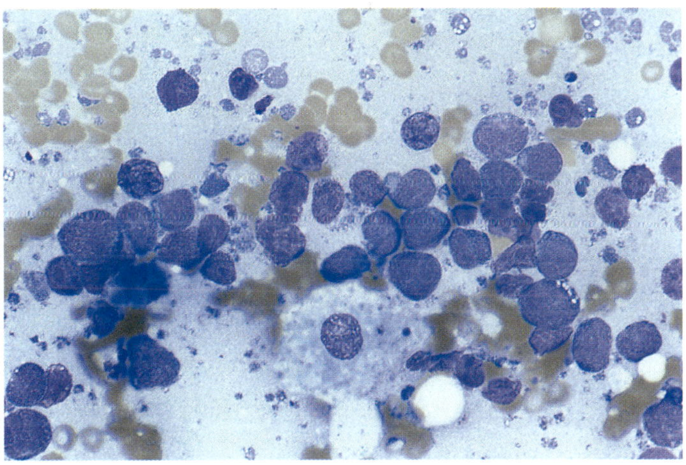

D

Figure 2.25 MALT lymphoma. **A.** 49 year old patient with a history of excision of MALT lymphoma of the right parotid some years ago. **B.** Now presenting with a swelling of the left lobe. **C.** FNAC from the left side showed dense lymphoid population with apparent residual follicle centre fragments overrun with small centrocyte-like cells (MGG ×100). **D.** Detail of lymphoid cells (×600 oil).

adenolymphoma (Warthin's tumour). Other types are much rarer and the clinical importance of FNAC in this case is to recognise them primarily as benign tumours. The cytological features described in this chapter serve to raise awareness of the different benign tumour types and the pitfalls in diagnosis. An awareness of the morphological variation present on cytological preparations and correlation with clinical findings should prevent erroneous interpretation in the FNAC setting.

Pleomorphic adenoma

Pleomorphic adenoma is the most common salivary gland tumour. It accounts for 60–70% of parotid, submandibular or accessory gland tumours while sublingual tumours are rare. Typically, it arises in the tail of the parotid gland and is slow growing. When resected, the vast majority are 2–6 cm in size, with exceptions up to 26 cm in diameter (giant pleomorphic adenoma).[88] Patients (average age 40–45 years, female predominance) present with a painless, well-defined, mobile, firm nodule of some months or years duration (Figs 2.26, 2.27, 2.29, 2.31 and 2.33). Rarely, it may be bilateral synchronous or familial.[89] Most unusually for a benign tumour, it sometimes gives rise to distant metastases.[90]

FNAC is a recognised method for preoperative diagnosis. With appropriate sampling, a high degree of accuracy can be achieved. The reliability of FNAC in diagnosing pleomorphic adenoma has been reported as 89.5–96.2.%.[91] Klijanienko & Vielh analysed 412 preoperatively diagnosed pleomorphic adenomas and found 95% concordance with postoperative histology. This applies particularly to the chondromyxoid histological type (cellular, myoepithelial

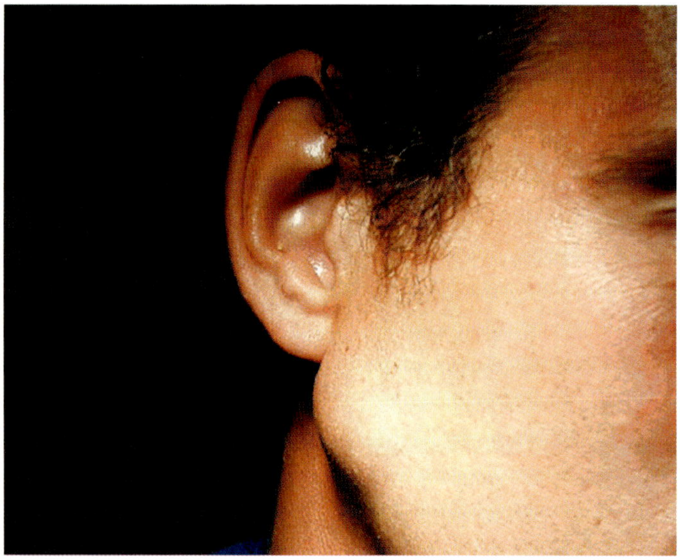

Figure 2.26 Pleomorphic adenoma. Patient presented with a typical, well-defined, firm, mobile lump at the angle of mandible. FNAC yielded dense, transparent material with particles. Microscopy was typical of pleomorphic adenoma.

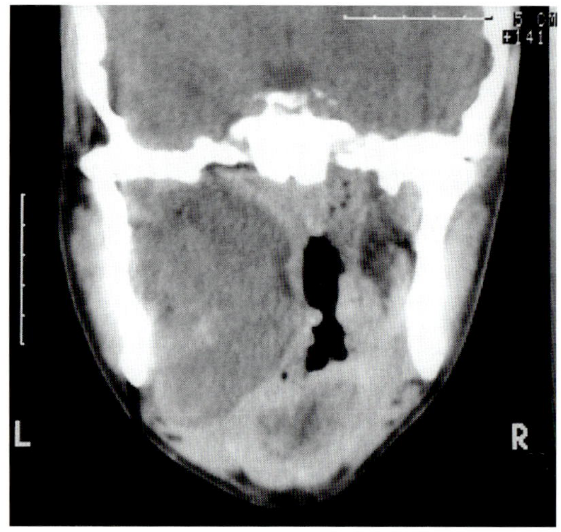

A

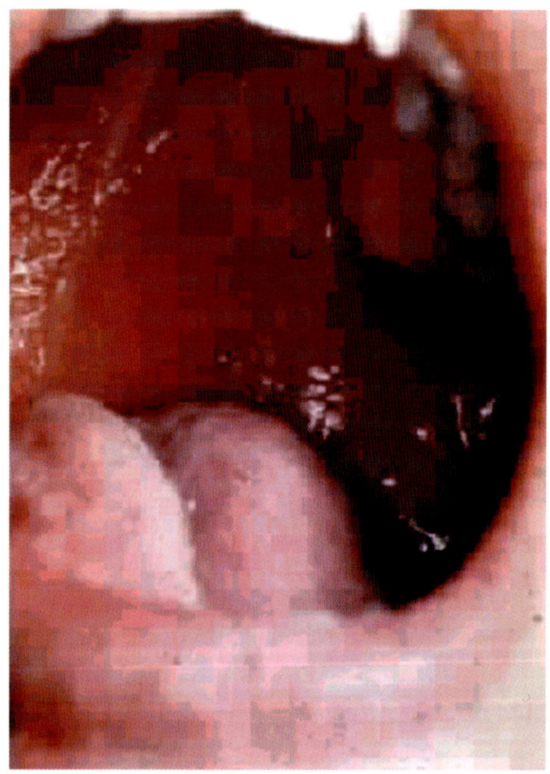

B

Figure 2.27 Pleomorphic adenoma. **A.** CT scan of the oropharynx in a 27-year-old patient with a large parapharyngeal mass. The tumour was of unusual size and presented at a young age. Clinically, malignant tumour was suspected. **B.** Same patient, mass viewed from the mouth. FNAC was performed from the inside of the mouth. Smears were typical of pleomorphic adenoma. Investigation allowed careful preoperative planning in order to achieve complete excision.

and metaplastic types of pleomorphic adenoma achieved 82% concordance).[92] Cytopathologists must be aware that the importance of preoperative diagnosis is to achieve complete resection, as incompletely resected tumours have a high recurrence rate.[93]

Cytological features classically present no difficulty in diagnosis of pleomorphic adenoma. They include variable cellularity, an extracellular myxoid stroma with uniform, cytologically bland epithelial cells arranged in cohesive clusters, individually or in a tubular arrangement (Fig. 2.28). The epithelial cells have plasmacytoid or spindle cell appearance. Peripherally located spindle-shaped myoepithelial cells mingle imperceptibly with the myxoid stroma giving the epithelium a 'sunburst' appearance.[94] Cytological features reflect considerable histological variation of the cellular composition within the same tumour, composed of different proportions of epithelial and myoepithelial cells and stroma. Klijanienko classifies tumours into chondromyxoid (70% of cases) and cellular types (26.9%) (Fig. 2.29) (Fig. 2.30A–C) with minority cases classified as myoepithelial or metaplastic.[92]

Minor variations in cytological presentation of pleomorphic adenoma consist of duct metaplasia mucinous, squamous (Figs 2.31, 2.32, Fig. 2.32C), oxyphilic (Fig. 2.34A) and sebaceous, variable stromal cellularity, tyrosine and

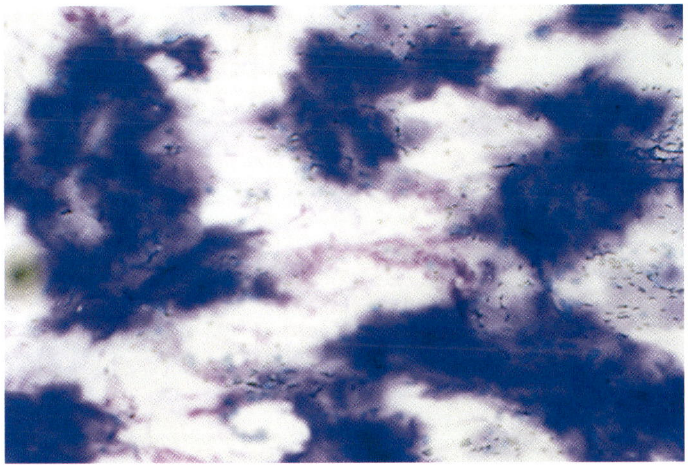

A

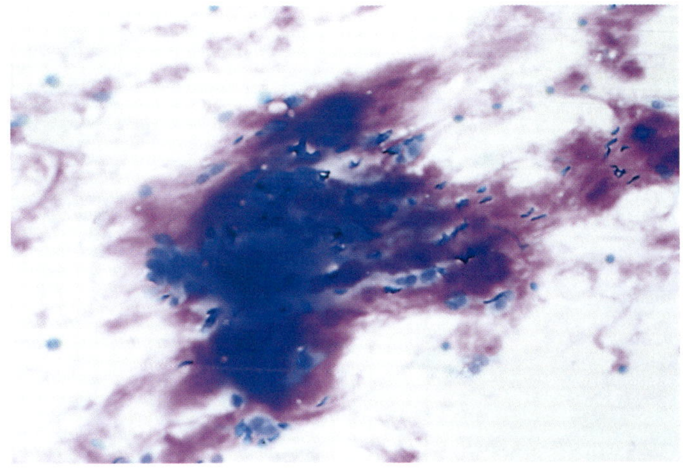

B

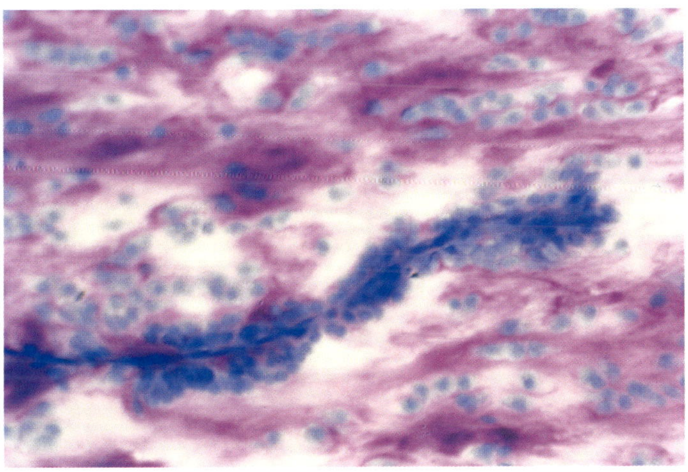

C

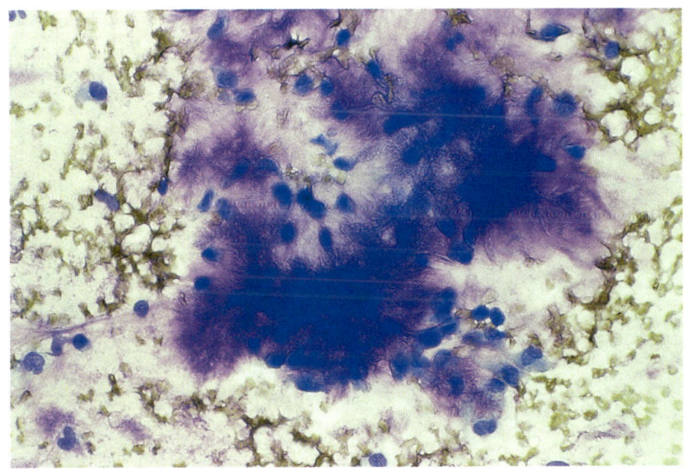

D

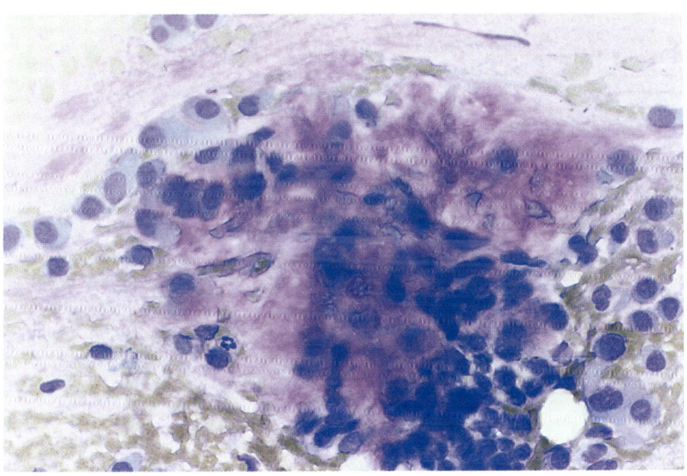

F

Figure 2.28 Pleomorphic adenoma. **A.** Typically, FNAC material shows a mixture of fibrillary myxoid ground substance in which spindle or rounded cells are found either in clusters or lying free (MGG ×200). **B,C.** Same case. Cells are often immersed within the chondromyxoid stroma and may appear poorly stained because of the reduced stain penetration (MGG ×400). **D,E.** Clusters of epithelial cells with 'sunburst' appearance imparted by the peripheral epithelial cells streaming into the fibrillary material (MGG ×400, ×600).

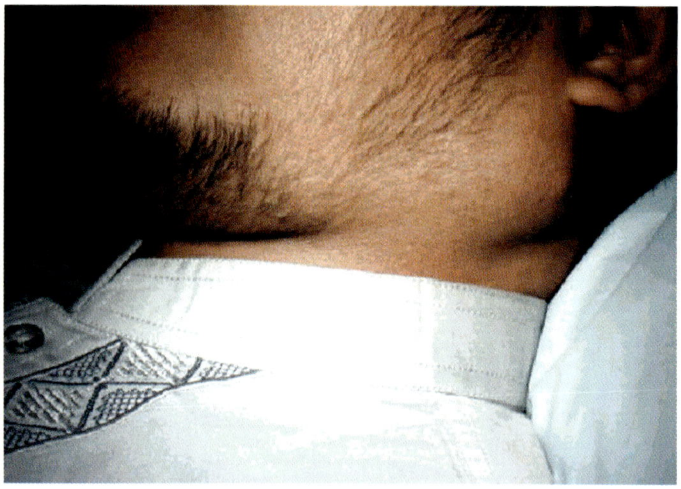

Figure 2.29 Pleomorphic adenoma. A 27-year-old patient presented with a solid, mobile, painless swelling at the angle of the mandible.

collagenous crystalloids deposition and intranuclear cytoplasmic inclusions. In most cases, these changes are found in material otherwise typical of pleomorphic adenoma. *Major cytological variations* are represented by cellular atypia, cystic transformation and the presence of a cylindromatous pattern resembling adenoid cystic carcinoma (Fig. 2.32D). These must be considered in order to avoid important errors in the preoperative management of and surgical approach to salivary gland lesions.[91]

Apart from pleomorphic adenoma, *cystic change* can be seen in low-grade mucoepidermoid carcinoma, Warthin's tumour, acinic cell carcinoma, metastatic squamous cell carcinoma and benign, non-neoplastic lesions (Box 2.2). Pleomorphic adenoma should be suspected when epithelial and stromal elements are seen within the mucinous material.

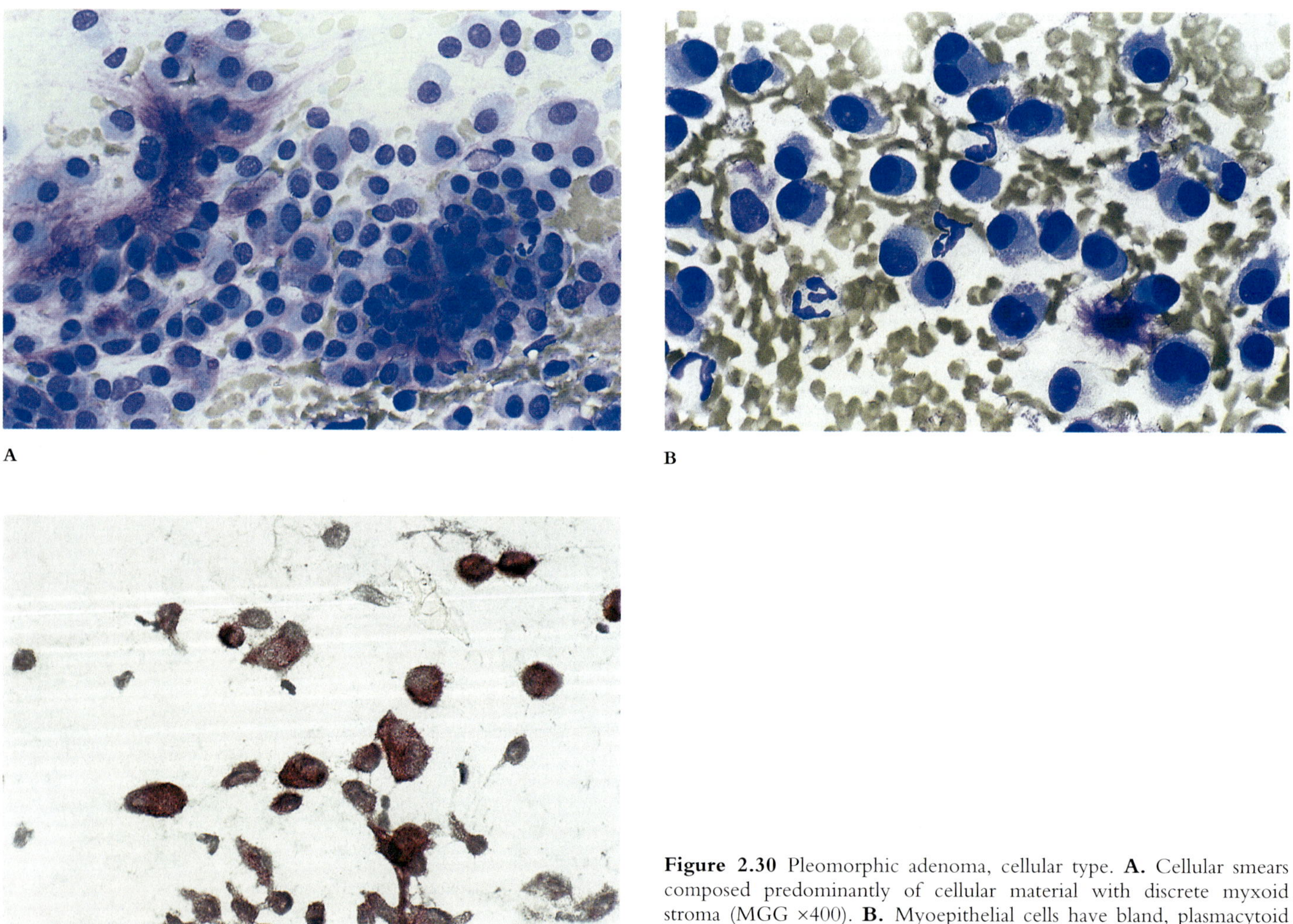

A

B

C

Figure 2.30 Pleomorphic adenoma, cellular type. **A.** Cellular smears composed predominantly of cellular material with discrete myxoid stroma (MGG ×400). **B.** Myoepithelial cells have bland, plasmacytoid appearance with oval or round nuclei (MGG ×600 oil). **C.** S-100 staining positivity in myoepithelial cells (anti-S-100, APAAP ×600).

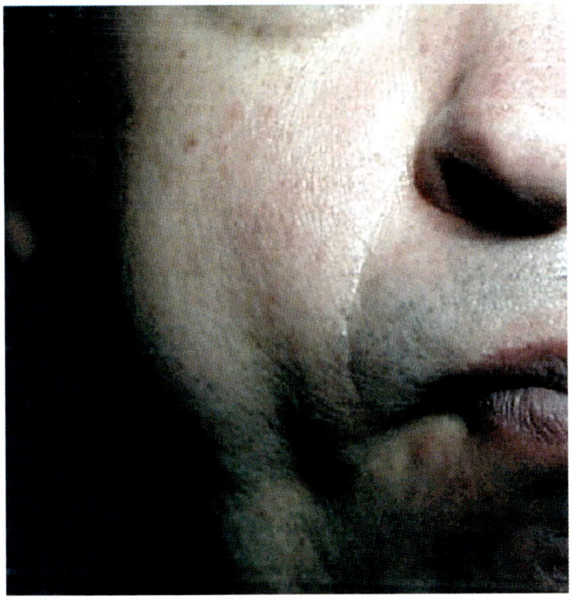

Differential diagnosis of *cellular pleomorphic adenoma* is wide: mucoepidermoid carcinoma, adenoid cystic carcinoma, acinic cell carcinoma, basal cell adenoma, myoepithelioma, spindle cell neoplasm, malignant myoepithelioma, all of which have cellular appearances.[95] The excess of mesenchymal mucinous stroma can be misinterpreted as mucin and pleomorphic adenoma may be mistaken for cyst fluid of low-grade mucoepidermoid carcinoma. For diagnosis of mucoepidermoid carcinoma, the presence of squamous, intermediate and vacuolated cells is necessary. Pleomorphic adenoma with a *cylindromatous* pattern should not be mistaken for adenoid cystic carcinoma. In adenoid cystic cell

Figure 2.31 Pleomorphic adenoma. The patient presented with swelling within the cheek, most prominent when muscles were tense. Pleomorphic adenoma of the accessory parotid was found on FNAC.

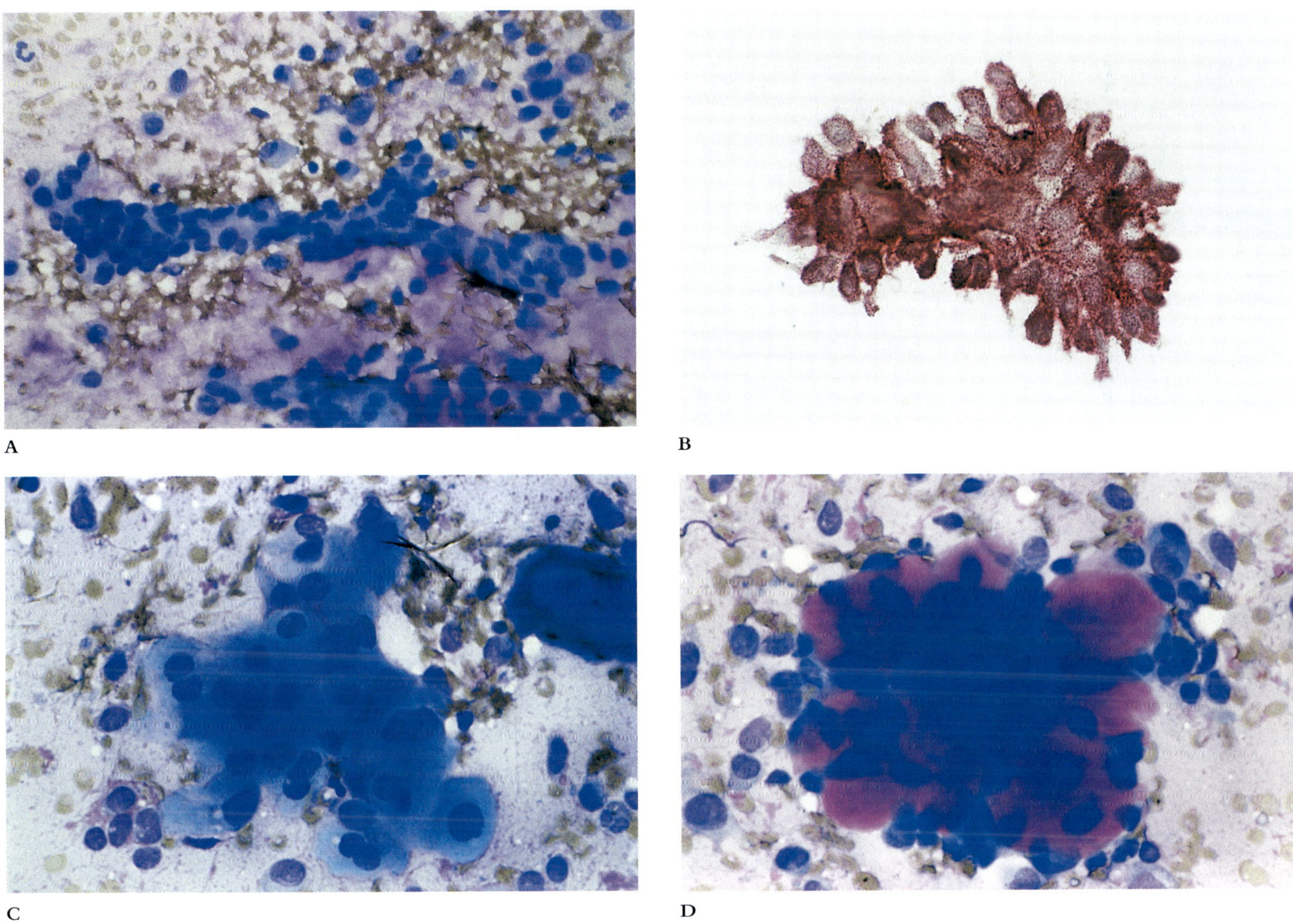

Figure 2.32 Pitfalls in diagnosis of pleomorphic adenoma. **A.** Predominance of epithelial cells forming ducts and tubules (MGG ×600). **B.** Epithelial markers confirm epithelial origin (anti-CAM 5.2, APAAP ×600 oil). **C.** Squamous metaplasia within a pleomorphic adenoma. Keratinisation may be misleading diagnosis of mucoepidermoid carcinoma (MGG ×600 oil). **D.** Cylindromatous pattern. Spherical balls of stroma are surrounded by epithelial cells. Note the presence of cytoplasm and bland nuclei of epithelial cells (MGG ×600 oil).

carcinoma, cells are usually smaller and hyperchromatic. Stroma may be present but is usually homogenous as opposed to the fibrillary stroma of pleomorphic adenoma. Although there are cytological features common to both tumours, each has a unique relationship of epithelial cells to stroma. Aspirates in pleomorphic adenoma show cell clusters with a 'sunburst' appearance caused by peripheral spindled cells streaming into a fibrillary myxoid stroma. In adenoid cystic carcinoma, well-delineated, tightly cohesive basaloid cells surrounding mucoid/hyaline globules or clear spaces in a honeycomb pattern are seen. The cytological distinction between pleomorphic adenoma and acinic cell carcinoma is sometimes difficult, particularly if the epithelial cells of pleomorphic adenoma show 'plasmacytoid' appearance and are scattered singly and in clusters. These cells have eccentrically placed, oval to round nuclei with finely granular chromatin, inconspicuous nucleoli and dense cytoplasm, sometimes containing hyaline globules.[94]

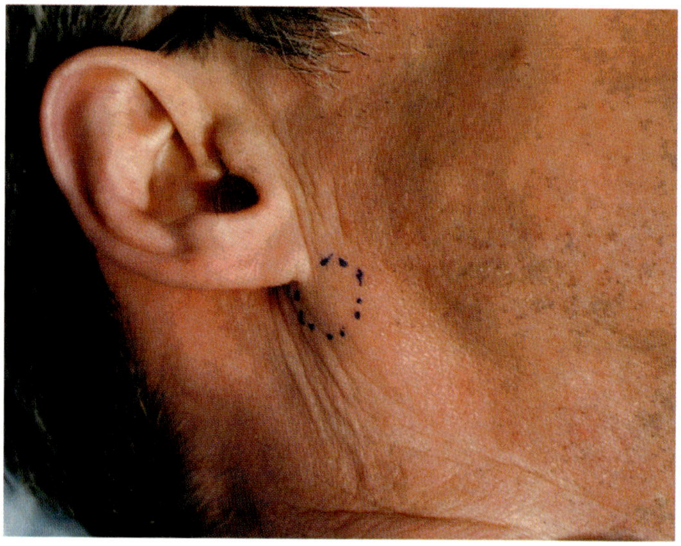

Figure 2.33 Pleomorphic adenoma. The most common presentation is that of a discrete swelling at the angle of mandible, barely visible but readily palpable. Patients often say that they have had the lump for many years. Only rarely do they appear to have noticed it recently. In both instances, the lesion warrants investigation.

Benign primary neoplasms of the salivary gland such as monomorphic adenoma and myoepithelioma can be easily mistaken for pleomorphic adenoma on cytology. The distinction is of little practical importance since the treatment is the same. The similarity of pleomorphic adenoma to benign neurilemoma is particularly prominent with the spindle type of pleomorphic adenoma. Intranuclear cytoplasmic inclusions are relatively common in pleomorphic adenoma, and nuclear grooves have been described. Diagnosis should not be confused with papillary carcinoma of the thyroid. Intravenous pyogenic granuloma is a rare, benign lesion occurring usually as a subcutaneous mass in the neck or upper extremity. Cytologically it may mimic pleomorphic adenoma.[96] In all cases where morphological diagnosis is difficult on FNAC, the case should be discussed with a surgeon.

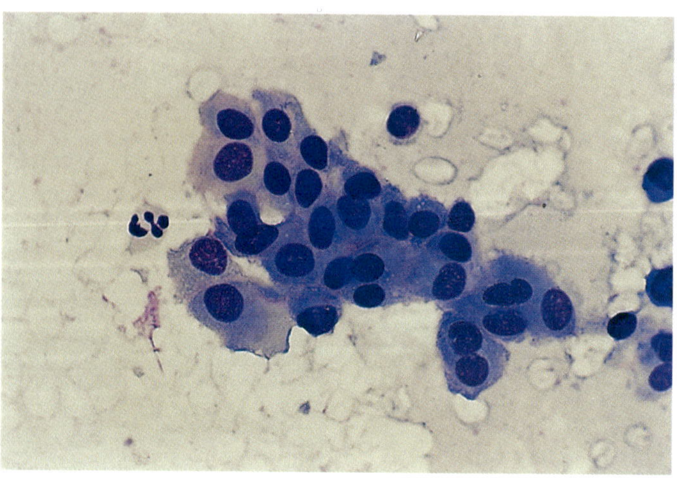

A

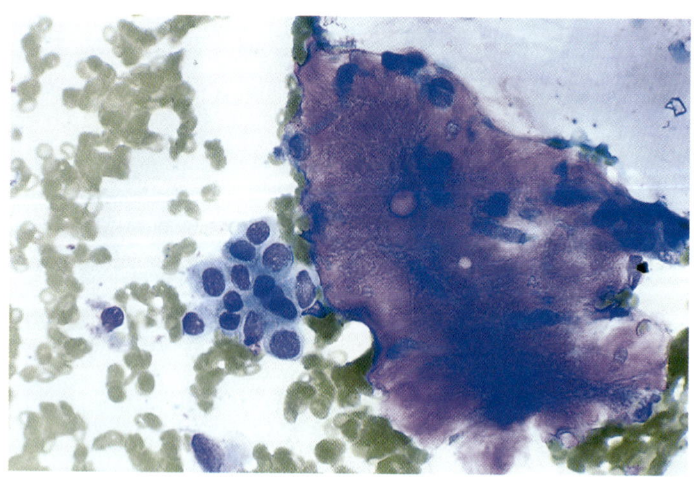

B

Figure 2.34 Pitfalls in diagnosis of pleomorphic adenoma. **A.** Metaplastic pleomorphic adenoma. Predominantly oncoytic cells may be mistaken for Warthin's tumour or oncocytoma (×600 oil). **B.** Cellular atypia in pleomorphic adenoma can be seen. It should not be overinterpreted as malignant (MGG ×600 oil).

Carcinoma ex pleomorphic adenoma

Epithelial atypia within an otherwise typical pleomorphic adenoma should not generally be interpreted as indicating malignancy (Fig. 2.34B). Enlarged, irregular, even bizarre nuclei of stromal cells are sometimes found in the smears of benign tumours. The abnormal cells are most likely degenerative in nature. On the other hand, obviously atypical epithelial cells showing nuclear enlargement, hyperchromasia and nucleoli found side by side with the usual pleomorphic adenoma cells is suspicious of carcinoma ex pleomorphic adenoma (Fig. 2.58). Definitive diagnosis is deferred because invasive growth is a necessary criterion. In an attempt to analyse which, if any, features might indicate a greater likelihood of malignant transformation of pleomorphic adenoma (13.8%),[97] Auclair & Ellis[97] studied the atypical histological features of pleomorphic adenoma: hypercellularity, capsule violation, hyalinisation, necrosis and cellular anaplasia. The mitotic rate was also analysed. Benign mixed tumours that showed prominent zones of hyalinisation or at least moderate mitotic activity were more likely to develop carcinoma than those that did not. Clinical findings at the initial diagnosis that indicated a greater likelihood of malignant transformation were: occurrence in the submandibular gland, older patient age and large tumour size.[97] A sudden increase in the growth rate of a tumour that has been present for many years gives clinical support to the diagnosis.[21]

Accurate diagnosis of malignancy on FNAC is achieved in high-grade tumours; low sensitivity may cause interpretative difficulties in low-grade tumours.[90]

Myoepithelial carcinoma with predominance of plasmacytoid cells arising in a pleomorphic adenoma of the parotid gland has been described.[98]

Rare cases of benign salivary gland pleomorphic adenoma metastatic to bone (benign-metastasising pleomorphic adenomas and not carcinoma ex pleomorphic adenoma or carcinosarcoma) diagnosed by fine needle aspiration biopsy have been described.[99] The metastatic lesions contained benign epithelial, myoepithelial, and stromal components. No evidence of malignancy was observed on cytology smears or histology sections in any of the cases. The differential diagnosis is primary bone tumours. Clinically, metastasising pleomorphic adenomas may represent unrecognised malignancy, because the biological course of the tumours may lead to fatal outcome.[100]

Adenolymphoma (Warthin's tumour)

This is the second most common benign salivary gland tumour. It represents approximately 5–6% of salivary gland lesions, arises most commonly within the parotid gland, grows slowly and is typically detected at around the age of 55 years (Fig. 2.35). There is a male predominance. Histologically, the tumour consists of a double layer of oncocytic epithelium with lymphoid stroma containing lymphoid follicles and cystic spaces containing inflammatory/necrotic material (Fig. 2.36F).

Cytological features include 3 distinct components: oncocytic cells in flat sheets or papillary structures, lymphoid stroma and contents of the cystic spaces with inflammation/necrosis (Fig. 2.36A–F). Oncocytic cells are round or polyhedral with centrally placed nuclei and dense, well-outlined cytoplasmic borders. Nucleoli are usually not prominent but may be conspicuous. Epithelial cells are characteristically associated with mast cells that may be detected on the MGG stain.[101,102] Lymphoid cells represent follicle centre cells and range from mature lymphocytes to blasts and plasma cells. Cystic debris contains macrophages and may contain polymorphs and crystals.[62] All 3 components are present in about 28% of cases, 2 components in 55% (oncocytes and necrosis or oncocytes and lymphocytes) and 17% show 1 component only.[103] Diagnosis of Warthin's tumour is easily made when all 3 components are present, or even 2 components, since the oncocytes are obvious in

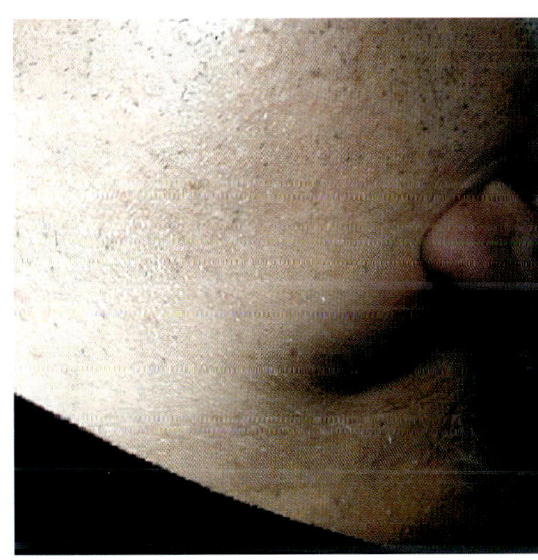

Figure 2.35 Warthin's tumour. Patients present with several months or years history of a soft swelling which does not vary in size. FNAC may yield turbid fluid. In this case it is advisable to sample the wall of the lesion to avoid sampling errors.

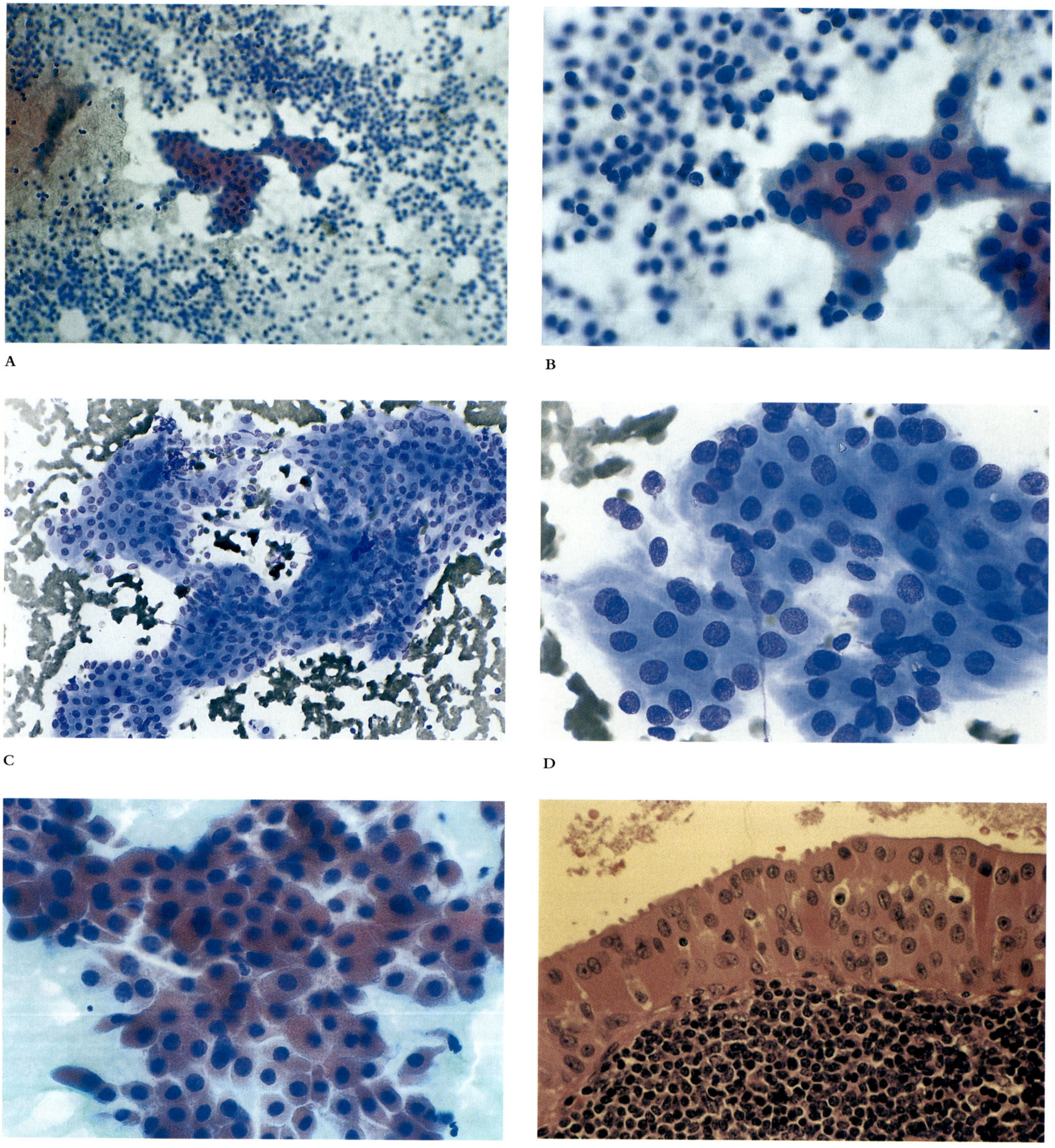

Figure 2.36 Warthin's tumour. **A.** Typical cytological appearance of Warthin's tumour. Islands of oncocytes are arranged in flat sheets surround by lymphoid cells (PAP ×200). **B.** Same case. Oncocytic epithelium has centrally placed nuclei and dense eosinophilic cytoplasm in alcohol-fixed smears (PAP ×400). **C.** Oncocytic epithelium may be sparse or, as in this case, may dominate the FNAC. Differential diagnosis is oncocytoma (MGG ×200). **D.** Oncocytes in air-dried smears are often associated with mast cells. This may be helpful in distinguishing this tumour from other oncocyte containing tumours (MGG ×600 oil). **E.** PAP stain may show intracytoplasmic granules in oncocytic epithelium (PAP ×600). **F.** Histology of adenolymphoma shows that lymphoid cells in the wall of the cyst are lined by oncocytic epithelium (H&E ×400).

most cases. If a smear shows a single component, diagnosis is more difficult and differential diagnosis should include oncocytoma, intraparotid lymphadenitis, salivary gland cyst or low-grade mucoepidermoid carcinoma.

Diagnostic errors may be caused by a lack of typical features and the presence of individual atypical squamous cells in a necrotic background mimicking carcinoma, particularly in cases where there is *squamous metaplasia* and mucinous content of the cystic space.[104] In this case, a low-grade mucoepidermoid carcinoma should be considered. This is particularly true of the metaplastic (or infarcted) variant of Warthin's tumour. It is characterised by replacement of much of the original oncocytic epithelium by metaplastic squamous cells, along with areas of extensive necrosis, fibrosis and inflammatory change. The pathogenesis is unknown, but it is most likely to be vascular in origin. An association with a previous fine needle aspiration (1–4 months presurgery) has been suggested.[39] Another possible association with the previously performed FNAC of Warthin's tumour is the finding of multiple sarcoid-like granulomas with multinucleate giant cells on tissue sections. These are probably caused by the exposure of lymphoid tissue to the contents of cystic spaces.[105] In addition to Warthin's tumour, a spectrum of neoplastic and non-neoplastic lesions of the salivary glands may contain squamous cells. These include chronic sialadenitis, lymphoepithelial cyst, pleomorphic adenoma, mucoepidermoid carcinoma and squamous cell carcinoma.[48] It is therefore important to recognise metaplastic Warthin's tumour, because the differential diagnosis of this benign neoplasm includes mucoepidermoid and squamous carcinoma, both primary and metastatic.

Oncocytic change, so typically a part of Warthin's tumour, may be seen in other tumours. Oncocytes are large, apparently swollen epithelial cells with cytoplasm densely filled with eosinophilic granules scattered amongst the ductal and acinar cells of the salivary gland cells. The name originates from the Greek word ονκοσ, meaning 'to swell' or 'to gain in size'. Hürthle first described them in 1894.[106] They are mitochondria-rich epithelial cells characterised by the presence of granules in the cytoplasm. The granules sometimes coalesce so that the cytoplasm appears homogeneous. The cell of origin is though to be the multipotential cell of intercalated ducts, as evidenced by the transition of small basophilic cuboidal cells into swollen acidophilic granular cells. They are not typically a prominent feature of mucoepidermoid carcinoma of the salivary glands, and only 5 such cases have been reported.[107] Because most salivary gland lesions with oncocytic change are benign, it is important to distinguish mucoepidermoid carcinoma from other entities that may show prominent oncocytic change.

The recently described phenomenon of electrocautery-induced oncocytic change deserves the attention of histopathologists. This is believed to occur as a consequence of electrothermal discharge.[108] Oncocytic change can also be seen in multifocal oncocytic adenomatous hyperplasia.[109]

Lymphoid cells within Warthin's tumour may be mistaken for an intraparotid lymph node or a lymphoma (Fig. 2.37; Box 2.3).[2] Follicle centre non-Hodgkin's lymphoma and

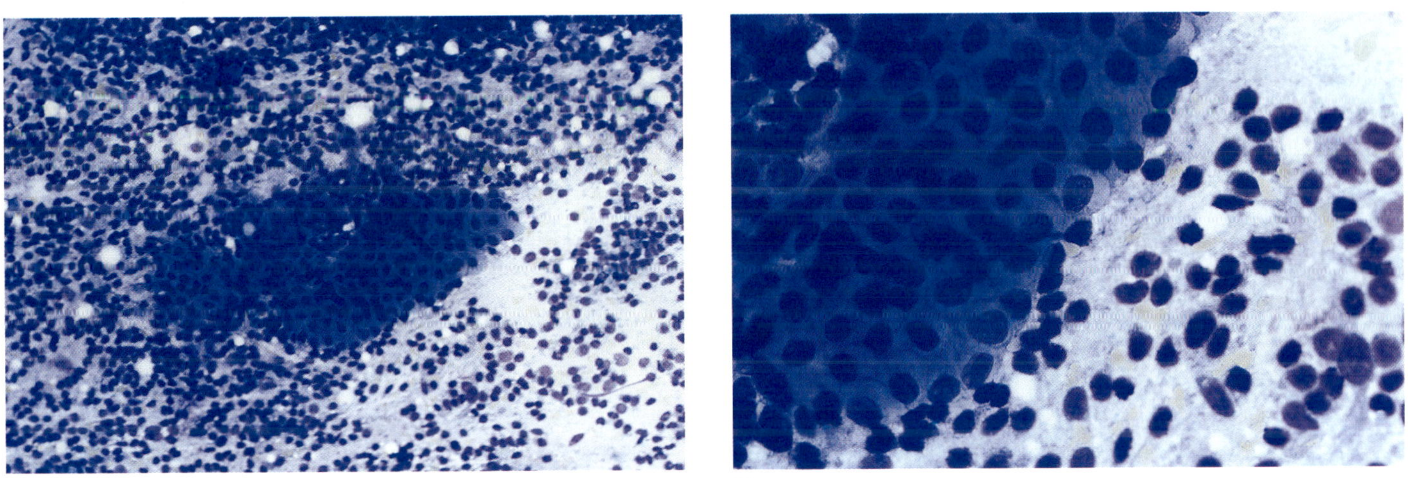

A B

Figure 2.37 Warthin's tumour. **A.** FNAC material can sometimes have a dominant lymphoid component with only occasional islands of epithelium, and may be difficult to distinguish from ductal epithelium of lymphoproliferative conditions including myoepithelial sialadenitis and MALT lymphoma.

Warthin's tumour involving the same site have been described.[110] The localised non-Hodgkin's lymphoma described suggests that it initially arose in the lymph node involved by Warthin's tumour and thus the Warthin's tumour may have provided a source of long-term antigenic stimulation from which a monoclonal B-cell population subsequently arose. These findings support the hypothesis that Warthin's tumour arises from heterotopic salivary gland ducts within lymph nodes.

Malignant transformation of Warthin's tumour is a rare event and very few cases of mucoepidermoid carcinoma arising in Warthin's tumour in the parotid gland have been described.[111,112] Extraparotid Warthin's tumours occasionally arise in the cervical region[113] or in the larynx.[71] Awareness of this may prevent diagnostic difficulties.

Monomorphic adenomas

Monomorphic adenomas are rare, benign tumours that do not recur or metastasise, hence they should be recognised and separated from other tumours. They have unique morphologic features, some of which can be recognised on FNAC, helping in further clinical management.

Basal cell adenoma

Basal cell adenoma is an uncommon salivary gland tumour and makes up approximately 1.2% of all salivary gland tumours.[114] Histologically, basal cell adenomas are subdivided into solid, tubular, trabecular and membranous variants.

Cytological features are those of small clusters of branching cords composed of small, uniform cells with round to oval nuclei and scanty cytoplasm looking like naked nuclei. Sparse homogenous background material is seen (Fig. 2.38). The trabecular variant contains hyaline globules and membranous variant contains membranous material around the cell groups.[114] The solid variant contains very little apart from basaloid cells.

Differential diagnosis of basal cell adenoma on FNAC material includes pleomorphic adenoma, basal cell adenocarcinoma, adenoid cystic carcinoma and metastatic basal cell carcinoma. The cells of pleomorphic adenoma tend to be less cohesive, with cell aggregates appearing to fall apart at the edges. The cells of basal cell adenoma tend to adhere to sheets of basement membrane. Basal cell adenocarcinomas are similar to basal cell adenomas but usually contain some cell pleomorphism, occasional mitoses and/or focal necrosis (Figs 2.50 and 2.51). A review of 6 major studies encompassing 10 cases of basal cell adenocarcinoma diagnosed on FNAC show cumulatively 100% sensitivity and specificity.[115]

Cytological features of the cell–stroma interface are useful in distinguishing between monomorphic adenomas of the basal cell type and adenoid cystic carcinoma. In basal cell adenomas, the collagenous stroma interdigitates with adjacent cells, whereas in adenoid cystic carcinoma the two are

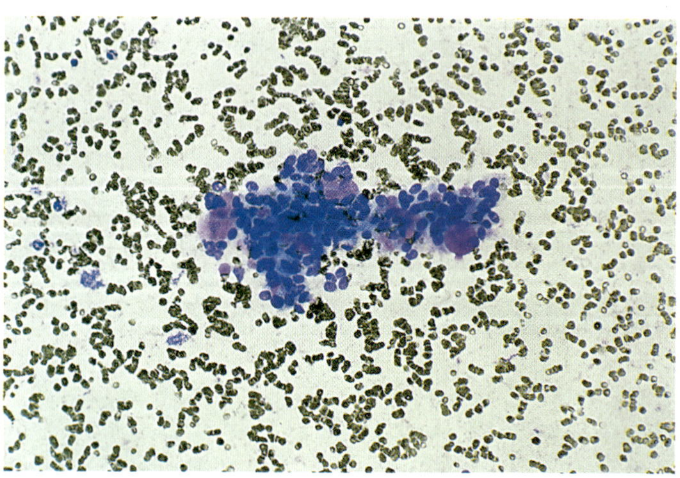

A

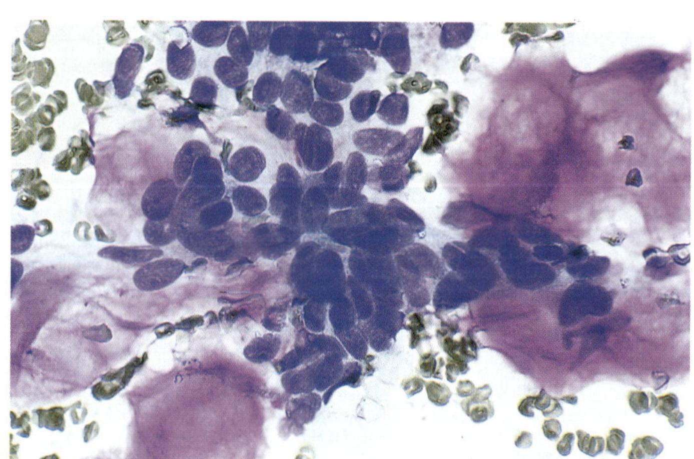

B

Figure 2.38 Basal cell adenoma. **A.** Tightly cohesive clusters of small uniform cells with round or oval nuclei and scanty cytoplasm (MGG ×200). **B.** Sparse homogenous background material (MGG ×600 oil).

separated by a sharp, smooth border. Furthermore, the stroma of basal cell adenomas can contain rare spindle cells or capillaries, but the cylinders of adenoid cystic carcinoma are acellular. Occasionally, however, adenoid cystic carcinoma shows the small blue cell pattern and cell–stroma interface features of basal cell adenoma and does not contain smooth-bordered cylinders typical of adenoid cystic carcinoma. These may be incorrectly interpreted as benign at the time of fine needle aspiration. Stanley et al[116] suggest that the stroma aspirated from solid adenoid cystic carcinoma represents desmoplastic tumour stroma which mimics the pattern of basal cell adenoma in smear material. Occasionally hyaline globules in the trabecular type of basal cell adenoma may be misinterpreted as adenoid cystic carcinoma.[115] Close attention should be paid to the appearance of the epithelial nuclei. These are bland with a finely granular chromatin and no or inconspicuous nucleoli in basal cell adenoma and hyperchromatic and coarse in adenoid cystic carcinoma. Distinction between basal cell adenoma and adenoid cystic carcinoma (particularly the solid type) at the time of fine needle aspiration remains a difficult problem.[116]

Oncocytoma

Oncocytomas are rare, benign salivary gland neoplasms that represent approximately 1.5% of all salivary gland tumours. The parotid gland is most commonly involved; the submandibular gland is very rarely the site of this tumour. Males and females are affected equally and the age range is 21–88 years. Clinically, the tumours are generally asymptomatic, well-circumscribed masses that increase in size over a period ranging from several weeks to 20 years and which are occasionally associated with pain. Histologically, the tumours are characterised by large epithelial cells with eosinophilic, granular cytoplasm. The cytoplasm stains positively with stains used to demonstrate mitochondria (phosphotungstic acid-hematoxylin, Novelli, Cresylecht violet V, and Kluver Barrera Luxol fast blue stains). Immunohistochemical reactions demonstrate an epithelial origin (keratin and epithelial membrane antigen), whereas markers for myoepithelial derivation (S-100 protein, actin and glial fibrillary acidic protein) are not identified.[117] Surgical resection is the only treatment.

Cytological features include cohesive multilayered sheets of oncocytic cells with small, regular, round nuclei and abundant, well-outlined cytoplasm. There is absence of cystic change, lymphoid cells and debris (Fig. 2.39).

Differential diagnosis includes Warthin's tumour and other salivary gland tumours in which cells resemble oncocytes; for example, oncocytic carcinoma (Fig. 2.53), acinic cell carcinoma (Fig. 2.41A,B), intermediate-grade mucoepidermoid carcinoma and adenocarcinoma cells all have these appearances occasionally (see *Oncocytic change*, page 39). Oncocytic cells in Warthin's tumour are usually monolayered, and in oncocytoma they are multilayered.

Cases of benign parotid gland oncocytoma with pseudomalignant change that mimics acinic cell carcinoma have been described. In histological sections there are clusters of pigmented cells with PAS-positive foamy to finely granular cytoplasm similar to those seen in salivary gland acinic cell carcinomas. This is a diagnostic pitfall that may be observed in histological tissue specimens removed after FNAC of oncocytic tumours.[118] Malignant oncocytoma of the parotid has been described (Fig. 2.53).[119]

Rare benign tumours

Myoepithelioma

Of all salivary gland tumours, myoepithelioma accounts for less than 1%. Myoepithelial tumours affect patients of both sexes equally. The mean age of the patients is 54 years. It involves the parotid but also the submandibular glands. Rare cases have been found to involve the sinonasal tract, lacrymal gland and larynx. Myoepitheliomas also occur in the breast. Myoepithelioma is benign and has a good prognosis. Conservative surgical management is curative[120–122] Malignant variant of the tumour (malignant myoepithelioma) usually develops in a pre-existing salivary gland tumour, usually pleomorphic adenoma but also myoepithelioma.[123,124] Histologically, myoepithelial tumours are composed of epithelioid, plasmacytoid, spindle, or clear cell types, and they show a solid or myxoid pattern of growth.

Cytological features show a uniform population of small spindle cells with elongated oval nuclei with evenly distributed, homogenous chromatin, inconspicuous nucleoli with cytoplasm that forms thin bipolar wispy processes (Fig. 2.40A–E). Occasionally cells have a plasmacytoid appearance, similar to plasmacytoid cells of pleomorphic adenoma. The diagnosis can be confirmed by ultrastructural and

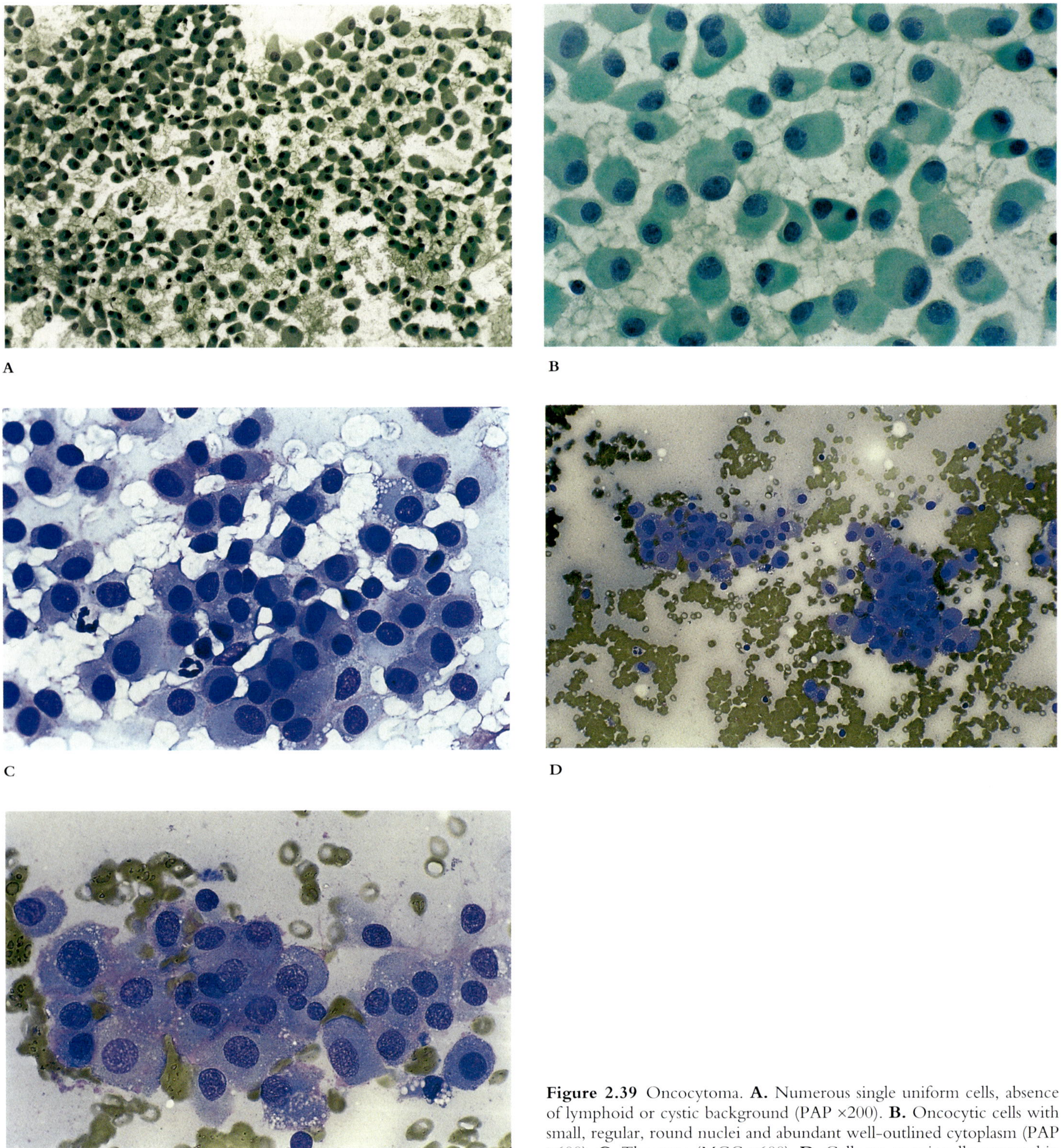

Figure 2.39 Oncocytoma. **A.** Numerous single uniform cells, absence of lymphoid or cystic background (PAP ×200). **B.** Oncocytic cells with small, regular, round nuclei and abundant well-outlined cytoplasm (PAP ×600). **C.** The same (MGG ×600). **D.** Cells are occasionally arranged in multilayered sheets (MGG ×400). **E.** The same (MGG ×600).

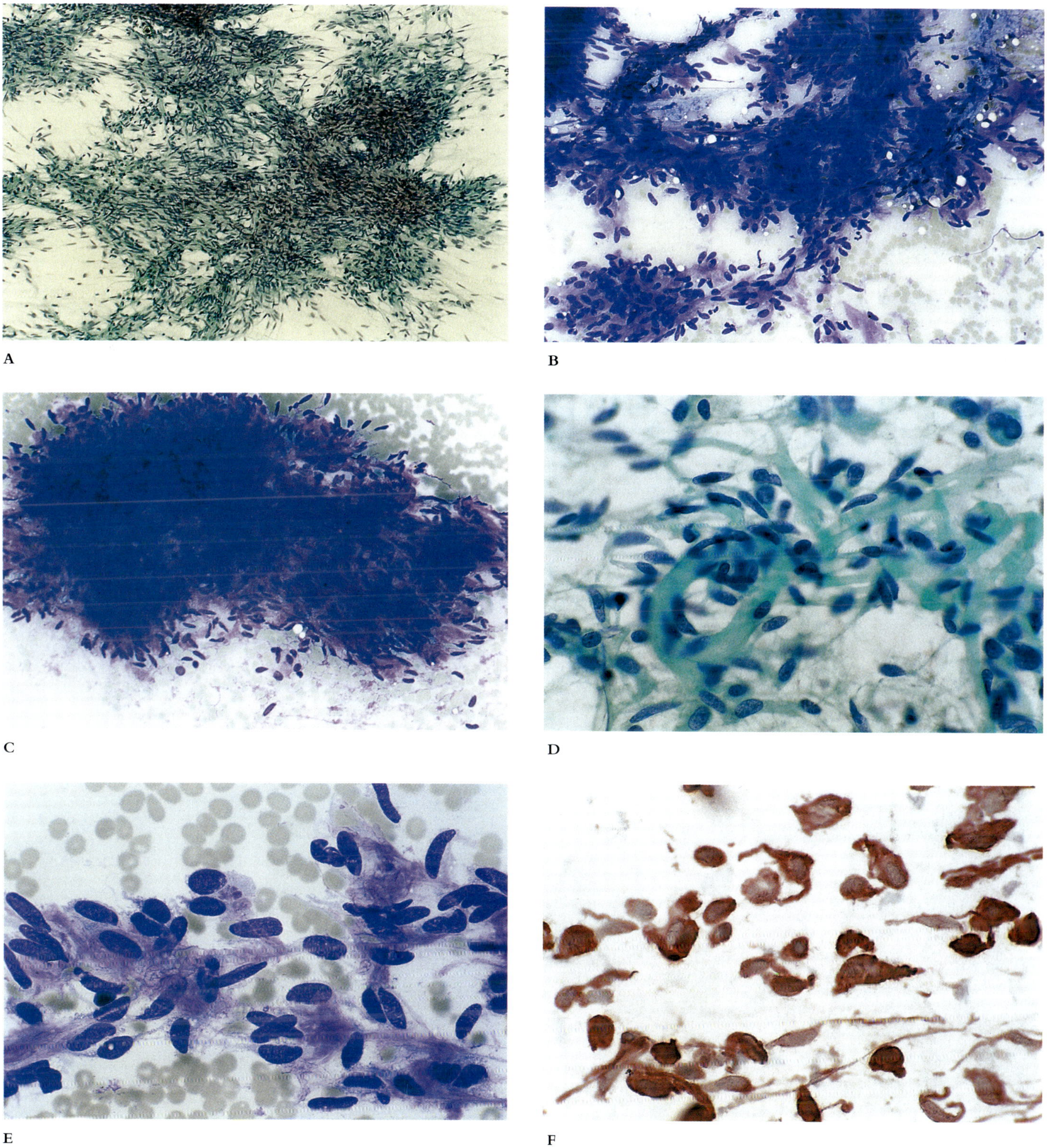

Figure 2.40 Myoepithelioma. **A.** FNAC yields cellular smears composed of interconnected aggregates and single cells (PAP ×100). **B,C.** Medium-power view is that of a spindle cell tumour with cells immersed in background material. No pleomorphism or mitoses are seen (PAP ×600 oil). **E.** Plump nuclei of myoepithelioma may be mistaken for leiomyoma or nerve sheath tumour (MGG ×600 oil). **F.** Antibodies against cytokerotin are positive as well as S-100 (×600 oil, APAAP anticytokeratin)

immunohistochemical analysis demonstrating myofilaments aggregation pattern and positive staining for S100-protein, vimentin and keratin antibodies (Fig. 2.40F). Glial fibrillary acidic protein is positive in 53%, and muscle-specific actin and smooth-muscle actin are positive in only 20%. Desmin is negative in both benign and malignant tumours.

Myoepithelioma composed of bland spindle cells is difficult to distinguish from soft tissue lesions, e.g. nodular fasciitis, leiomyoma, nerve sheath tumour or haemangiopericytoma (Fig. 2.61).[125]

Given the relative rarity of the tumour, most cytopathologists will not be familiar with the entity and will report a 'spindle cell neoplasm' that needs excision.

Intraductal papilloma

Intraductal papilloma of the salivary gland is an extremely rare benign tumour that occurs most commonly in the minor salivary glands. They are cystic, solitary neoplasms that arise from ductal epithelium and produce painless swellings from which fluid is usually aspirated. Excision is curative and recurrences are rare.

Cytological features of intraductal papilloma are three-dimensional epithelial clusters, some with a papillary configuration and histiocytes. The majority of cells shows oncocytic differentiation; however, benign-appearing ductal cells in honeycomb sheets can also be present.[126] Sebaceous differentiation may be seen.[127]

Other salivary gland tumours with *papillary* components include inverted duct papilloma, sialadenoma papilliferum, papillary cystadenoma and Warthin's tumour. Polymorphous low-grade adenocarcinoma, cystic mucoepidermoid carcinoma and the papillary variant of acinic cell carcinoma can all have papillary structures.[127]

A malignant counterpart of intraductal papilloma, intraductal papillary adenocarcinoma, has only recently been described.[128] It is architecturally similar to intraductal papilloma with the addition of cytological atypia, intraductal extension, microinvasion and lymph node metastases.

Sebaceous adenoma,[129] cystadenoma,[130] pleomorphic lipoma,[131] collagenous fibroma[132] and nodular fasciitis[133] are rare benign lesions that may present within the salivary glands.

MALIGNANT TUMOURS OF THE SALIVARY GLANDS

FNAC allows distinction between neoplastic and non-neoplastic salivary gland lesions (Table 2.1). Within the neoplasms, if established diagnostic criteria are present, FNAC can separate benign from malignant tumours with a high level of accuracy.[32] Malignant parotid tumours are uncommon and present a significant management challenge. Cytology can correctly diagnose malignancy with 88–100% sensitivity.[134] More precise tumour typing, together with other prognostic factors (age, sex, grading, TNM and pTNM, facial nerve involvement) means that a radical parotidectomy is required in a proportion of patients, the rest undergoing superficial parotidectomy.[135] The crude 5- and 10-year survival rates are 68–75% and 49–67% respectively while the locoregional control rate at 10 years is 79%.[134,136] Radical surgery with appropriate reconstruction followed by planned postoperative adjuvant radiotherapy gives effective control of malignant parotid tumours.

In an attempt to find a useful *ancillary technique* to help distinguish benign and malignant neoplasms, the expression and mutation patterns of p53 were studied in a series of benign pleomorphic adenomas and malignant salivary gland tumours.[137] P53 overexpression (nuclear staining exceeding 10%) was detected in 20% of the malignant salivary gland tumours, with the highest prevalence observed in polymorphous low-grade adenocarcinoma, squamous cell carcinoma and carcinoma ex pleomorphic adenoma, and the lowest in adenoid cystic carcinoma and acinic cell carcinoma. In contrast, none of the benign pleomorphic adenomas had nuclear staining exceeding 10%. p53 may be a useful marker to help discriminate between benign and malignant salivary gland tumours.[137]

Immunohistochemical evaluation of salivary gland lesions with monoclonal antibodies PC10 and MIB-1 shows that proliferating cell nuclear antigens (PCNA) (PC10) and Ki-67 (MIB-1) indices are reliable markers for discriminating between benign and malignant tumours of the parotid gland.[138] The values of MIB-1 and PC10 parameters increase progressively in benign lesions in comparison with the normal salivary gland and in malignant neoplasms in comparison with non-neoplastic groups and benign lesions. Values in benign salivary tumours are significantly lower than in malignant groups. Flow cytometry evaluation of DNA ploidy and S-phase fraction shows that all benign salivary tumours and low-grade carcinomas have a DNA diploid pattern. Some high-grade carcinomas exhibit DNA aneuploidy. Mean S-phase fraction values show a statistically significant difference between the benign and malignant tumours, diploid and aneuploid tumours, and low- and high-grade carcinomas. There is a potential utility of flow cytometry in evaluating DNA ploidy and S-phase fraction in evaluating the clinical behaviour of salivary gland neoplasms.[139]

Acinic cell carcinoma

Acinic cell carcinoma is considered the third most common primary salivary gland carcinoma after adenoid cystic and mucoepidermoid carcinoma, with incidence ranging from 2% to 19%. It arises mainly in the major salivary glands, can be bilateral[140] and shows a preponderance of females, age range 10–84 years. Familial occurrence has been described.[141] Tumour sizes range from 1 cm to 8 cm, although giant acinic cell carcinomas have been reported.[142] In the majority of cases patients present with a painful swelling as a main symptom.[143] It is locally recurrent in 18–42% of cases with 5% local lymph node metastases.[143] The interval between the primary and recurrent cancer ranges between 17 and 24 years.[144] It is therefore currently considered as a low-grade malignancy with unpredictable local recurrences and lymph node metastases. Management of acinic cell carcinoma is based on reports of small numbers of cases accrued over several decades. The National Cancer Data Base identified 1353 cases of acinic cell carcinoma. Five-year survival was 83.3% (observed) and 91.4% (disease specific). Worse survival was associated with high grade, age ≥ 30 years, and the presence of metastatic disease.[145] An aggressive subset of acinic cell carcinoma which is characterised by high grade and advanced stage rarely occurs in patients under the age of 30 years. Although better outcome was not statistically demonstrated for combined therapy, surgery with irradiation is the most common management in the USA for cases with regional metastases, high grade and microscopic positive margins.[145]

Histologically, acinic cell carcinomas can be solid, microcystic, papillary cystic and follicular. According to cell morphology, they can also be classified as: well differentiated, composed predominantly of acinic cells; moderately differentiated, containing duct-like, vacuolated or clear cells; and poorly differentiated, showing undifferentiated cells. About half of acinic cell carcinomas exhibit more than one cell pattern. The grade of differentiation influences prognosis. Well-differentiated acinic cell carcinoma is the most common histological type and also has better prognosis (2-year overall survival, 100%; 5-year overall survival, 83%; 10-year overall survival, 50%) than poorly differentiated tumours (2-year overall survival, 70%; 5-year overall survival, 50%; 10-year overall survival, 30%).[143]

Cytological features of a well-differentiated acinic cell carcinoma show a characteristic bland picture of cohesive clusters of cells with abundant, fragile, finely vacuolated or granular cytoplasm and an acinar architectural pattern (Fig. 2.41). The cells are similar to acinar cells of normal salivary gland. Cytoplasmic granules are purple with Papanicolaou staining, red with MGG, stain with alcian blue and are PAS positive. Many bare nuclei are often seen in the background. In addition to these diagnostic clue cells, other types of neoplastic cells including vacuolated cells, clear cells, cells resembling oncocytes and non-specific glandular cells may be encountered. A pronounced lymphocytic reaction is a hallmark in some acinic cell carcinomas.[146] Macrophages and debris may be seen in the papillary cystic type. Both the varieties of tumour cell differentiation and the pronounced lymphocytic reaction observed in acinic cell carcinoma might result in confusion with other salivary gland lesions.

The differential diagnosis of acinic cell carcinoma encompasses normal salivary gland, epithelial myoepithelial carcinoma, adenocarcinoma, adenoid cystic carcinoma, clear cell mucoepidermoid carcinoma, cellular pleomorphic adenoma, oncocytic neoplasms, sebaceous adenoma and metastatic renal cell carcinoma.[144] Differentiation from normal salivary gland and acinic cell hyperplasia is by the abundance of acinic cells and the absence of adipocytes, ductal epithelium and the presence of numerous naked nuclei. In the presence of vacuolated/clear acinic cells, epithelial-myoepithelial carcinoma presents the main differential diagnosis. In epithelial-myoepithelial carcinoma there is a bimodal population of large 'clear' myoepithelial cells and clusters of small cuboidal epithelial cells (Fig. 2.48) Acinic cell carcinoma with duct-like glandular structures may resemble adenocarcinoma. In poorly differentiated carcinomas, only a diagnosis of malignancy can be made. Cytoplasmic granules of acinic cell carcinoma may help to distinguish the two tumours of different prognosis. Although these are prominent in some tumours, they are not always seen. Small, purple (MGG) intracytoplasmic granules can be seen in cellular pleomorphic adenoma and mucoepidermoid carcinoma. Differentiation from the clear

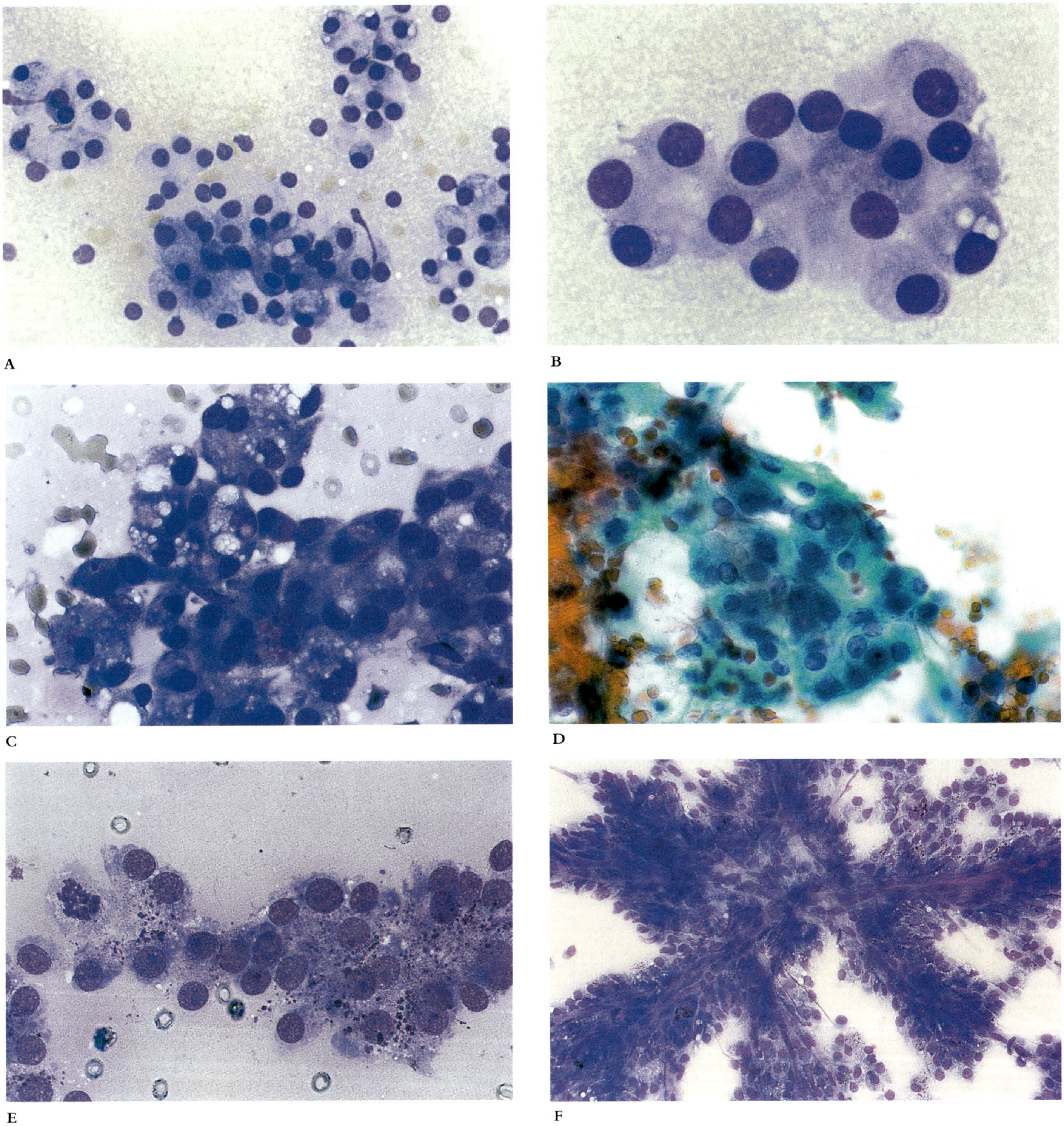

Figure 2.41 Acinic cell carcinoma. **A.** Well-differentiated acinic cell carcinoma. Abundant cohesive cell clusters with cells mimicking normal salivary gland cells. Nuclei are small and regular, cytoplasm fragile, relatively abundant and finely vacuolated (oncocyte-like) containing granules. However, the smears are more cellular than normal salivary gland, nuclei larger and less evenly distributed and the nuclear:cytoplasmic ratio is higher (MGG ×400). **B.** Resemblance of acinic carcinoma cells to oncocytes can cause difficulty in distinguishing them from oncocytoma and Warthin's tumour, particularly if there is a prominent lymphoid cell infiltrate in some of the acinic cell carcinomas (MGG ×600 oil, courtesy of Dr A. Rubin). **C.** Abundant, sometimes vacuolated cytoplasm may be confused with mucoepidermoid carcinoma or adenocarcinoma. Acinic cell carcinoma lacks the cell pleomorphism of adenocarcinoma and variability of mucoepidermoid carcinoma (MGG ×600 oil). **D.** Fairly uniform cells in aggregates (PAP ×400). **E.** Intracytoplasmic purple granules may be barely visible or marked as in this case (MGG ×600 oil). **F.** Low-power view shows capillary meshwork with acinic cells giving an impression of papillary structures (×400 MGG).

cell variant of mucoepidermoid carcinoma can be achieved by confirming the intra- and extracellular mucin in the former. Differentiation from oncocytic-type neoplasm, including Warthin's, can be made through analysis of cell borders that are not as sharp in acinic cell carcinoma, by the cell arrangement in acinar structures rather than in flat sheets and by the absence of amorphous debris in acinic cell carcinoma. Cystic variants of acinic cell carcinoma have to be differentiated from other tumours with cystic components: Warthin's, pleomorphic adenoma, intraduct papilloma and mucoepidermoid carcinoma.

Mucoepidermoid carcinoma

Mucoepidermoid carcinoma represents 4–9% of all salivary gland tumours.[23] It occurs most frequently in the sixth and seventh decades of life (average age 48.9 years). Patients present with an average of 6 months to 2 years history of painless swelling, slowly increasing in size. There is a slight predisposition of females. Nearly all mucoepidermoid carcinomas are localised in the major salivary glands with the parotid being the most common, followed by the palate. Histologically, there are 3 grades of differentiation as well as variants: cystic, clear cell and oncocytic. The therapy of choice is radical ablative surgery of the primary tumour and resection of the related lymphatic system in patients suspected of having metastases of the regional lymph nodes. The prognosis is excellent in patients with a localised manifestation of the disease only. Patients who died for reasons of tumour metastases had all been classified as stage III or IV at the time of initial diagnosis. Distant metastases are rarely found even decades after surgical therapy, so a long-term follow-up is recommended.[147]

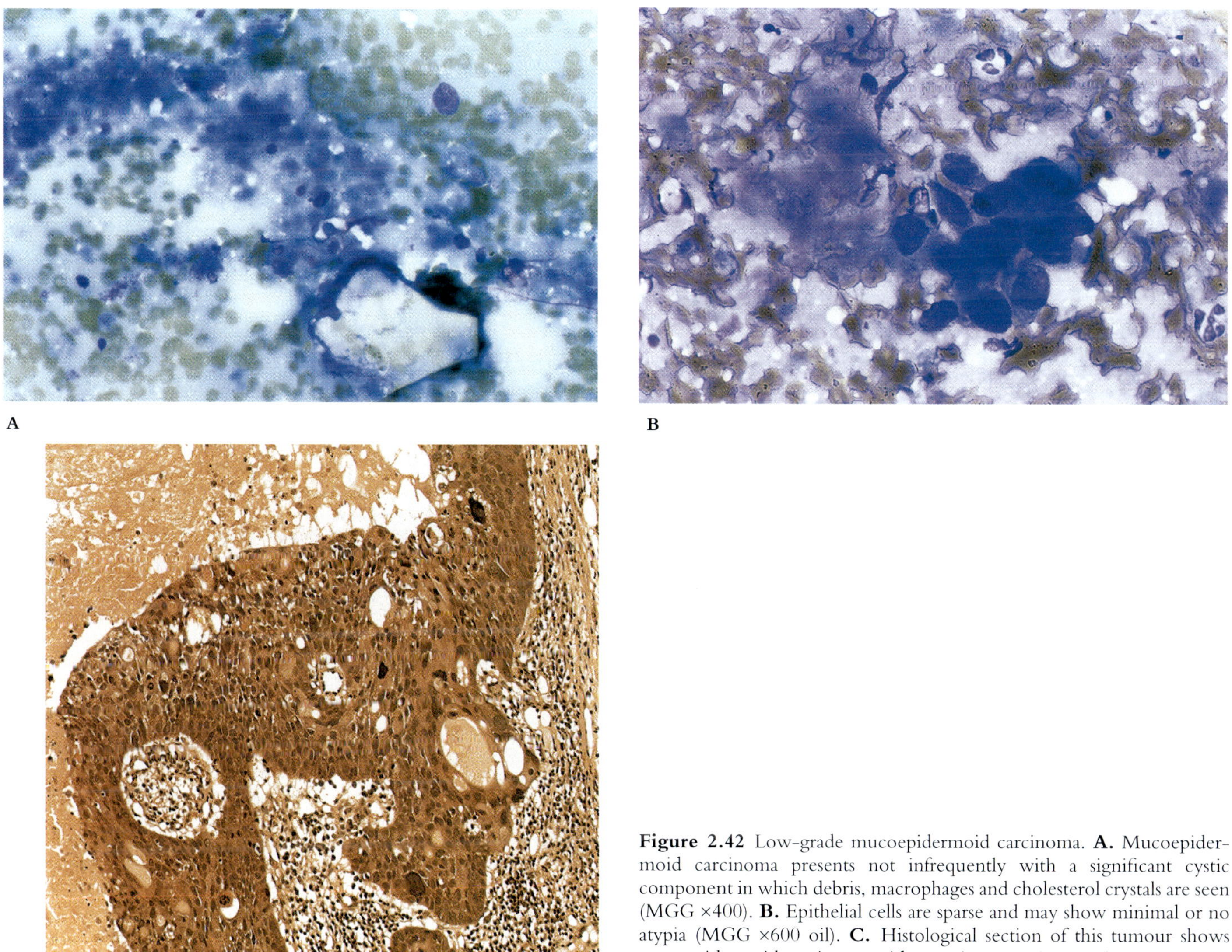

A B C

Figure 2.42 Low-grade mucoepidermoid carcinoma. **A.** Mucoepidermoid carcinoma presents not infrequently with a significant cystic component in which debris, macrophages and cholesterol crystals are seen (MGG ×400). **B.** Epithelial cells are sparse and may show minimal or no atypia (MGG ×600 oil). **C.** Histological section of this tumour shows mucoepidermoid carcinoma with prominent cystic areas (H&E ×400).

Cytological features. Of the common salivary gland tumours, mucoepidermoid carcinoma is probably the most difficult to diagnose accurately by FNAC. Different cell types and degrees of differentiation make for a variety of cytological presentations with a result that there are no specific diagnostic features of mucoepidermoid carcinoma but rather a combination of cellular and background features that may lead to a correct diagnosis. A combination of squamous and mucin-secreting epithelium is thought to be diagnostic of mucoepidermoid carcinoma. However, this may sometimes be difficult to prove, especially in cystic lesions. Cohen et al[148] used 3 cytological features as most predictive of mucoepidermoid carcinoma: intermediate cells; squamous cells; and overlapping epithelial groups. Using these three features together, they achieved the sensitivity and specificity of accurately diagnosing mucoepidermoid carcinoma of 97% and 100% respectively.[148] Other reports differentiate between the sensitivity of FNAC diagnosis for high- and intermediate-grade (87% and 85% respectively) and low-grade tumours where sensitivity is lower (68%).[149]

The presence of intermediate, squamous and vacuolated, mucin producing cells in flat sheets or clusters against a background of mucus and debris is usually found in low-grade tumours (Fig. 2.42). Cells may look bland and if there is predominance of intermediate (metaplastic) cells they may look rather oncocytic, therefore the features may be mistaken for a benign cystic lesion such as Warthin's tumour. High-grade tumours have more obvious features of malignancy with overlapping, crowding and prominent nucleoli, but they may be difficult to type (Fig. 2.43). Cells are variably squamoid, vacuolated or have clear cytoplasm, probably due to glycogen. Intermediate cells from tissue sections correspond to the metaplastic-looking cells in smears.

Differential diagnosis includes other squamous lesions, oncocytic tumours, acinic cell carcinoma and other cystic tumours. High-grade tumours are difficult to distinguish from other poorly differentiated primary or metastatic tumours. The nuclei of salivary duct carcinoma have abundant, dense eosinophilic cytoplasm, which can be mistaken for squamous differentiation. Cystic mucoepidermoid carcinoma may resemble benign lesions, e.g. retention cysts, inflammatory processes with squamous metaplasia, mucus and debris. Lymphocytic infiltrate may be prominent within mucoepidermoid carcinoma, making distinction from benign conditions difficult. Oncocytic change within mucoepidermoid carcinomas is rare and only a few cases have been reported.[107,150] Oncocytic change is not typically a prominent feature of mucoepidermoid carcinoma of the salivary glands. Because most salivary gland lesions with oncocytic change are benign, it is important to distinguish mucoepidermoid carcinoma from other entities that may show prominent oncocytic change. Mucoepidermoid carcinoma arising in Warthin's tumour has been described.[111] Since oncocytic change is said to be occasionally a consequence of previous FNAC and/or electrocautery, caution in interpreting the oncocytic change in an inappropriate background is needed.[39,108]

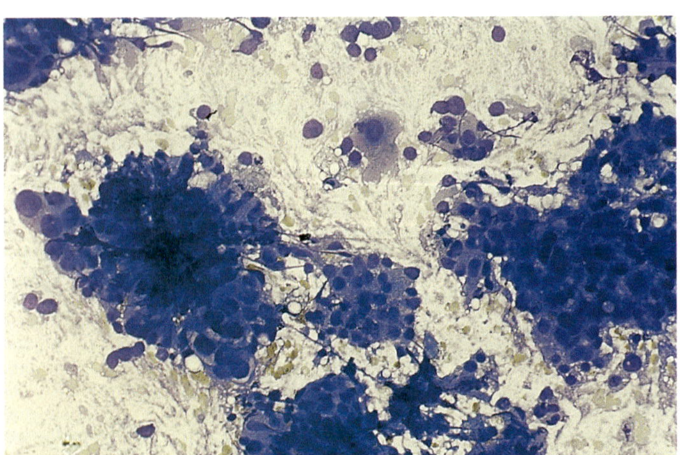

A

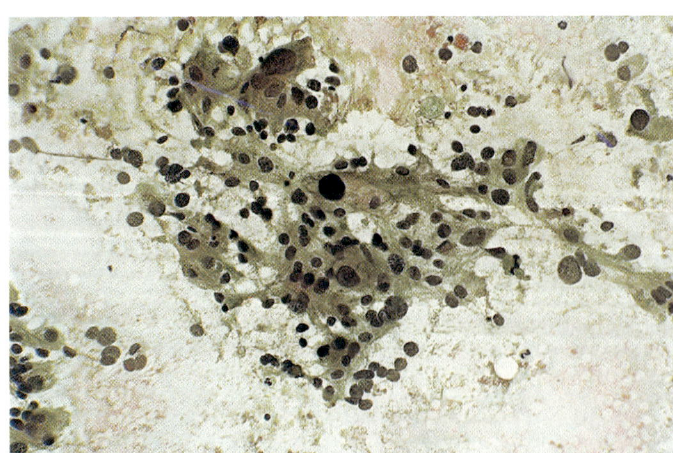

B

Figure 2.43 High-grade mucoepidermoid carcinoma. **A.** Low-power view shows obvious features of malignancy, pleomorphism, overlapping and crowding (MGG ×200). **B.** PAP ×200. ***(continued)***

Mucoepidermoid carcinoma ex pleomorphic adenoma

Mucoepidermoid carcinomas ex pleomorphic adenoma cytologically present as non-specific high-grade malignancies and consist of highly malignant cells, in clusters or isolated, rarely associated with intracellular and extracellular mucin. A background of cellular and stromal elements consistent with pleomorphic adenoma can be identified. Although it is nearly impossible cytologically to distinguish these lesions from other high-grade primary or metastatic carcinomas (such as poorly differ-

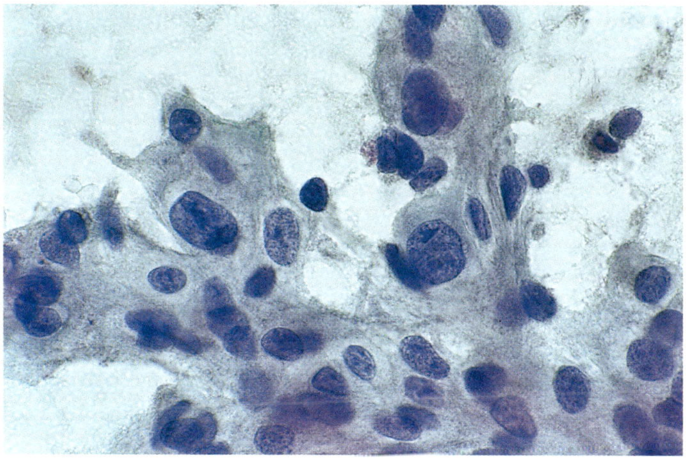
C

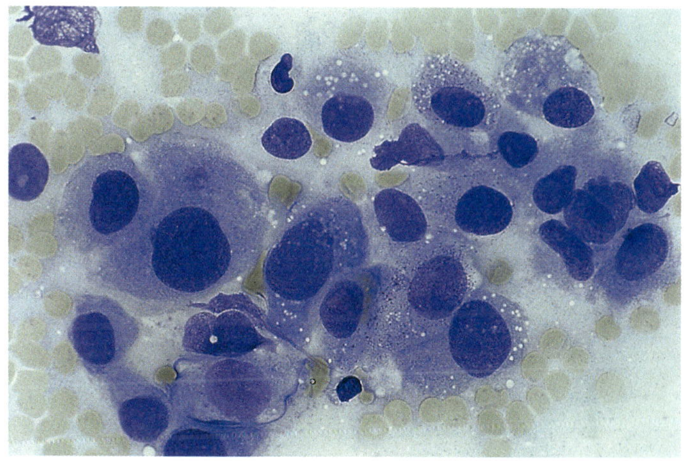
D

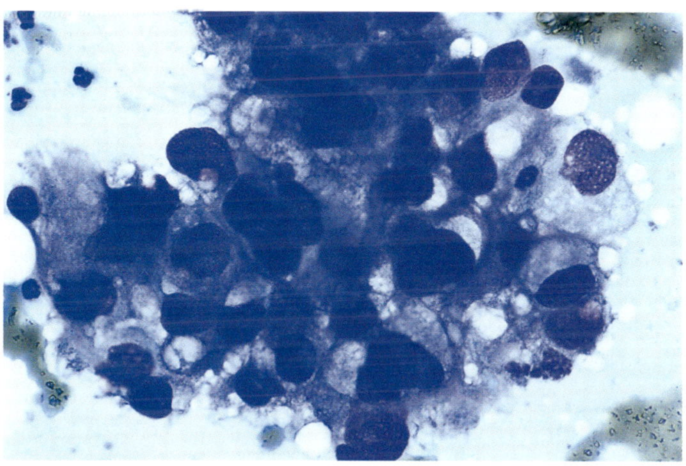
E

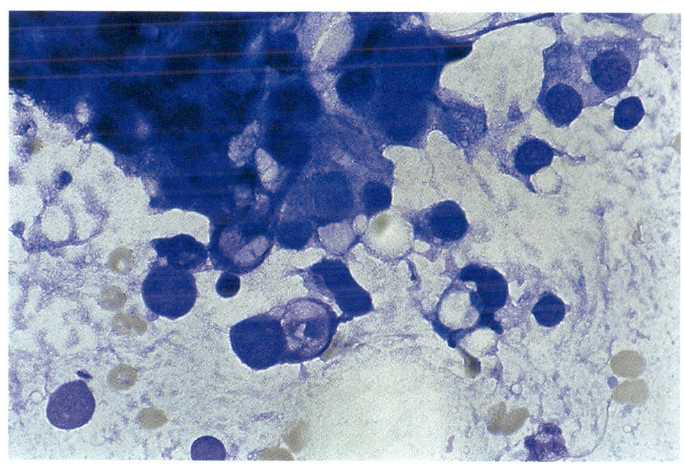
F

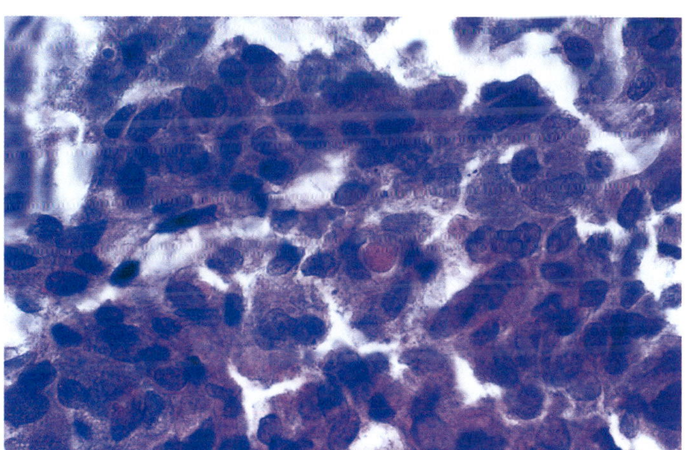
G

Figure 2.43 ***(continued)*** High-grade mucoepidermoid carcinoma. **C,D,E.** High-power view shows squamoid, intermediate and vacuolated cells with features of malignancy (PAP, MGG ×600 oil). **F.** Mucin secreting vacuolated cells are a useful pointer to the diagnosis in some cases (MGG ×600). Mucoepidermoid carcinoma. **G.** Intracytoplasmic mucin present in cells (PAS diastase ×600).

entiated squamous cell carcinomas, adenosquamous carcinomas and salivary duct carcinomas), this limitation is not dramatic. Cytological diagnosis of high-grade malignancy per se allows for proper preoperative patient management.[151,152]

Clinical features associated with metastasis or death are more advanced age, tumour size and preoperative symptoms. Histopathological features that correlate with poor outcome are a cystic component less than 20%, 4 or more mitotic figures per 10 high-power fields, neural involvement, necrosis and anaplasia. Patients with tumours of equal histopathological grade have a better prognosis when their tumours are in the parotid gland than when their tumours are in the submandibular gland.

Multivariate analysis indicates proliferating cell nuclear antigen (PC10) to be the most important parameter in predicting survival. Thus the measurement of proliferating cell nuclear antigen is a useful predictor of survival for patients with mucoepidermoid carcinoma.[153]

Although the role of the cytopathologist in the primary diagnosis may be difficult, knowledge of the possible pitfalls may prevent missing a neoplasm in the first instance, particularly with the low-grade tumours. In the cases of diagnostic staging or recurrence, FNAC diagnosis should not pose any problems. It can offer a valuable service ensuring that these relatively indolent tumours are cured.

Adenoid cystic carcinoma

Adenoid cystic carcinoma is one of the commonest primary salivary gland carcinomas, its incidence around 5% of salivary gland tumours.[154] Over half of these tumours arise in the major salivary glands (Fig. 2.44). The incidence of lymph node metastases is low, ranging from 5% to 15% of cases. Patients may present with facial nerve paresis since the tumour often involves the nerves (Fig. 2.47A). Histologically, two main patterns are recognised: tubulocribriform and solid.[20] The former type is thought to have a better prognosis.

Cytological features of adenoid cystic carcinoma are most characteristically seen as large hyaline globules of extracellular matrix (basement membrane material), staining red/magenta (MGG) or green (Papanicolaou), partially surrounded by basaloid tumour cells (Fig. 2.45A–E). The

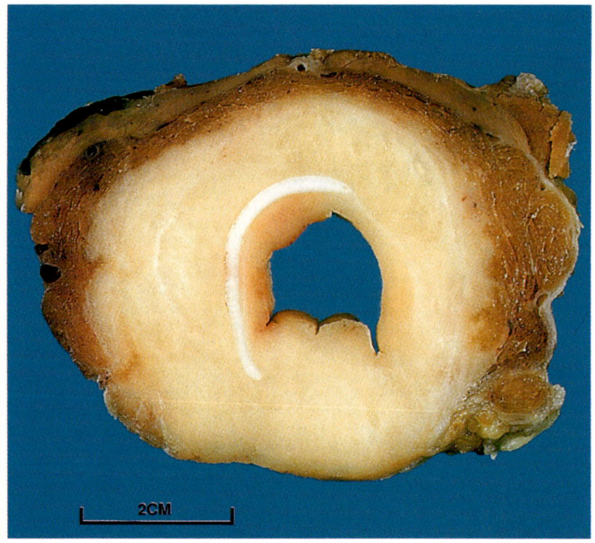

Figure 2.44 Section of larynx showing adenoid cystic carcinoma in a 27-year-old woman. CT scan suggested an unusual infiltrate in the larynx (soft tissue, amyloid). FNAC was performed transcutaneously tangential to trachea. A diagnosis of adenoid cystic carcinoma was made. The patient underwent laryngectomy in hope of a surgical cure.

hyaline globules may vary considerably in size. Basement membrane material, as well as in hyaline globules, is seen in finger-like structures with naked nuclei (Fig. 2.45E). Cylindrical structures containing naked nuclei, closely cohesive in the middle of the cylinder and dissociated at each end, are thought to be characteristic (Fig. 2.45D).[154] Basaloid cells are tightly cohesive or single, with uniform oval or round nuclei, coarse chromatin and very scanty or absent cytoplasm. Nuclei may be hyperchromatic with prominent nucleoli, particularly in the poorly differentiated tumours without hyaline globules (Fig. 2.46). When hyaline globules are present in large numbers, a diagnosis of adenoid cystic carcinoma can be made with confidence.[155] However, hyaline globules are not always present, particularly in the solid type (Fig. 2.47). Hyaline globules are not pathognomonic for adenoid cystic carcinoma. They can be seen in basal cell adenoma, epithelial-myoepithelial carcinoma, polymorphous low-grade carcinoma and pleomorphic adenoma. In FNACs with predominance of basaloid tumour cells but lacking characteristic globules, all other benign and malignant salivary gland tumours of epithelial-myoepithelial differentiation should be considered in the cytological diagnosis.[156]

Pleomorphic adenoma is most frequently confused with adenoid cystic carcinoma. The most consistent finding for differentiating adenoid cystic carcinoma from pleomorphic adenoma is the amount of cytoplasm of individual tumour cells. Plasmacytoid appearance is a reliable finding for pleomorphic adenoma, and it enables to rule out adenoid cystic carcinoma.[40] In contrast with pleomorphic adenoma, most adenoid cystic carcinomas show little cytoplasm. Hyaline spherical globules are sensitive but not specific for diagnosis of adenoid cystic carcinoma. They are found in 80% of adenoid cystic carcinomas but only rarely in pleomorphic adenoma.[154] Fibrillary chondromyxoid ground substance and a mixture of epithelial cells with stroma are found in the

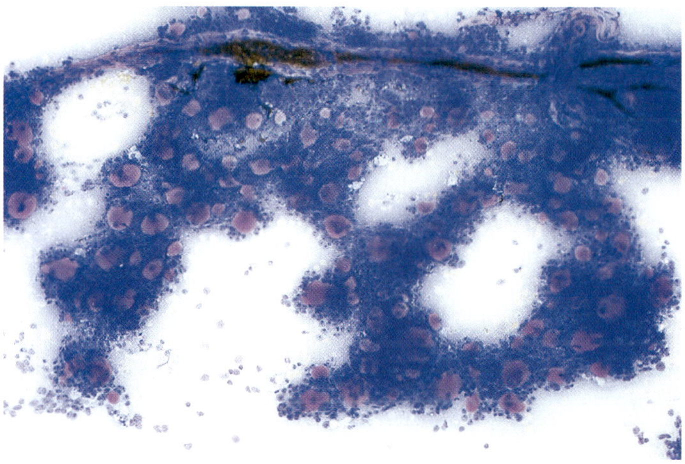
A

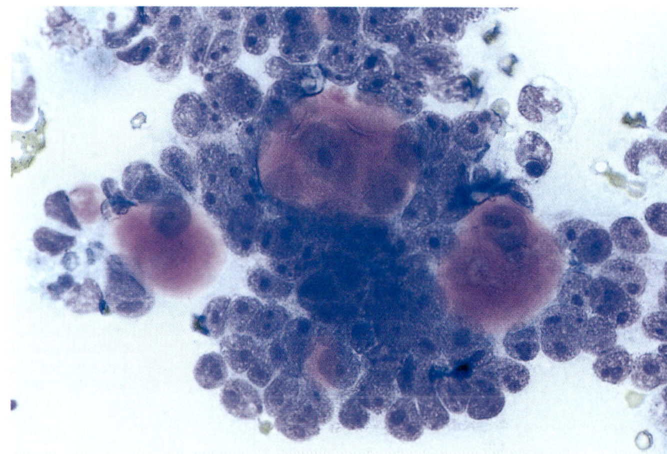
B

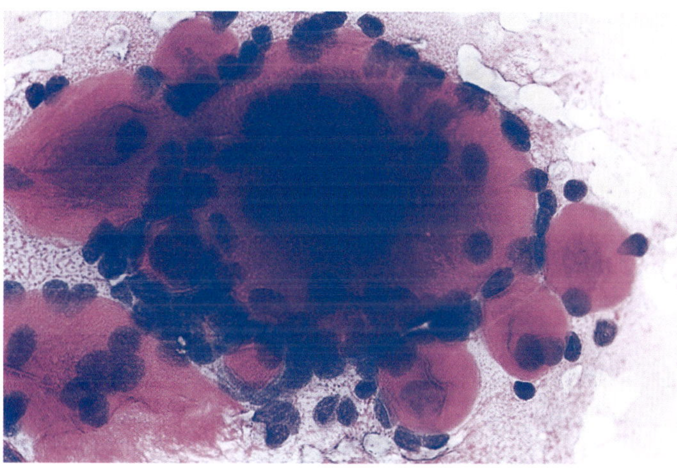
C

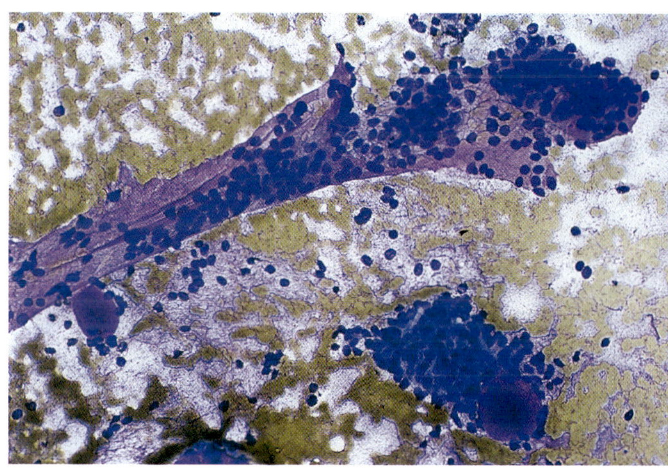
D

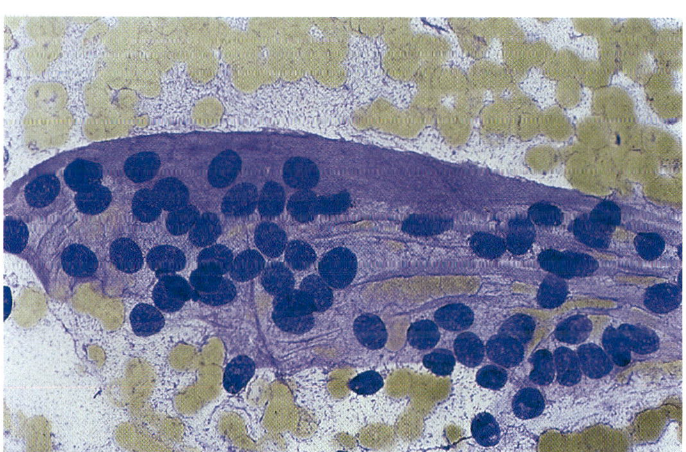
E

Figure 2.45 Adenoid cystic carcinoma case shown in Figure 2.44. **A.** Sieve-like arrangement of basaloid tumour cells and medium-sized globules equivalent to the cribriform histological pattern. **B.** Basaloid tumour cells arranged in rosette-like formations surrounding small homogenous globules (MGG ×100). **C.** Globules of hyaline material of various size presenting as a matrix structure. **D.** Another case. Cylindrical structures with concentrations of nuclei at either end representing stromal fragments, partially surrounded and containing basaloid tumour cells (MGG ×400). **E.** Finger-like reddish structures with low concentration of naked nuclei (MGG ×1000, oil).

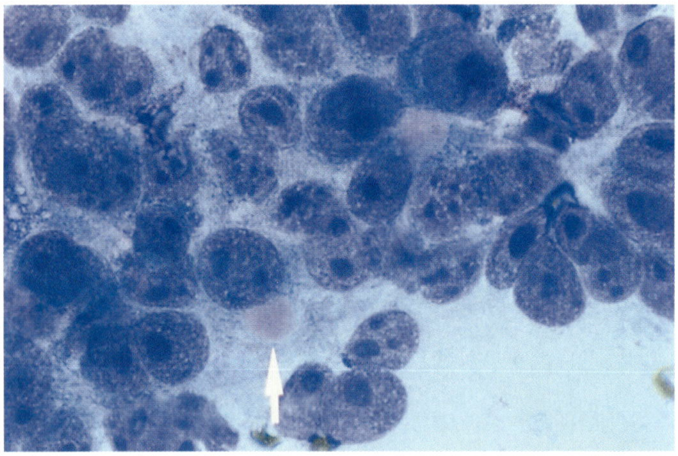

Figure 2.46 Adenoid cystic carcinoma. Poorly differentiated malignant cells with nucleoli are a rare presentation of the disease but may be seen in recurrent tumours. Note the intracytoplasmic vacuole (arrow) (MGG ×600 oil).

majority of pleomorphic adenomas. The pattern of cell clusters is helpful to differentiate pleomorphic adenoma from adenoid cystic carcinoma. Large, loose clusters with a spindle cell core suggest pleomorphic adenoma. Small, dense trabeculae with a smooth margin and dense clusters containing clear, round spaces are more suggestive of adenoid cystic carcinoma. Overall cellularity, proportion of isolated cells, orientation of cellular clusters and degree of cellular overlapping give almost no help in making the distinction between the lesions.

Distinction from rare neoplasms of salivary glands with epithelial-myoepithelial cell differentiation, including basal cell adenoma and carcinoma, epithelial-myoepithelial

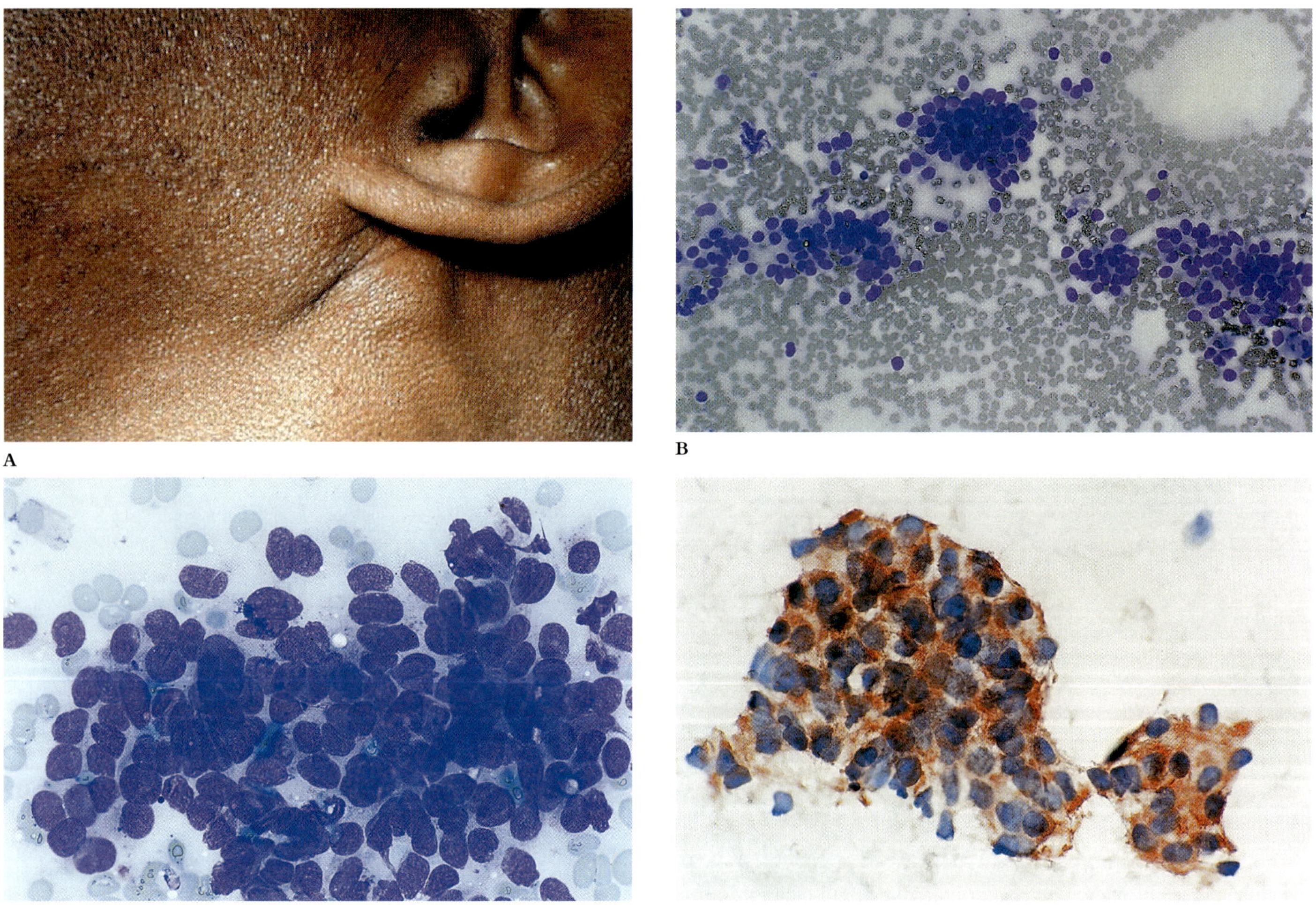

A B C D

Figure 2.47 **A.** Salivary gland malignant tumour. A 4-month history of swelling at the left angle of the mandible. The mass is adherent to surrounding tissues with skin pulling facial nerve paralysis present. **B.** FNAC reveals adenoid cystic carcinoma. Basaloid tumour cells with no globules or hyaline stroma (MGG ×400). Clinical features were helpful in diagnosing malignancy. **C.** Basal cells show overlapping and crowding and irregular chromatin pattern but these features are subtle and may be difficult to distinguish from other tumours containing basal cells (see text) (MGG ×600 oil). **D.** Laminin positivity of the intercellular matrix substance in adenoid cystic carcinoma (IP, ×600,oil immersion)

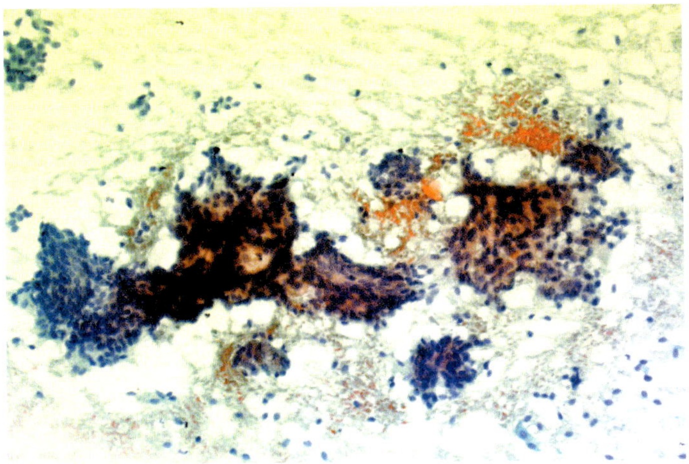

A

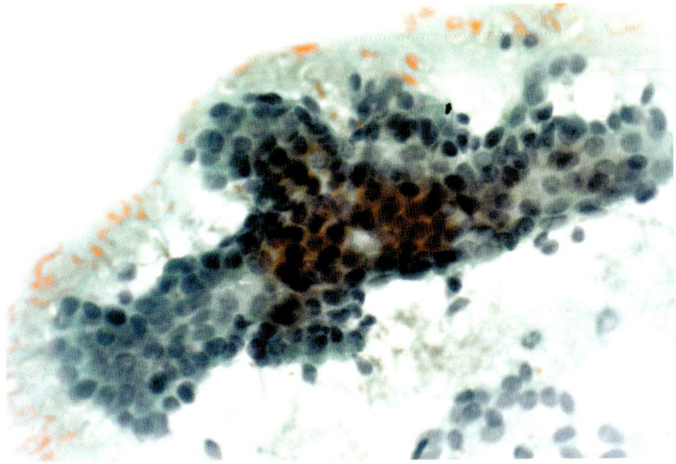

B

Figure 2.48 Polymorphous low grade carcinoma. **A.** Hypercellular smear with branching papillae, sheets and clusters composed of bland uniform cells with round-to-oval nuclei, dispersed chromatin, and absent or inconspicuous nucleoli (PAP ×400).**B.** The cells have a scant-to-moderate amount of eosinophilic cytoplasm. Mitoses and nuclear pleomorphism are absent. These cells form tubular structures containing hyaline globules and often a dispersed myxohyaline stroma. Short, spindle shaped myoepithelial-like cells with ill-defined cell borders may be present in the background (PAP ×600,oil immersion) (Courtesy of Dr I. Robinson)

carcinoma and polymorphous low-grade adenocarcinoma, as well as some non-salivary gland neoplasms presenting an adenoid cystic pattern (e.g. dermal sweat gland tumours), must be considered in differential diagnosis of adenoid cystic carcinoma. Distinction from basal cell adenoma may be difficult and includes cell arrangement and the features of the background. Hyaline globules can be present in both tumours (trabecular type of basal cell adenoma).[115] Differentiation from epithelial-myoepithelial tumour is made on the basis of the characteristic appearance of epithelial-myoepithelial carcinoma with three-dimensional cellular aggregates of basaloid cells, which are clear at the periphery. Given the ultrustractural similarities between epithelial-myoepithelial carcinoma and adenoid cystic carcinoma (both tumours produce excess basal lamina at the margins of cellular nests and widened intercellular spaces contain reduplicated basal lamina and accumulations of glycosaminoglycans) as well as not infrequent histomorphological 'hybrid' tumours, the distinction may be difficult on cytology alone.[157] Distinction from polymorphous low-grade carcinoma may be difficult since the tumour has small- to medium-sized, regular cells without nuclear atypia. It occurs more frequently in the palate. Although both tumours are malignant, adenoid cystic carcinoma has a more aggressive behaviour. Immunocytochemistry for smooth muscle and calponin markers may be helpful in distinguishing the two. Poorly differentiated adenoid cystic carcinoma can be mistaken for anaplastic carcinoma and metastatic carcinoma.

Myoepithelial differentiation

Immunocytochemistry using 3 novel smooth muscle-specific proteins, alpha-smooth muscle actin, smooth muscle myosin heavy chains, and calponin, may be helpful in cases where myoepithelial differentiation needs to be established in benign and malignant salivary gland tumours. In adenoid cystic carcinomas and epithelial-myoepithelial carcinomas, all 3 markers exclusively highlight the myoepithelial cell components and the epithelial cells are entirely negative. No immunostaining is detected in canalicular adenomas, oncocytomas, Warthin's tumours, acinic cell carcinomas, mucoepidermoid carcinomas, squamous cell carcinomas and polymorphous low-grade adenocarcinomas. Salivary duct carcinomas and adenocarcinomas not otherwise specified have a distinctive pattern of uniform periductal staining of reactive myofibroblastic cells, and in salivary duct carcinomas some ducts retain a peripheral immunoreactive myoepithelial cell layer. Immunoreactivity for these 3 smooth muscle-specific proteins confirms the known neoplastic myoepithelial component of adenoid cystic carcinomas and epithelial-myoepithelial carcinomas. The consistently positive staining pattern in adenoid cystic carcinomas may be diagnostically useful in discriminating histologically and cytologically similar but consistently negative polymorphous low-grade adenocarcinomas. Periductal linear staining in adenocarcinoma not otherwise specified and salivary duct carcinomas is distinctive and appears to represent a tight cuff of myofibroblasts associated with the infiltrating glands.[158]

The diagnostic accuracy of FNAC of adenoid cystic carcinoma, as analysed in several large studies, is 84% with 13.7% of tumours diagnosed as benign.[154]

Polymorphous low-grade adenocarcinoma

Polymorphous low-grade adenocarcinoma of the salivary glands is a low-grade neoplasm that occurs almost exclusively in the oral cavity.[159] In this site it is amenable to biopsy and histological diagnosis. However, experience with fine FNAC findings in these tumours is limited. Although they are well circumscribed and appear clinically benign, they lack capsule and show local invasion.[160] The rate of local invasion and lymph node metastases is 17% and 9% respectively.[161] Histologically, polymorphous low-grade carcinoma is composed of a variety of morphological patterns, including tubular, solid, fascicular and cribriform areas.[162] Tumour cells are regular with small cuboidal and short spindle cells and exhibit variation of both cellular nature and architecture between and within the tumours.

Cytological features, originally described as terminal duct carcinoma, show hypercellular smears with branching papillae, sheets and clusters composed of bland uniform cells with round to oval nuclei, dispersed chromatin and absent or inconspicuous nucleoli (Fig. 2.48). The cells have a scant to moderate amount of eosinophilic cytoplasm. Mitoses and nuclear pleomorphism are absent. These cells form tubular structures containing hyaline globules and often a dispersed myxohyaline stroma. Bare nuclei frequently appear in the background.[163,164] In addition, short, spindle-shaped myoepithelial-like cells with ill-defined cell borders may be present . Stromal fragments may be present. Cytological diagnosis of malignancy can be established in 83% of cases.[165] Tyrosine-rich crystalloids may be seen.[166]

Differential diagnosis includes pleomorphic adenoma and myoepithelioma. The cellular variant of pleomorphic adenoma is the one that is most difficult to distinguish from polymorphous low-grade carcinoma. Both tumours have cuboidal and spindle-shaped cells with various amounts of myxoid but not chondromatous material. The nuclear atypia of cellular pleomorphic adenoma may be the same or greater than in polymorphous low-grade carcinoma. The finding of pallisading short spindle cells around myxoid material may be pointing towards polymorphous low-grade carcinoma because the myxoid material of pleomorphic adenoma is conventionally present around the cell clusters or intimately intermingled with the tumour, sometimes as hyaline globules.[167] Myoepithelioma is composed mainly of spindle and plasmacytoid cells. The nuclei of myoepithelioma are more elongated and smaller than those in polymorphous low-grade carcinoma. Clusters of cuboidal cells are not seen in myoepithelioma.

Epithelial-myoepithelial carcinoma

Epithelial-myoepithelial carcinoma is a rare low-grade salivary gland neoplasm, with an incidence of less than 1%, that occurs in both major and minor salivary glands. The majority of these tumours arise in the parotid with a peak incidence from the 6th to the 8th decade.[168] There is preponderance of females. Although they are thought to be of low-grade malignancy, epithelial-myoepithelial carcinomas are locally aggressive, with a recurrence rate of 37%, and fatal courses have been described.[169,170]

Histologically, epithelial-myoepithelial carcinoma shows a high degree of differentiation. It typically has a multinodular growth pattern with islands of tumour separated by dense, fibrous connective tissue. These tumour masses are composed of well-defined tubules lined by two layers of cells: outer cells are large and clear with variable amounts of glycogen; inner cells are small, cuboidal and eosinophilic. Perineural invasion and necrosis are seen occasionally. In some cases, this biphasic pattern is less apparent with solid masses of clear cells. Electron microscopic and immunohistochemical studies confirm the epithelial and myoepithelial differentiation.[171] Immunoreactivity of smooth muscle-specific proteins, alpha-smooth muscle actin, smooth muscle myosin heavy chains and calponin, to assess myoepithelial differentiation show that in adenoid cystic carcinomas and epithelial-myoepithelial carcinomas, all 3 markers exclusively highlight the myoepithelial cell components and the epithelial cells are entirely negative. No immunostaining is detected in canalicular adenomas, oncocytomas, Warthin's tumours, acinic cell carcinomas, mucoepidermoid carcinomas, squamous cell carcinomas and polymorphous low-grade adenocarcinomas. Salivary duct carcinomas and adenocarcinomas not otherwise specified have a distinctive pattern of uniform periductal staining of reactive myofibroblastic cells.[158]

Cytological features. The usual type of epithelial-myoepithelial carcinoma is characterised by bimodal population dominated by large, 'clear' myoepithelial cells and clusters of small, cuboidal ductal cells (Fig. 2.49). The myoepithelial

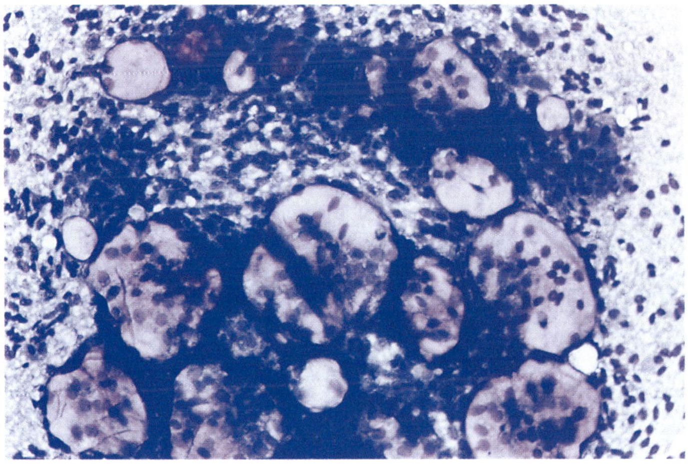

A

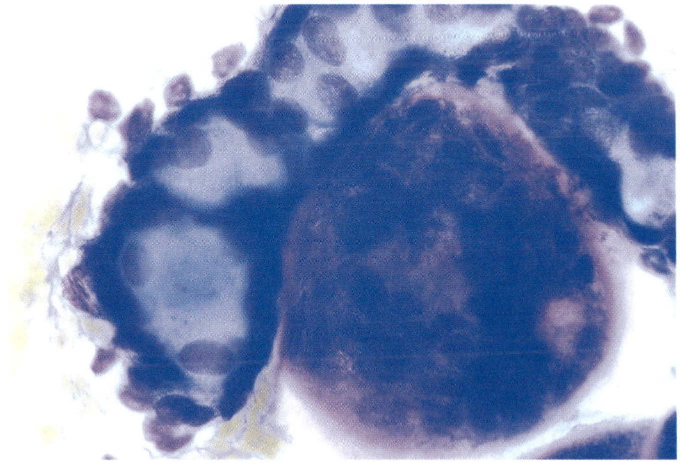

B

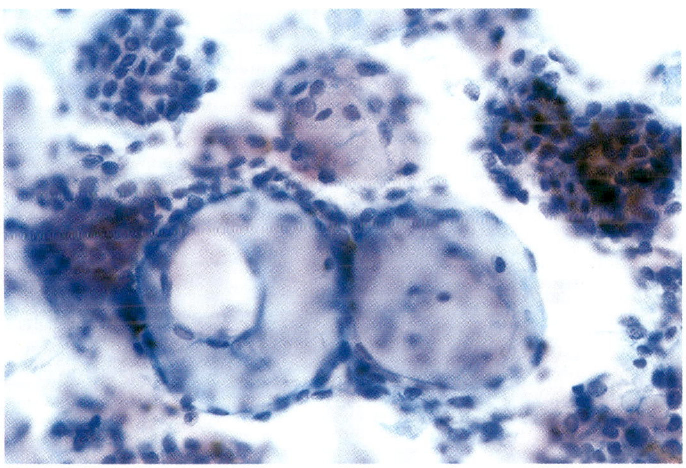

C

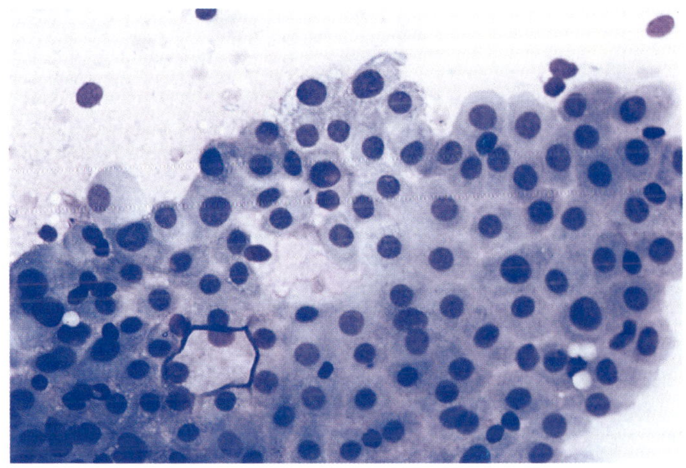

D

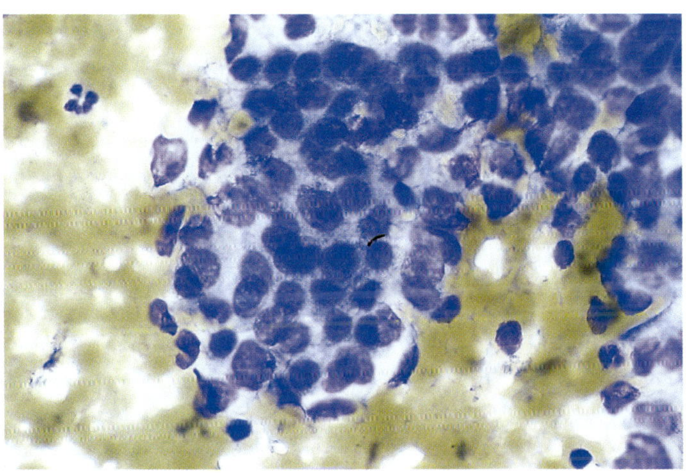

E

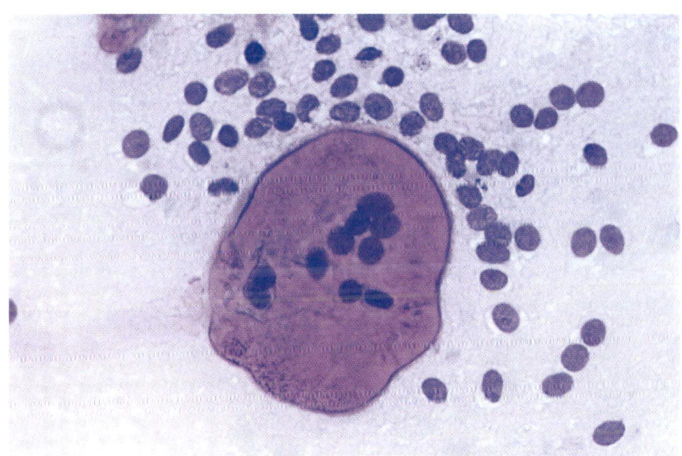

F

Figure 2.49 Epithelial-myoepithelial carcinoma. **A.** Low-power view shows cellular smears with characteristic bimodal pattern dominated by large 'clear' myoepithelial cells and clusters of small cuboidal cells (MGG ×200, courtesy of Dr T. Levine). **B,C.** Pale homogenous material corresponding to the cytoplasm of myoepithelial cells with distinct cell borders often surrounds tubules of ductal cells (MGG, PAP ×600 oil). **D.** Epithelium may have oncocytic appearance (MGG ×600 oil). **E.** Another case. Epithelium shows cytological atypia (MGG ×600). **F.** Hyaline globules reminiscent of adenoid cystic carcinoma may be seen (MGG ×600).

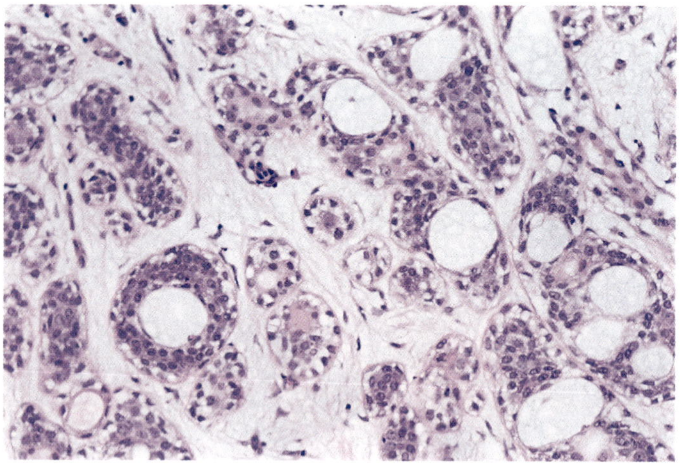

G

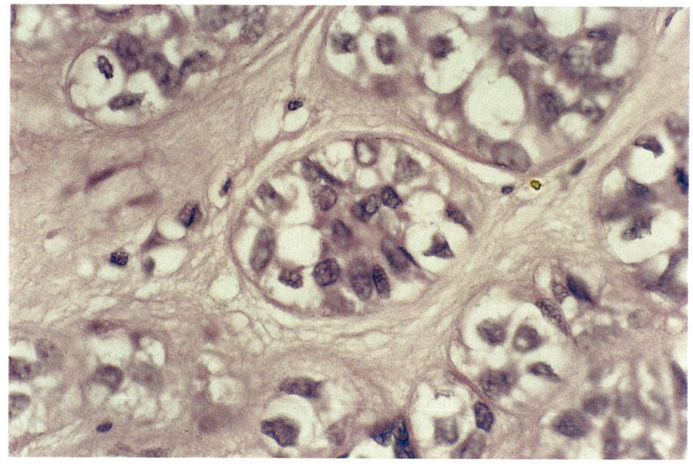

H

Figure 2.49 ***(continued)*** Epithelial-myoepithelial carcinoma. **G.** Histological section showing well-defined tubules lined by two layers of cells (H&E ×200, courtesy of Dr T. Levine). **H.** High-power view, different case. Tubules are lined by outer cells which are large and contain variable amounts of glycogen, and inner cells which are cuboidal and eosinophilic (H&E ×600 oil).

cells have small, uniform nuclei, ample, clear cytoplasm and distinct cell borders. Ductal cells tend to form tubules among background sheets of clear myoepithelial cells. This feature, if present, is an important diagnostic clue.[172] Hyaline, pale homogeneous acellular material surrounding cell clusters is another diagnostic clue.[173] Focal adenoid cystic carcinoma-like areas with hyaline globules are commonly present. Immunocytochemistry positivity for S-100 would confirm the nature of 'clear' cells. Recently the cytological features of ductal predominant-type epimyoepithelial carcinoma have been described.[174] Depending on the ratio of ductal to myoepithelial cell components, epithelial-myoepithelial carcinoma has different cytological presentations.

The differential diagnosis includes pleomorphic adenoma, adenoid cystic carcinoma, and 'clear cell' tumours of the salivary gland: acinic cell carcinoma, clear cell oncocytoma, sebaceous carcinoma, mucoepidermoid carcinomas, primary clear cell carcinoma, basal cell adenomas and metastatic renal cell carcinoma.[124]

Epithelial-myoepithelial carcinoma is a tumour of low-grade malignancy of duct origin, which should be differentiated from salivary duct carcinoma. While the cytological appearances may closely mimic that of other salivary gland tumours, certain peculiar cytological features may allow a distinction to be made on fine needle aspiration biopsy.[175]

Basal cell adenocarcinoma

Basal cell adenocarcinoma was first introduced as an entity in the 2nd edition of The World Health Organization's *Histological Typing of Salivary Gland Tumours* in 1991. Basal cell adenocarcinoma accounts for about 2.9% of all salivary gland malignancies. More than 90% of the tumours are situated in the parotid gland. Intraoral manifestations are known from case reports only. Tumours of the palate have been mentioned in 3 cases.[176] Basal cell adenocarcinoma of the parotid gland is a low-grade malignant neoplasm. It has cytological features of basal cell adenoma and a histologically infiltrative growth pattern of malignant tumours with perineural and vascular invasion. Histologically this tumour can be easily confused with basal cell adenoma and the solid basaloid subtype of adenoid cystic carcinoma (Fig. 2.51).

Cytological features are those of cohesive, focally papillary and filiform groups of neoplastic cells, which are highly reminiscent of basal cell adenoma on low-power examination (Fig. 2.50).[177] Higher power reveals significant cytological atypia and mitotic activity. No single cytological feature is thought to unequivocally distinguish this lesion from basal cell adenoma and/or solid-variant adenoid cystic carcinoma (Figs 2.38 and 2.47). Therefore, for diagnostic purposes, Moroz et al[178] group all 3 lesions under the term *basal cell tumours*. Other differential diagnoses include epithe-

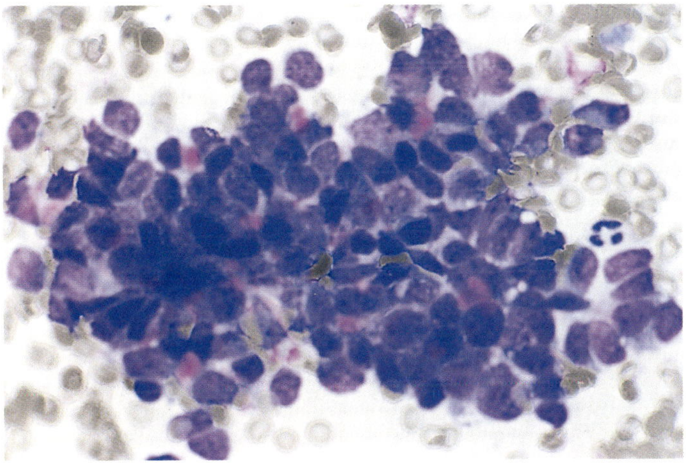
A

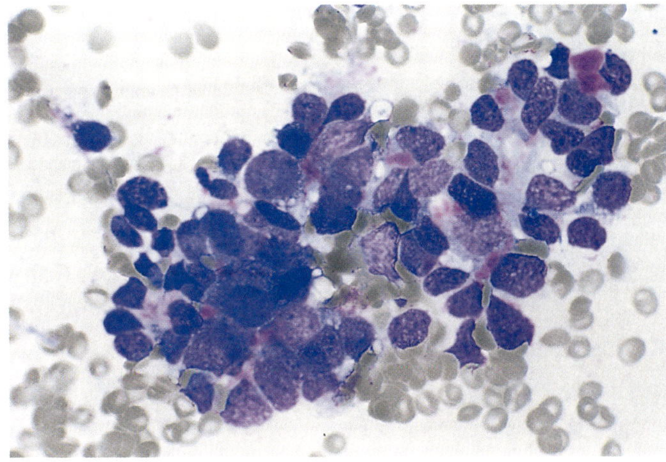
B

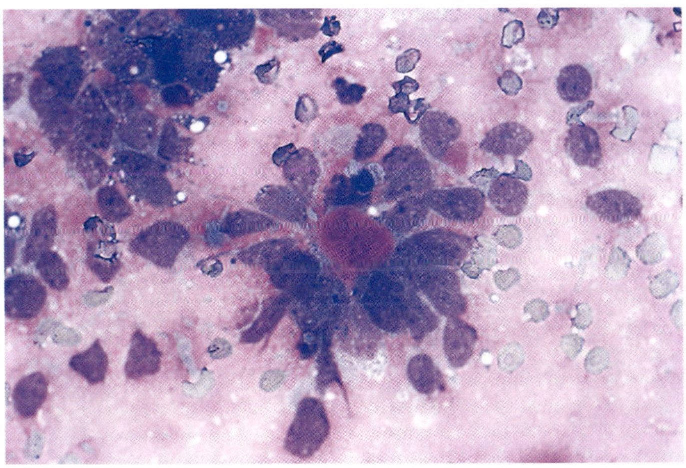
B

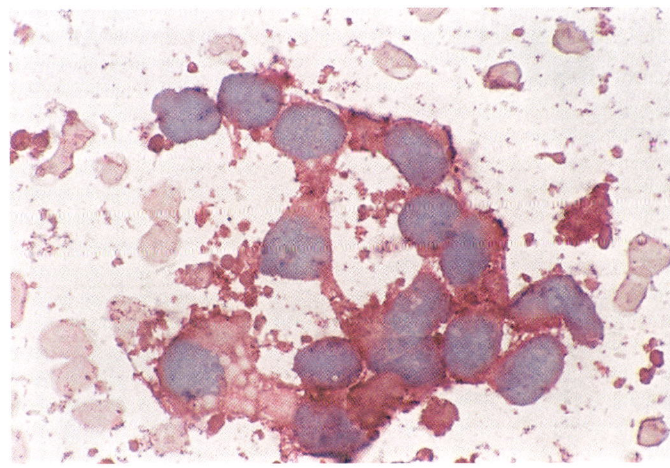
C

Figure 2.50 Basal cell carcinoma. **A.** Basal cell carcinoma cells are small, often tightly cohesive and morphologically similar to basal cell adenoma and solid variant of adenoid cystic carcinoma (MGG ×600 oil). **B.** Cell detail in less cohesive clusters usually permits diagnosis of malignancy on the basis of mitoses, irregular chromatin and irregular nuclear outline (MGG ×600 oil). **C.** Globules of hyaline material may be found surrounded by basaloid cell showing nuclear pleomorphism (×600 oil). **D.** Cells are laminin positive (APAAP, antilaminin ×600 oil).

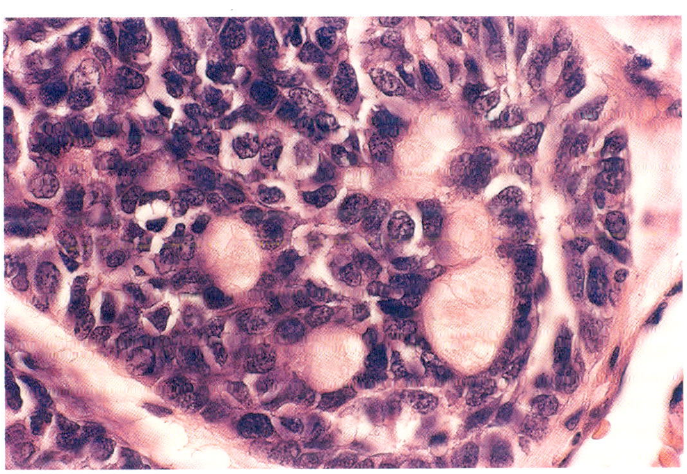
A

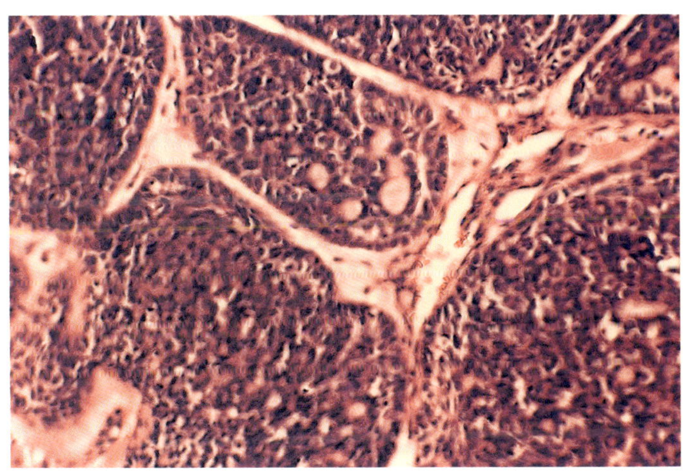
B

Figure 2.51 Basal cell adenocarcinoma. Histological section of the case in Figure 2.50. **A.** Basal cell adenocarcinoma has cytological features of basal cell adenoma but an infiltrative growth pattern (H&E ×200). **B.** High-power view shows tubular structures with peripheral pallisading. Cytological detail shows atypia similar to that seen in Figure 2.50. (H&E ×600 oil).

lial-rich pleomorphic adenoma, myoepithelial lesions, small cell undifferentiated carcinoma and metastatic carcinoma. Evaluation of the DNA content of tumour cells reveals diploid histograms in both cytological material and paraffin-embedded tissue. Infiltrative tumour nests, the histological basis for differentiating basal cell adenocarcinoma from adenoma, showed the same diploid pattern. Though DNA quantitation may not discriminate basal cell adenoma from basal cell adenocarcinoma, it may prove useful in separating them from adenoid cystic carcinoma, which is considered to be a tumour with high malignant potential.[178]

Papillary cystadenocarcinoma

Salivary gland cystadenocarcinomas represent a distinct group of malignancies that have an indolent biological behaviour.[179] Current classification schemes for salivary gland neoplasms categorise cystadenocarcinomas on the basis of a recurring morphological pattern of cystic, and often papillary growth without features of other specific types of salivary gland tumours. The tumour affects patients aged between 20 and 86 years, and patients aged over 50 years account for 71% of cases.[179] The majority of tumours occur in major salivary glands. Grossly, the lesions are cystic or multicystic masses that range in size from 0.4 to 6.0 cm. Histologically, tumours demonstrate an invasive cystic growth pattern and have a conspicuous papillary component. The predominant cell type varies among tumours and includes small cuboidal cells, large cuboidal cells and tall columnar cells (Fig. 2.52). Ruptured cysts with haemorrhage and granulation tissue are common. The tumour may recur locally or (rarely) metastasise to regional lymph nodes.

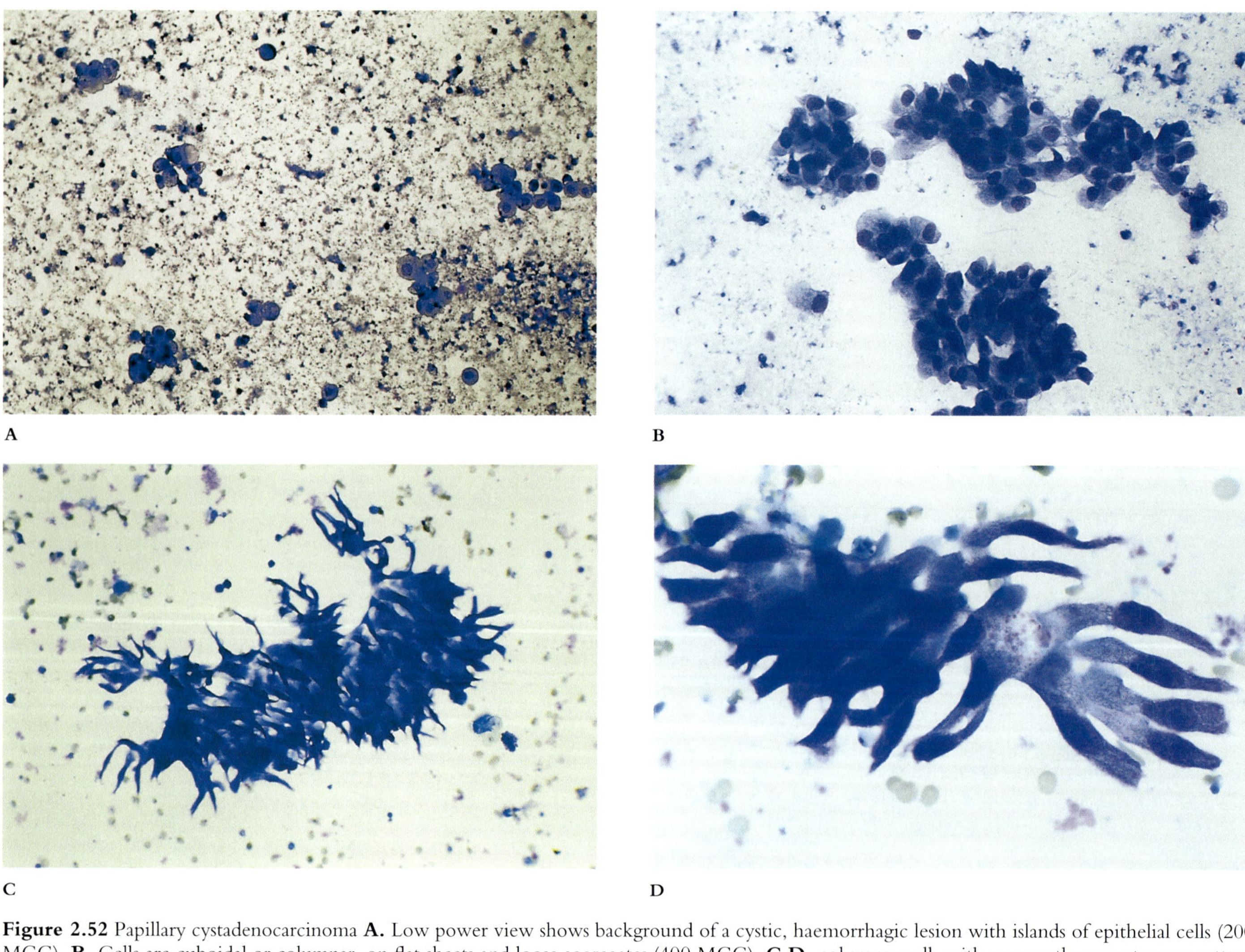

A B C D

Figure 2.52 Papillary cystadenocarcinoma **A.** Low power view shows background of a cystic, haemorrhagic lesion with islands of epithelial cells (200 MGG). **B.** Cells are cuboidal or columnar, on flat sheets and loose aggregates (400 MGG). **C,D.** columnar cells with apparently monotonous pattern (400, 600 MGG). ***(continued)***

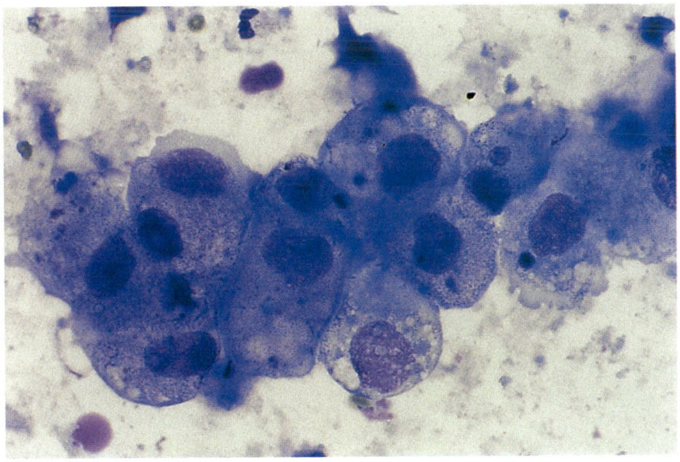

E

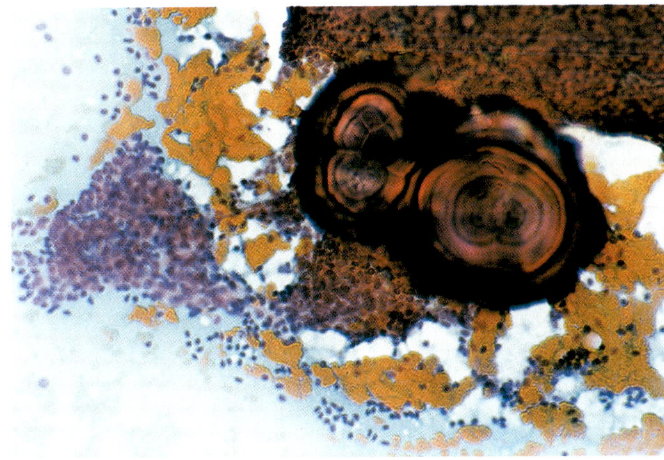

F

Figure 2.52 (*continued*) Papillary cystadenocarcinoma **E.** High power view of the cell detail reveals anisonucleosis, irregular chromatin pattern and cytopharmic vacuolation (1000 MGG). **F.** Psanomoma bodies may be seen occasionally but are not pathognomanic of this lesion (400, PAP).

Mucinous adenocarcinoma

Mucinous adenocarcinoma rarely arises as a primary tumour within the parotid gland, and only one case report of cytological features has been described.[180] The tumour was cystic on CT. FNAC yielded monomorphic, moderately atypical cells, both single and clustered, associated with abundant mucoid material and focal necrosis. Tumour cells had eccentric nuclei, prominent nucleoli and occasional cytoplasmic vacuolisation. A few binucleated and multinucleated tumour cells were present. Histological sections of the resected gland showed mucinous adenocarcinoma. The differential diagnoses on cytology included other primary tumours of the parotid gland producing mucin or a mucoid matrix and metastatic mucinous adenocarcinomas.

Oncocytic carcinoma

Malignant oncocytoma is an exceedingly rare type of salivary gland tumour.[181] Oncocytes are large, apparently swollen epithelial cells with cytoplasm densely filled with eosinophilic granules (see p. 39) Oncocytic carcinomas appear to arise from benign oncocytomas, or may also arise *de novo*. In oncocytic carcinoma of the head and neck, the presence of distant rather than local lymph node metastasis is the most important prognostic indicator.[182]

Cytological features show numerous, predominantly dissociated cells with nuclear enlargement and anisonucleosis, prominent nucleoli, multinucleation and abundant homogeneous cytoplasm (Fig. 2.53), in contrast with benign oncocytoma in which cells occur in cohesive clusters with well-defined cell borders, small nuclei, bland chromatin pattern and inconspicuous nucleoli (Fig. 2.39).

In the FNACs of oncocytoma, differential diagnosis includes Warthin's tumour and malignant oncocytoma. The morphological difficulty in oncocytic lesions is distinguishing between benign and malignant tumours. In a review of literature including 34 malignant or locally aggressive oncocytomas, Gray et al[183] set the histological criteria for malignancy as cellular pleomorphism, frequent mitoses, local lymph node metastases and distant metastases.

Salivary duct carcinoma

Salivary duct carcinoma is an uncommon and highly aggressive neoplasm. It represents between 2.8% and 8.3% of primary salivary gland malignancies. The tumour has preponderance for males, median age 69 years. It usually occurs in the parotid. Patients usually have symptoms of high grade malignancy at presentation (Fig. 2.54), with a high proportion of facial paralysis. A history of chronic sialadenitis preceding salivary duct carcinoma has been described in 1 case.[59] Tumour has a tendency for early metastases and often fatal outcome. Brandwein et al[184] reported 45% of local recurrences, 54% of metastases and 45% patients dead of disease within 10 years of diagnosis.

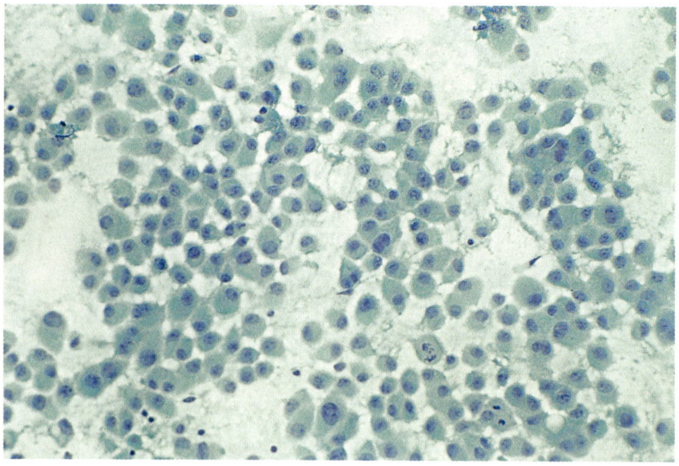

A

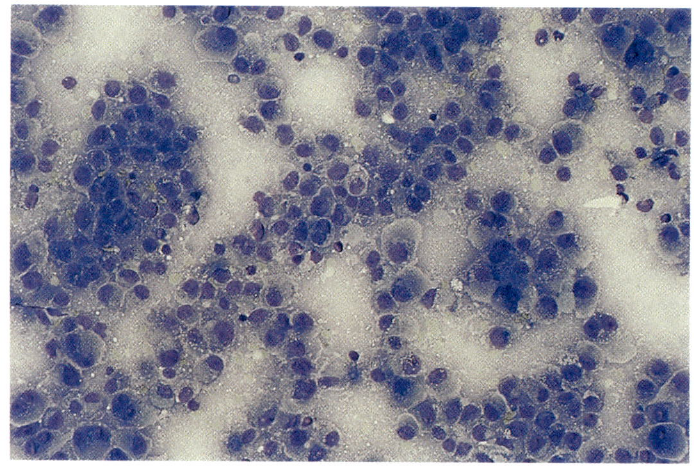

B

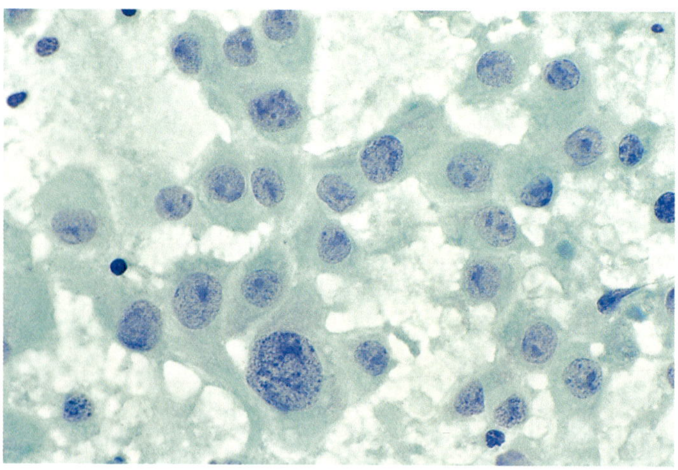

C

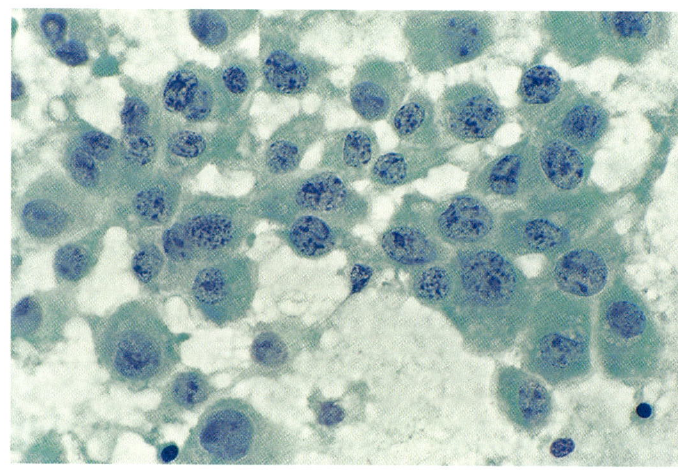

D

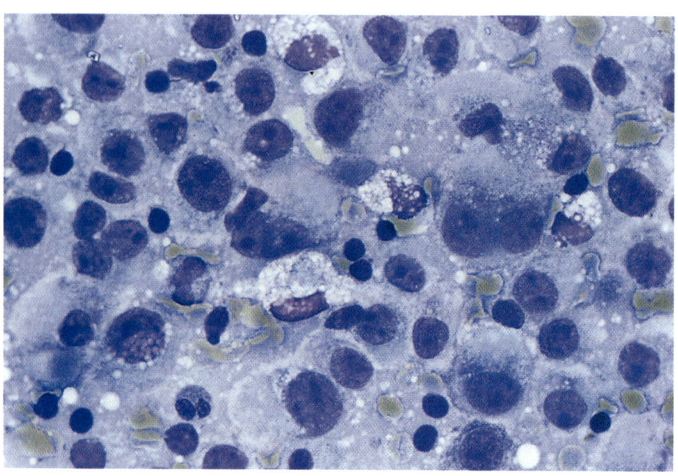

E

Figure 2.53 Oncocytic carcinoma. **A.** Low-power view showing numerous single cells, similar to that in oncocytoma (see Fig. 2.39A) (PAP ×200). **B.** Low-power view revels oncocytic cells with characteristics eccentric nuclei and dense cytoplasm (MGG ×200). **C,D.** Distinction from benign oncocytoma can be made by careful scrutiny of cytological detail which reveals anisonucleosis, irregular chromatin pattern and prominent multiple nucleoli (PAP ×600 oil). **E.** Similar features on air-dried material are more difficult to appreciate (MGG ×600 oil).

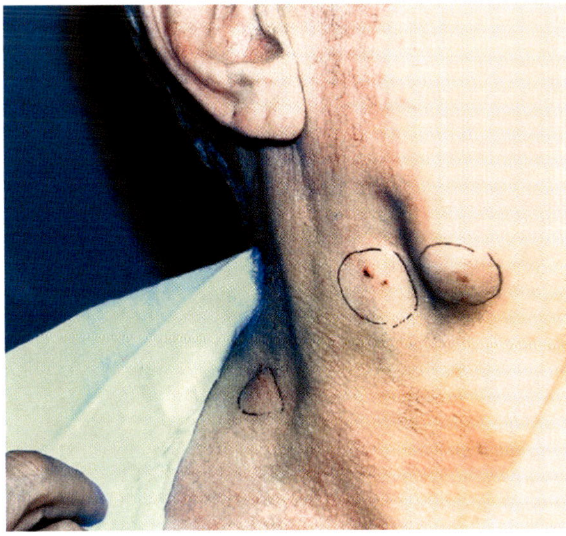

Figure 2.54 Salivary duct carcinoma. This patient presented with a 4-month history of submandibular swelling. On examination, regional lymph nodes were found to be enlarged and extra material was taken from these sites.

Histologically, this tumour is similar to intraductal breast carcinoma and may display a cribriform or papillary pattern as well as necrotic areas such as comedocarcinoma variant.

Cytological features can be observed in highly cellular samples. Typically, cells are arranged in clusters or flat sheets with a cribriform pattern and eccentric, round hyperchromatic nuclei, abundant finely granular cytoplasm and necrosis in the smear background (Fig. 2.55).[185–187] They are similar to comedo-type breast carcinoma but may also have predominantly oncocytic features. Cribriform and papillary patterns with necrosis and cystic change are often present. The cytoplasm of well-preserved cells is polygonal, well outlined, basophilic and may contain vacuoles. Oncocytic-type cells have ill-defined eosinophilic cytoplasm and usually do not show necrosis. Nucleoli may be prominent.[188] The recently described variant of 'low-grade salivary duct carcinoma' shows cells arranged in individual papillary clusters or in complex branching papillae. Cells are medium sized and show no cytological atypia. The tumour, in contrast to the salivary duct carcinoma, seems biologically indolent.

Differential diagnosis includes high-grade mucoepidermoid carcinoma with necrotic background and vacuolated cells, squamous cell carcinoma, metastatic breast carcinoma and oncocytic carcinoma. FNAC can exclude the solid type of adenoid cystic carcinoma, carcinoma ex pleomorphic adenoma, undifferentiated carcinoma, myoepithelial carcinoma and adenosquamous carcinoma.[189] Squamous cell carcinoma with much keratinisation excludes both salivary duct carcinoma and mucoepidermoid carcinoma. Oncocytic carcinoma, apart from being very rare, usually does not exhibit such nuclear atypia as salivary duct carcinoma. Salivary duct carcinoma arising on the basis of pleomorphic adenoma has been described.[190]

Immunocytochemistry shows diffuse positivity for epithelial membrane antigen (100%), keratin (AE1/AE3) (88%), Ber-EP4, alpha-lactalbumin (88%), GCDFP-15 (76%) and carcinoembryonic antigen (72%); S-100 protein is rarely detected (4%). Stains for oestrogen receptor are uniformly negative.[191] Overexpression of c-ERB B-2 is absent and <5% show immunoreactivity for p53.[192] Prasad et al[158] used alpha-smooth muscle actin, smooth muscle myosin heavy chains and calponin to assess myoepithelial differentiation. They found periductal linear staining in adenocarcinoma not otherwise specified and salivary duct carcinomas, which is distinctive and appears to represent a tight cuff of myofibroblasts associated with the infiltrating glands (see epithelial myoepithelial carcinoma).[158]

Cerilli et al[193] made analysis of chromosome 9p21 deletion and p16 gene mutation in salivary gland carcinomas. Seven of 9 salivary duct carcinomas showed loss of heterozygosity of 1 or more polymorphic markers. Loss of heterozygosity was found in 1 of 10 adenoid cystic carcinomas and 1 of 8 mucoepidermoid carcinomas, and was absent in the remaining subtypes. No mutations in exon 1 or exon 2 or homozygous deletion of p16 were found in these 2 particular neoplasms with loss of heterozygosity. These results suggest that inactivation of p16 is important in the development or progression of at least some salivary duct carcinomas.[193] When studying prognostic markers, Felix et al[194] found that tumour size, distant metastasis and C-erbB2 amplification are independent prognostic parameters in patients with salivary duct carcinoma. Female gender is thought to be a negative prognostic factor.[191]

Although the cytological appearances may vary and sometimes be difficult in terms of tumour type, diagnosis of malignancy is rarely in doubt. Cumulative diagnostic accuracy of cytological diagnosis of salivary duct carcinoma, as suspicious of malignancy or malignant, in the studies published up to date, is 94.3%. The false-negative rate is 6.7% (3 out of 40).[188] The 3 false-negative diagnoses were in the

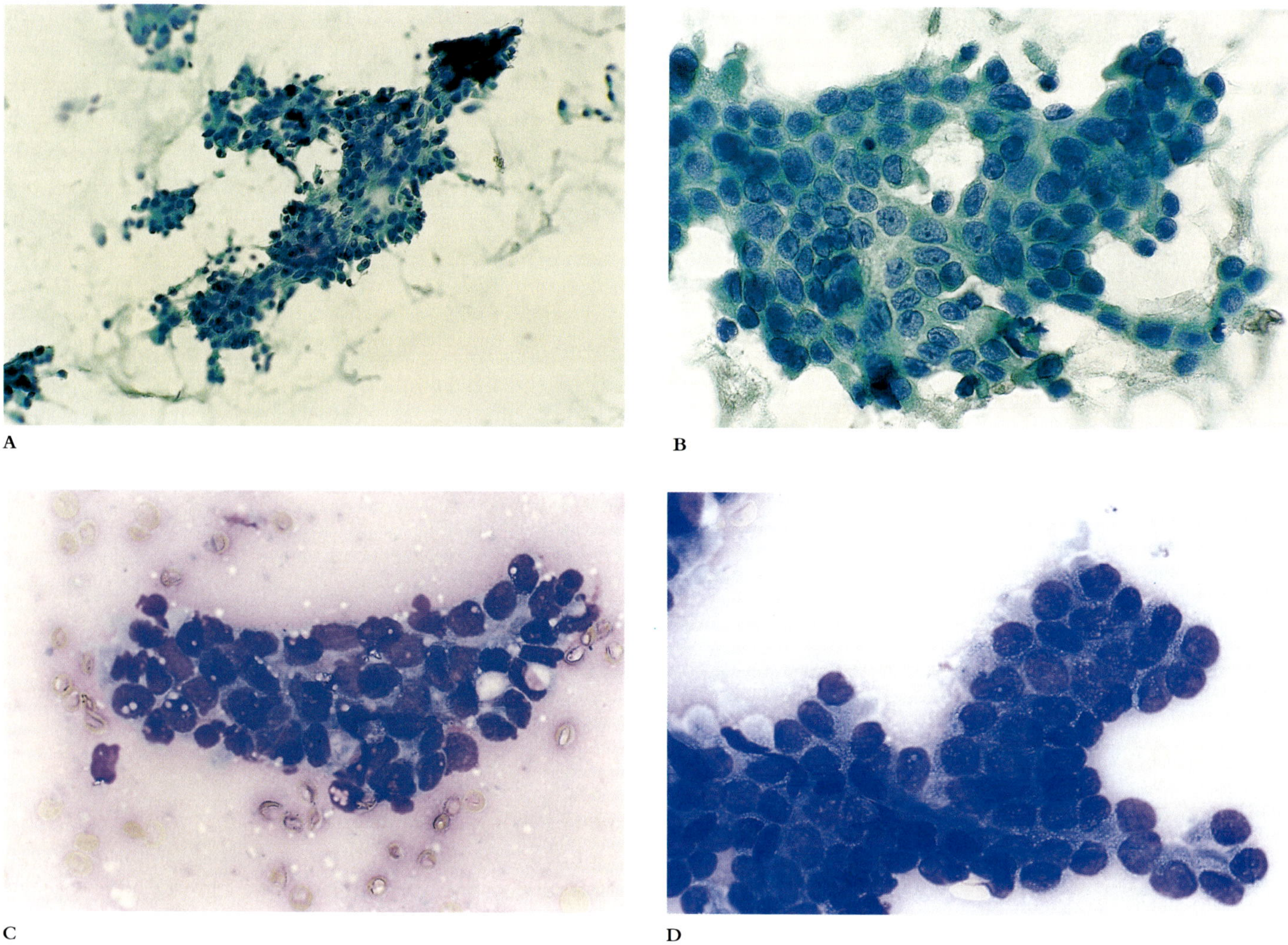

Figure 2.55 Salivary duct carcinoma. **A.** Low-power view of salivary duct carcinoma shows cellular sample with cells arranged in sheets with cribriform pattern (PAP ×200). **B.** Cells have round, oval irregular nuclei and may have abundant granular cytoplasm (PAP ×600 oil). **C,D.** Cytoplasm of the cells may contain vacuoles making the distinction from mucoepidermoid carcinoma difficult (MGG ×600 oil).

low-grade salivary duct carcinoma and in 2 other salivary duct carcinomas with low-grade areas. 'Low grade salivary duct carcinoma' is a new and challenging entity, as evidenced by the high rate of false-negative cytological diagnoses.[195]

Adenocarcinoma not otherwise specified

Adenocarcinoma includes several entities ranging from the relatively indolent polymorphous low-grade adenocarcinoma to the usually fatal salivary duct carcinoma. Cytologically, it is usually possible to diagnose malignancy and, in the absence of any specific features, to indicate the degree of differentiation (Fig. 2.56).

Carcinoma ex pleomorphic adenoma

Secondary malignant change occurs in approximately 3–4% of pleomorphic adenomas. The risk increases with the duration of the tumour and in 15 years is at 9.5%. Malignancy may take 1 of 4 forms: carcinoma, malignant myoepithelioma,[98] carcinosarcoma[196] and metastasising pleomorphic adenoma. The commonest patterns are poorly differentiated ductal and undifferentiated carcinomas. Acinic carcinoma does not arise in the pleomorphic adenoma and adenoid cystic and mucoepidermoid carcinoma do so rarely.

Cytological features of epithelial atypia within an otherwise typical pleomorphic adenoma should not be overinterpreted. Occasional irregular, large cells may be seen in

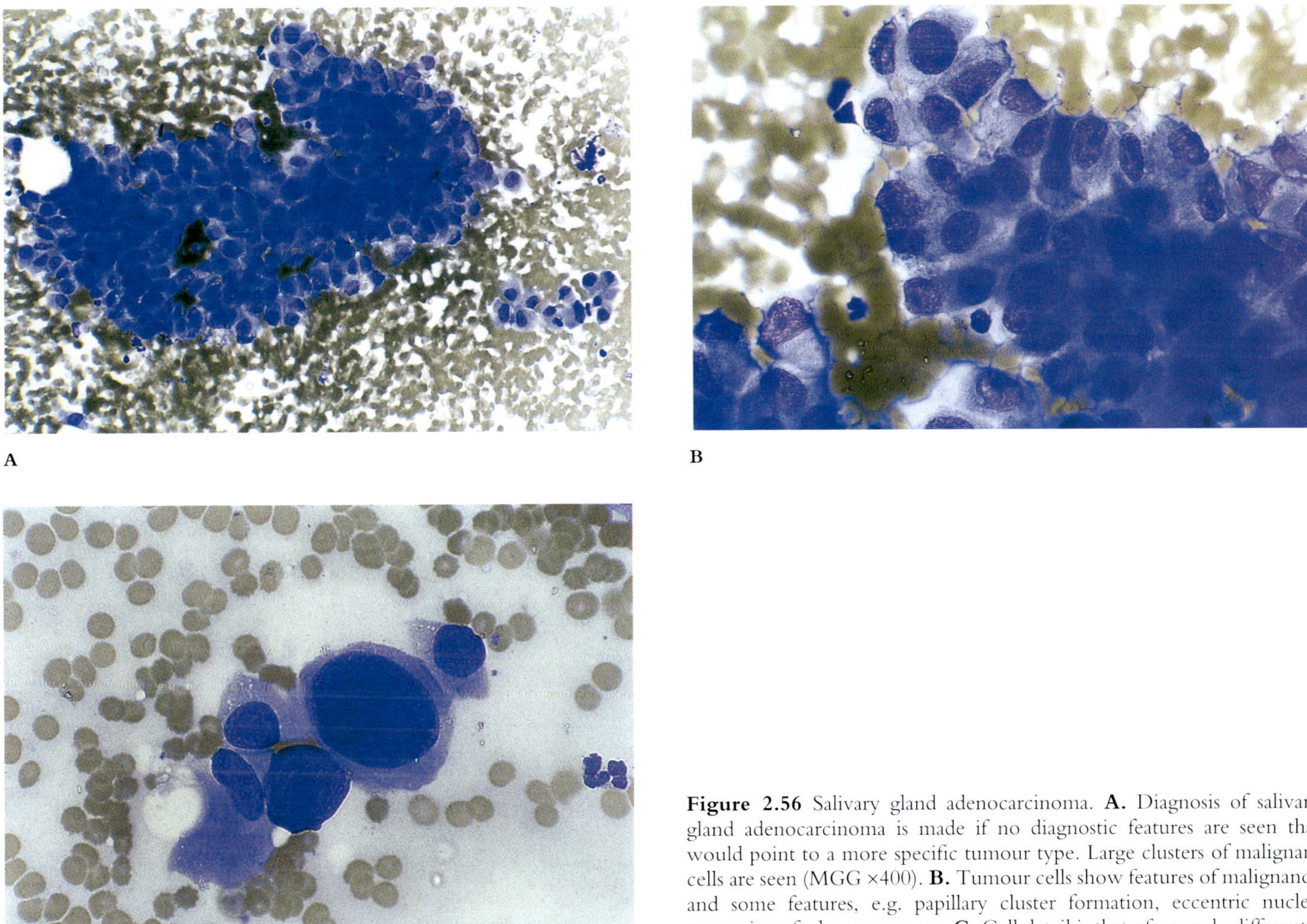

A

B

C

Figure 2.56 Salivary gland adenocarcinoma. **A.** Diagnosis of salivary gland adenocarcinoma is made if no diagnostic features are seen that would point to a more specific tumour type. Large clusters of malignant cells are seen (MGG ×400). **B.** Tumour cells show features of malignancy and some features, e.g. papillary cluster formation, eccentric nuclei, suggestive of adenocaronoma. **C.** Cell detail is that of a poorly differentiated carcinoma (MGG ×100 oil).

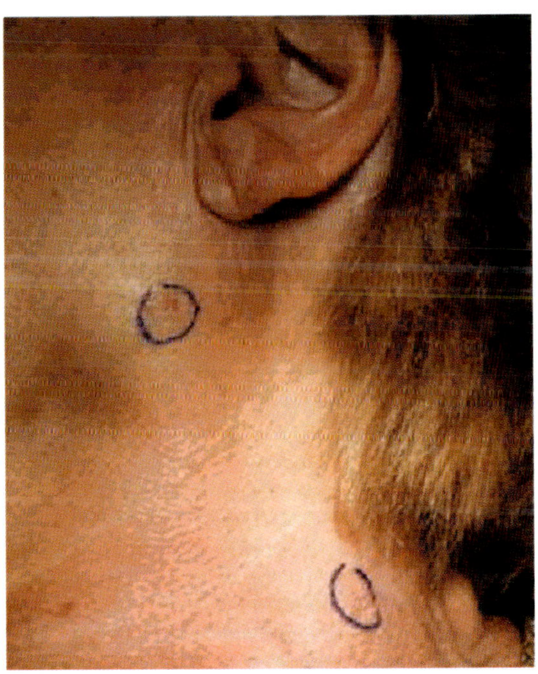

Figure 2.57 Salivary swelling and regional lymph node enlargement. Patient has a pleomorphic adenoma and a reactive lymph node hyperplasia unrelated to the salivary pathology. Without the FNAC result, it would have been tempting to assume malignancy with regional spread.

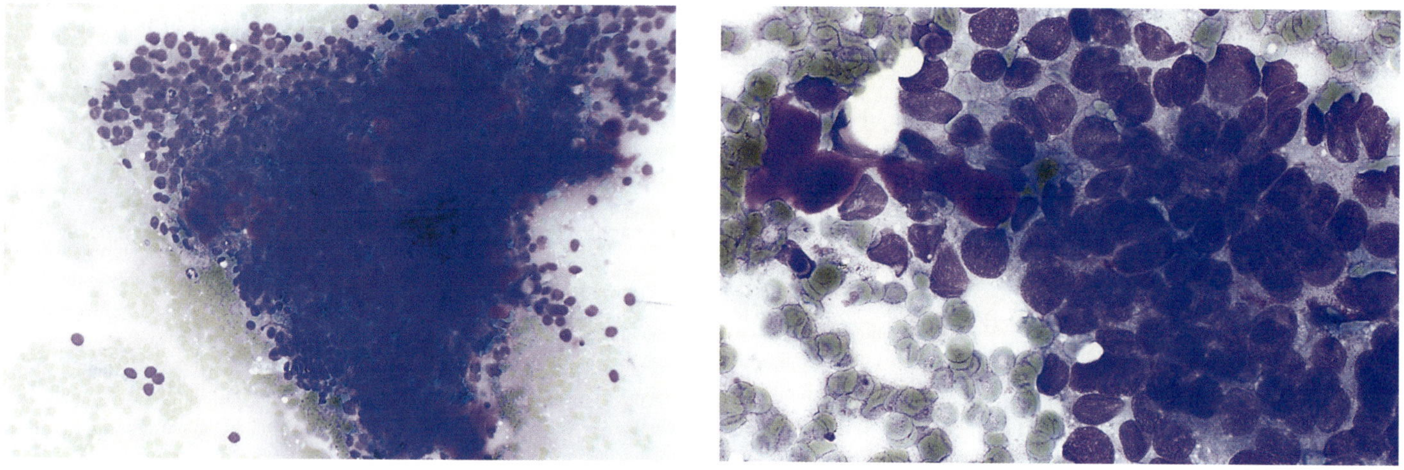

A B

Figure 2.58 Carcinoma ex pleomorphic adenoma. **A.** Large cellular clusters intermixed with myxoid stroma (MGG ×400). **B.** High-power view reveals marked cytological atypia, overlapping and crowding. Myxoid stroma is noted (MGG ×600 oil).

pleomorphic adenoma and unless a substantial number of malignant cells is seen, malignancy should be reported with caution in the context of pleomorphic adenoma. In the material that is obviously malignant, it is sometimes possible to find areas reminiscent of pleomorphic adenoma and postulate its origin (Fig. 2.58). A cytological diagnosis of malignancy can be established in 76.5% of high-grade malignancy. Most negative results are encountered in low-grade carcinomas.[90]

Primary squamous cell carcinoma

Primary squamous cell carcinoma of the salivary glands is an uncommon, aggressive malignancy with a poor prognosis. It repesents 2% of malignant salivary gland tumours[197] and is localised predominantly in the major salivary glands. Patients usually present in advanced stage and with facial nerve involvement or cervical metastases. Prognosis is poor even with radical surgery and adjunctive radiotherapy (Fig. 2.59).

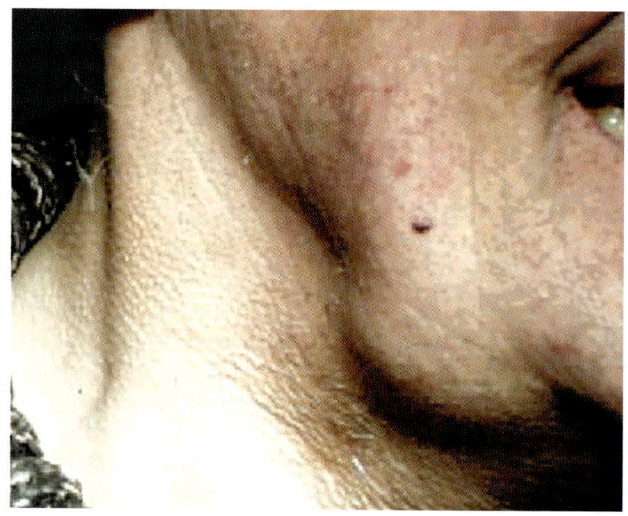

Figure 2.59 Primary squamous cell carcinoma. The patient presented with a 3-month history of painless, non-mobile, hard swelling in the submandibular area. There was no history of other regional or systemic disease.

As the primary squamous cell carcinoma of the salivary glands is rare, it must be distinguished from metastases of extraglandular squamous cell carcinoma of the skin, especially of the head and neck area. Squamous cell metaplasia in non-tumourous diseases of the salivary gland (e.g. necrotizing sialometaplasia) as well as in benign or malignant salivary gland tumours (e.g. metaplastic Warthin's tumour) can simulate squamous cell carcinoma. Other differential diagnostic problems are the structural variants of squamous cell carcinoma that develop predominantly in the minor salivary glands, but not in the major salivary glands. Special types include the very rare adenoid squamous cell carcinoma with pseudoglandular structures as the result of acantholysis, the biphasic adenosquamous carcinoma with differentiation as squamous cell carcinoma and adenocarcinoma, the biphasic basaloid squamous carcinoma with a structure as squamous cell carcinoma, solid basaloid carcinoma (analogous to the solid type of adenoid cystic carcinoma) and the poorly differentiated mucoepidermoid carcinoma (grade III) with biphasic structure of undifferentiated epidermoid and intermediate cells as well as inclusion of small groups of mucus-producing goblet cells.[198]

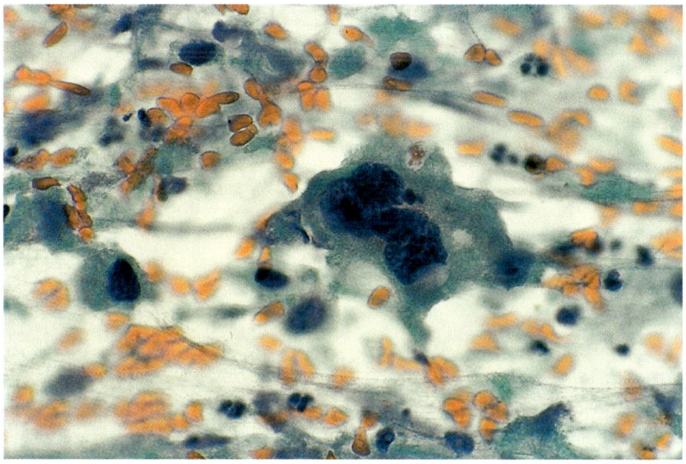

Figure 2.60 Squamous cell carcinoma. Malignant cells show keratinisation, surrounded by necrotic debris. Diagnosis of primary squamous cell carcinoma is made by exclusion of any other primary site in the head and neck or elsewhere.

Cytological features are similar to those of sqamous cell carcinoma elsewhere (Fig. 2.60). Cytological diagnosis of malignancy has been possible in 95% of squamous cell carcinomas.[199] A spectrum of neoplastic and non-neoplastic lesions of the salivary glands may contain squamous cells. These include chronic sialadenitis, lymphoepithelial cyst, pleomorphic adenoma, Warthin's tumour, mucoepidermoid carcinoma, as well as squamous cell carcinoma. The squamous cells may be a defining feature of the lesion, or an occasional and thus unexpected finding with a consequent potential for misdiagnosis. Clinical management of these lesions differs significantly, and careful evaluation of the squamous elements, along with attention to other cellular and background components, facilitates accurate diagnosis.[48]

Small cell carcinoma

Extrapulmonary small cell carcinoma is recognised as a clinicopathologic entity distinct from small cell lung cancer. Such carcinomas as primary tumours have been described in several locations in the head and neck, although most cases of metastatic tumour in the neck originate from a pulmonary primary. A review of the current literature shows that most small cell carcinomas in the head and neck are extrapulmonary primary tumours.[200] Since histological criteria are the same, a pulmonary neoplasm has to be excluded in every case. The differentiation between a primary head and neck tumour and metastatic disease as well as the location and staging are essential criteria for therapy and prognosis.[201]

Cytological features of small cell undifferentiated carcinoma show nuclear granularity and markedly angular nuclear moulding of numerous small cells that are usually present as large syncytia in an inflammatory background. Numerous mitotic figures are also present in this vascular lesion. Immunohistochemistry demonstrates positivity for neuroendocrine markers while transmission electron microscopy (TEM) demonstrates intracytoplasmic neurosecretory granules, indicating a neuroendocrine derivation for this neoplasm, instead of the more usual origin of salivary gland undifferentiated carcinoma in ductal epithelial or myoepithelial tissue.[202]

Undifferentiated carcinoma

Undifferentiated carcinoma of the salivary gland is a rare, high-grade neoplasm which accounts for a very small number (1–5.5%) of salivary gland tumours.[203] It may occur in parotid and in small salivary glands. There is no known sex predilection and middle-aged and elderly patients are most commonly affected. Grossly, large cell undifferentiated carcinoma is solid, poorly circumscribed, infiltrating with foci of necrosis and haemorrhage.

Undifferentiated carcinomas of salivary glands are those epithelial malignancies whose histopathological features are not sufficient to place them in other defined classes of carcinoma. They are ultrastructurally heterogeneous and can manifest neuroendocrine differentiation. With or without the latter, the carcinomas are biologically high grade and rank with salivary duct and high-grade mucoepidermoid carcinomas in terms of morbidity and mortality.[204]

Cytological features show isolated and loosely cohesive large cells with abundant cytoplasm, and variably pleomorphic nuclei with prominent nucleoli. Multinucleated tumour giant cells and macrophage polykaryons may be seen. There is no evidence of squamous, myoepithelial or widespread mucinous differentiation by morphological, cytochemical or immunohistochemical analyses (focal rare mucin production is identified on special stains occasionally).

The differential diagnosis is lengthy and consists of other high-grade primary salivary gland malignancies as well as metastatic adenocarcinoma, poorly differentiated squamous cell carcinoma, anaplastic lymphoma, high-grade sarcomas and metastatic melanoma. Differentiation from high-grade mucoepidermoid carcinoma may be difficult. In high-grade mucoepidermoid carcinoma, large cells of epidermoid differentiation are conspicuous in FNAC material and may resemble large cell undifferentiated carcinoma. However, mucoepidermoid carcinoma usually has an admixture of basaloid cells. A mixture of low- and high-grade appearances, common in mucoepidermoid carcinoma, is usually not seen in large cell undifferentiated carcinoma. Adenoid cystic carcinoma or adenocarcinoma not otherwise specified may contain foci of anaplastic large cells as well as non-epithelial, osteoclast-like giant cells. These, however, represent only a portion of tumour and should not be diagnosed as a large cell undifferentiated carcinoma. Distinction from salivary duct carcinoma may be difficult since the latter is also a high-grade tumour and has same age (old) and site (parotid) predilection. A characteristic feature differentiating the two tumours is the presence of cribriform, complex glandular architecture in salivary duct carcinoma. Malignant lymphoepithelial carcinoma can present in cytological preparations as a high-grade malignant tumour composed of syncitial islands of large malignant cells in a necrotic background.[205] A major clue as to its accurate diagnosis is the admixture of mature lymphocytes. Differentiation from oncocytic carcinoma may be difficult since the cells of large cell undifferentiated carcinoma may strongly resemble malignant oncocytes. Distinction from high-grade non-Hodgkin's lymphoma can usually be made on immunocytochemistry. The pattern of immunohistochemical reactivity (positive keratin, negative S-100, and HMB-45 antigens) and lack of conspicuous mucin production or significant lymphoid infiltrate are useful in establishing the correct diagnosis.

MISCELLANEOUS TUMOURS

Lymphoepithelial (nasopharyngeal) carcinoma

Lymphoepithelial carcinoma is a rare, undifferentiated epithelial malignancy with a predilection for Chinese and Eskimo populations, associated with Epstein-Barr virus. Most common is a rapidly growing nasopharyngeal neoplasm, it can arise in the salivary gland.

Cytological features show a highly malignant tumour in individual or cohesive clusters of medium to large polygonal and spindled cells with one or more prominent nucleoli intermingling with mature lymphocytes. These can be misinterpreted as lymphohistiocytic.[206] Sometimes much necrotic debris and only a few lym-

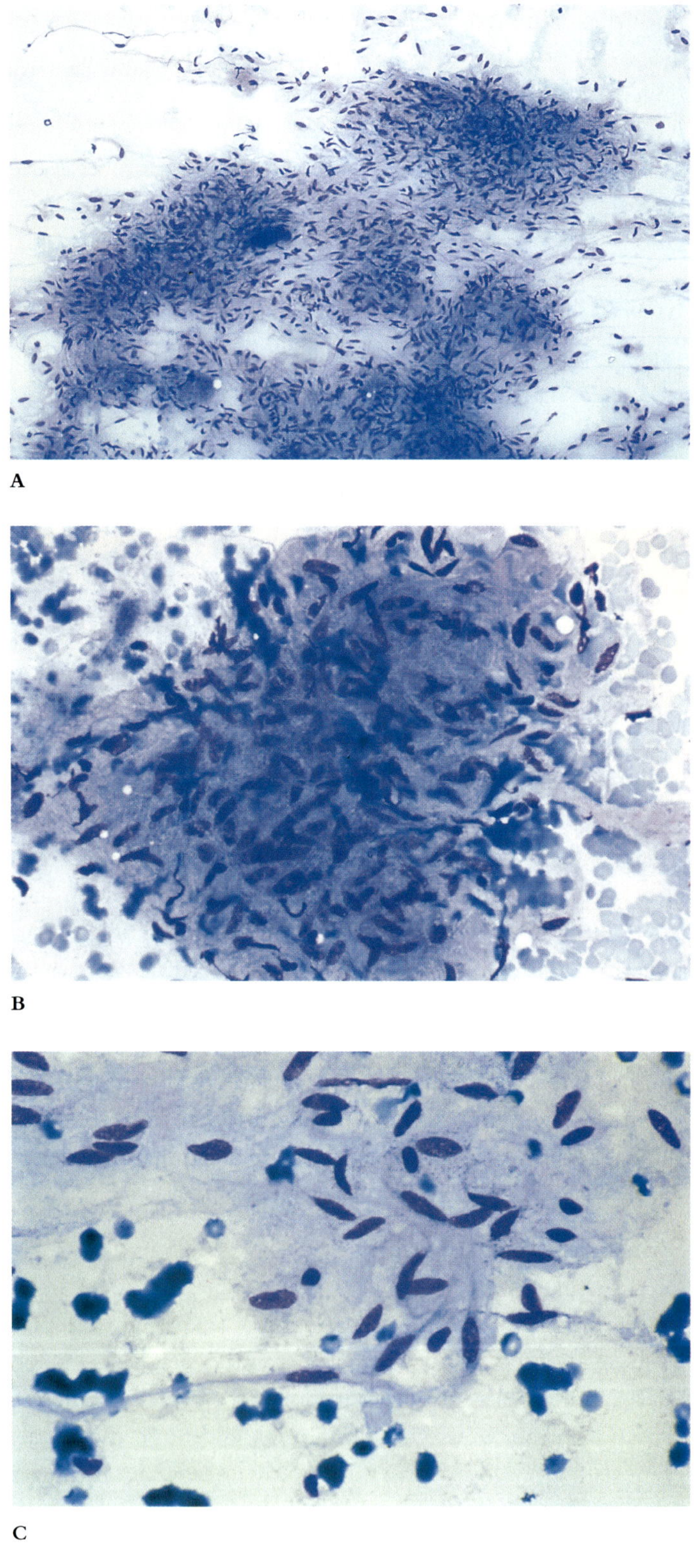

Figure 2.61 Benign nerve sheath tumour. **A.** Low-power view reveals cellular areas against a blue proteinaceous background material (MGG ×200). **B.** Cells have spindle-shaped nuclei streaming in all directions. Cytoplasm is poorly outlined (MGG ×400). **C.** High-power view reveals cytoplasmic processes in some of the cells. Immunocytochemistry is useful for distinction from myoepithelioma (see Fig. 2.40) (MGG ×1000).

phocytes admixed with tumour cells are seen. Neither cytology nor histology of the cervical lymph nodes is conclusive in establishing the primary site of a metastatic lymphoepithelioma-like carcinoma (MLEL). MLEL of the salivary glands must be included in the differential diagnosis (Chapter 4, Fig. 4.68).[205]

SOFT TISSUE LESIONS

Neurilemoma

Benign nerve sheath tumour can be found in the salivary glands and erroneously reported as pleomorphic adenoma or myoepithelioma[207,208] (Fig. 2.61, also Chapter 5, Fig. 5.7).

Sarcomas

Primary sarcomas of the major salivary glands are exceptionally uncommon.

Rhabdomyosarcoma

The head and neck region is one of the most common locations of rhabdomyosarcoma. Salivary gland involvement is usually secondary to advanced disease, and presentation as a primary salivary gland tumour is very rare. Patients are usually children and adolescents (although tumours can occur in adults) presenting with parotid gland enlargement. Clinically, the enlargements appear to be

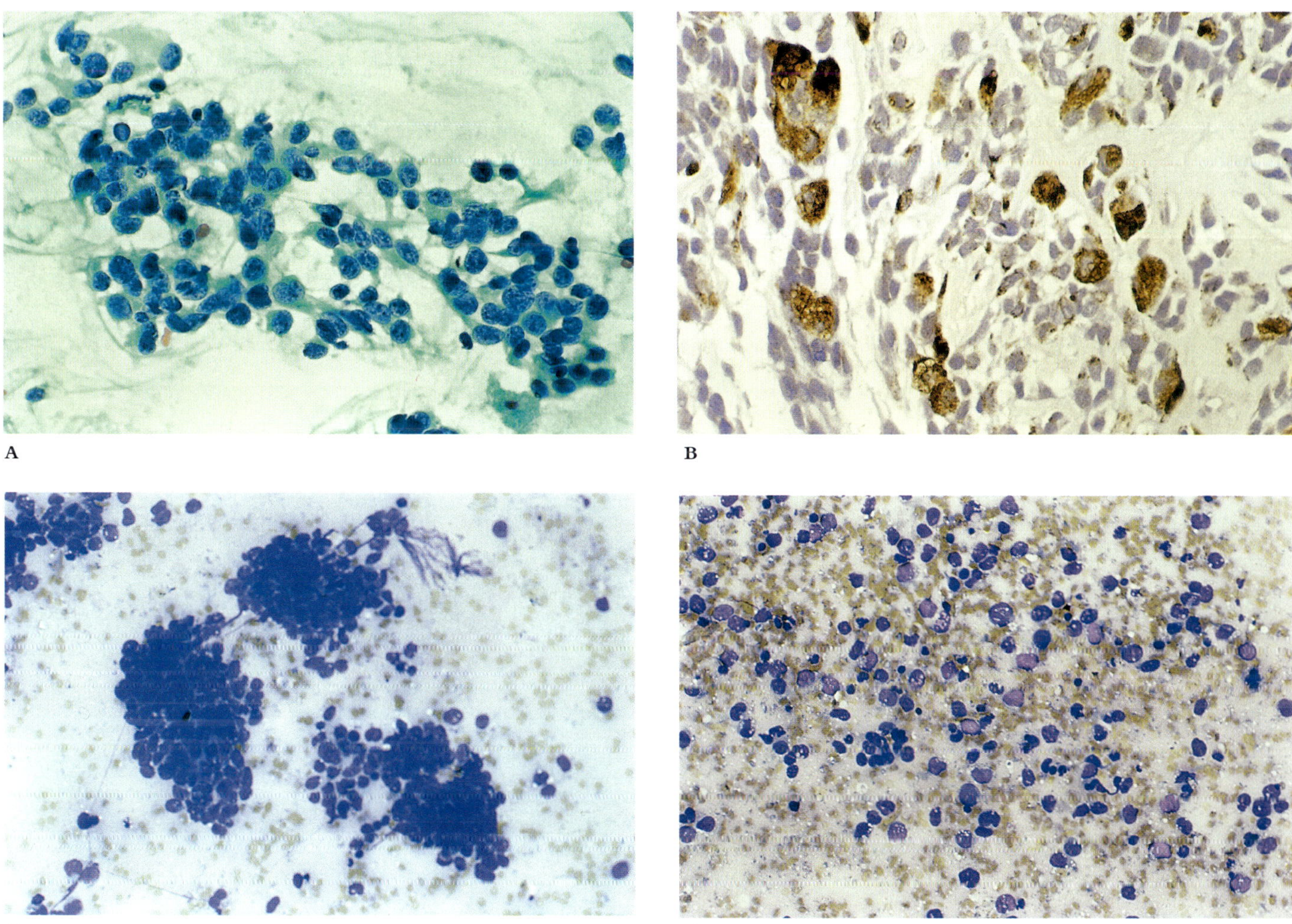

Figure 2.62 Rhabdomyosarcoma. **A.** FNAC from an adult with parotid swelling shows dispersed cuboidal and spindle cells with features of malignancy but not obviously of mesenchymal origin (PAP ×400). **B.** Desmin was positive on biopsy. **C.** Aggregates of small round blue cells in a parotid swelling of an adolescent. Cells were desmin positive, LCA and CD56 negative. Histology showed alveolar rhabdomyosarcoma (MGG ×400). **D.** Same case; a different field shows a more dispersed pattern (MGG ×400).

inflammatory, and they are often treated unsuccessfully with antibiotics.

Cytological features vary from those of a small round cell tumour to a monomorphic population of spindle cells in a metachromatic stroma or spindle cells with moderate cellular pleomorphism (Fig. 2.62 and also Chapter 5, Fig. 5.13). Immunohistochemical or ultrastructural studies confirm the diagnosis of rhabdomyosarcoma.[209]

Synovial sarcoma

Synovial sarcoma is a distinctive neoplasm that usually arises in the extremities in the region of the joints. Although synovial sarcomas arising in the head and neck region are well described, tumours actually originating in and around the major salivary glands are exceedingly rare (Fig. 2.63).[210]

Maligant haemangiopericytoma

The FNAC smear shows a spindle cell neoplasm with capillaries and benign endothelial cells. The spindle cells possess pleomorphic, hyperchromatic, elongated nuclei and a moderate amount of ill-defined cytoplasm. They show papillary clusters surrounded and encased by relatively small ovoid to short spindle cells.[211] Radiation-induced angiosarcoma has been described.[212]

Leiomyosarcoma

A primary leiomyosarcoma of the parotid gland has been reported only 3 times in the English literature.[213] This type of tumour represents an extremely rare group of salivary gland neoplasm. A review of the literature reveals that primary leiomyosarcoma and other sarcomas of the major salivary glands may share similar histogenesis and biological behaviour with their soft tissue counterparts.

Granulocytic sarcoma

Granulocytic sarcoma can on occasion infiltrate the parotid gland without the evidence of acute myeloid leukaemia or chronic myeloproliferative disease at time of diagnosis. The myeloid nature of the tumour can be discovered with the aid of immunocytochemistry. Granulocytic sarcoma should be considered in the differential diagnosis of malignant tumours of the parotid gland, although it is rare.[214] (Fig. 2.64).

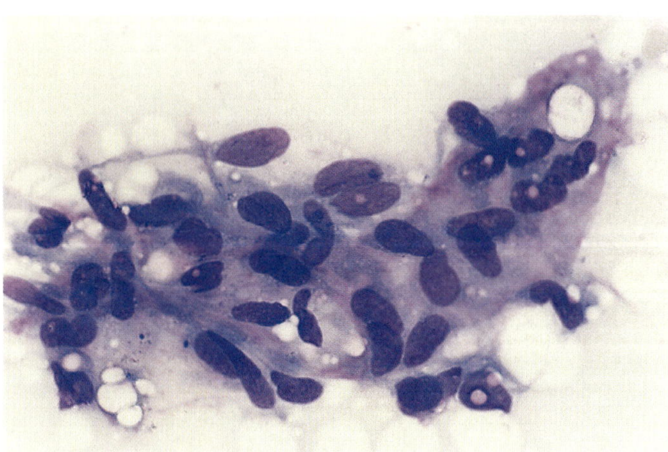

A

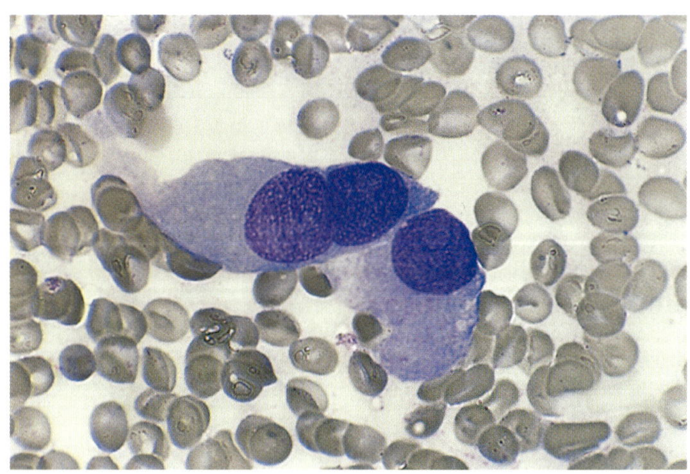

B

Figure 2.63 Synovial sarcoma. **A.** Spindle cells with blunt nuclei in an aggregate. Cytoplasmic processes. Diagnosis of a mesenchymal tumour, probably malignant, was made. Biopsy revealed synovial sarcoma (MGG ×600). **B.** Individual cell synovial sarcoma have oval or round nucleus and unipolar cytoplasm. Nucleoli are prominent. Features suggest malignancy but are not specific of synovial sarcoma (MGG ×1000).

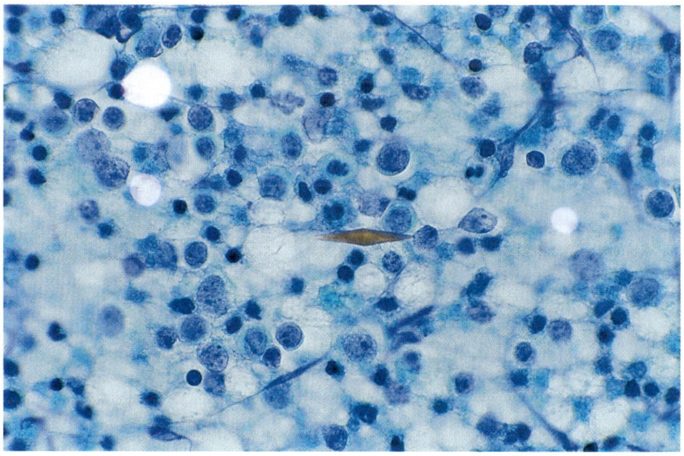

A

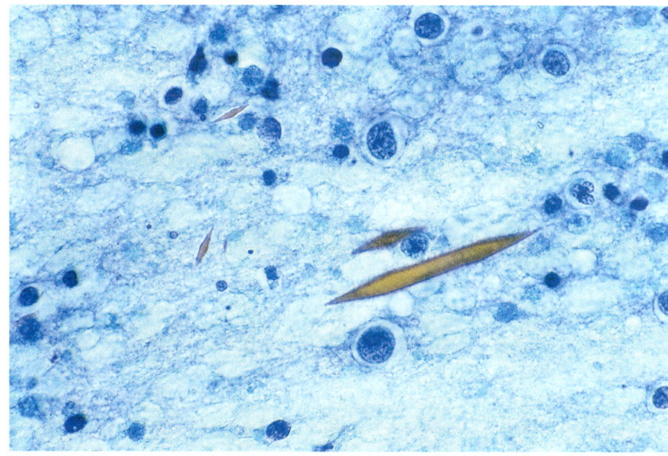

B

Figure 2.64 Acute myeloid leukaemia. First presentation in parotid. A 6-year-old child presented with unilateral diffuse swelling of 1 month duration which did not subside on antibiotics. **A.** Numerous single cells, some with blast features. Charcot Leiden crystals present (PAP ×400). **B.** High-power view of Charcot Leiden crystals and myeloid blasts. A diagnosis of haemopoietic disease was made. Bone marrow and peripheral blood showed acute myeloid leukaemia.

Paediatric lesions

Although paediatric parotid masses are unusual, they can represent a variety of pathological diagnoses, including malignancy. Orvidis et al[215] undertook a survey of nearly 30 years experience with parotid masses in patients aged 18 years and younger that were evaluated and treated at the Mayo Clinic, Rochester, Minnesota. Parotid masses were identified in 118 children (60 boys and 58 girls) most of which had an asymptomatic mass at presentation. Forty-three patients (36.4%) had infectious or inflammatory lesions, 56 (47.5%) had benign lesions and 19 (16.1%) had malignant lesions. The most common benign lesions were pleomorphic adenoma (22.9%) and haemangioma (10.2%).[215,216] The most common malignant lesions were mucoepidermoid carcinoma (6.8%) and acinic cell carcinoma (3.4%). The most common treatment was total parotidectomy (40.7%). Pleomorphic adenoma recurred in 4 (14.8%) of 28 patients and mucoepidermoid carcinoma in 3 (37.5%) of 8 patients. One patient with adenoid cystic carcinoma died of the tumour. The authors advocate prompt evaluation and treatment of these masses.

Lymphomas

Primary salivary gland lymphomas are rare. The low-grade extranodal non-Hodgkin's lymphomas of MALT type (marginal zone lymphoma) have been described earlier in this chapter (Figs 2.24, 2.25 and 2.65). Nodal lymphomas can occur in the salivary gland and the morphology is the same as in other lymph nodes (see Chapter 4) (Fig. 2.66, also Chapter 4, Fig. 4.55). Concurrent presentation of follicular and MALT lymphoma in the same salivary gland has been described[79]. High-grade non-Hodgkin's lymphoma presenting in the salivary gland is managed in the similar way as elsewhere (Fig. 2.67).

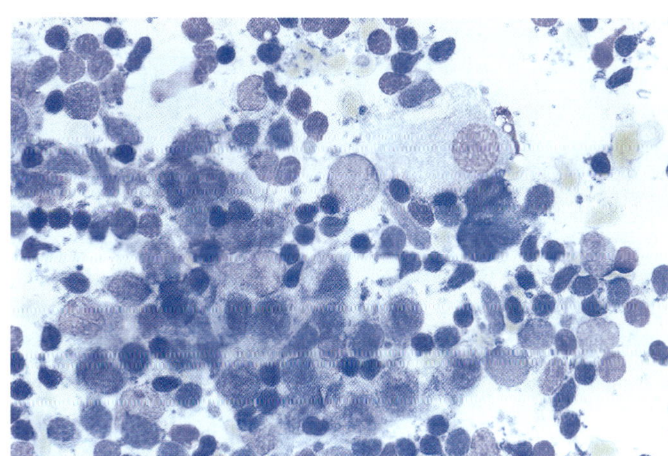

Figure 2.65 MALT lymphoma. As seen in Figures 2.24 and 2.25, MALT lymphoma may have a polymorphic cell population of small and medium-sized lymphocytes admixed with follicular dendritic cells. Lymphoepithelial lesions may be absent (MGG ×600).

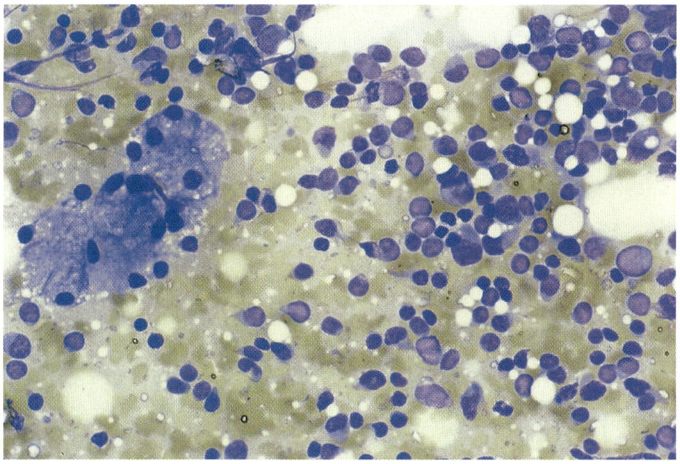

Figure 2.66 Parotid lymphoma. Polymorphic lymphoid infiltrate and salivary gland acini suggested lymphoid infiltration of parotid of uncertain nature. Biopsy was advised. Lesion was peripheral T-cell lymphoma (MGG ×400).

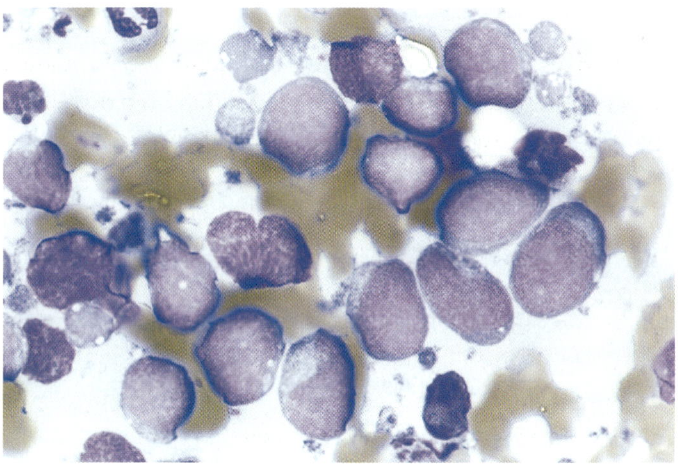

Figure 2.67 A 65-year-old woman presented with a 2-month history of diffuse painless parotid swelling. She was referred from an oncologist who was treating her breast cancer diagnosed some years previously. FNAC revealed a diffuse large B-cell lymphoma (MGG ×1000).

Primitive neuroectodermal tumour

Primitive neuroectodermal tumour is a malignant small round cell tumour that exhibits neuroepithelial differentiation. Isolated cases have been reported in visceral sites such as the kidney, uterus, ovary, testis, urinary bladder and pancreas. Deb et al.[217] were the first to report the tumour occurring in the parotid. They postulate the origin to be from the facial nerve.

Cytological features show a highly cellular, poorly cohesive smear pattern exhibiting small round cells, with scanty cytoplasm forming occasional rosette-like structures (Fig. 2.68,

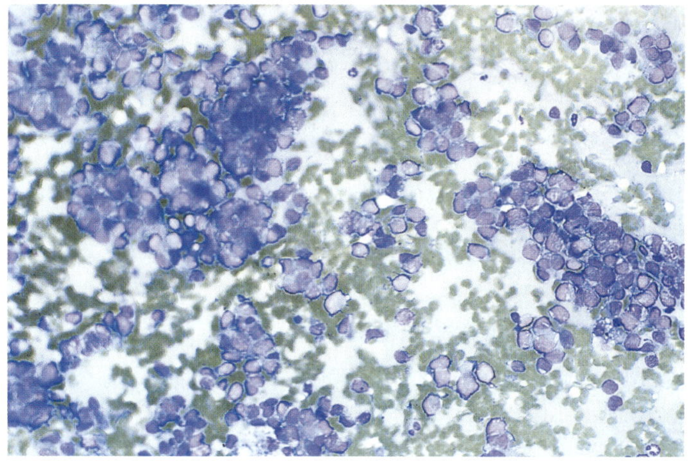

A

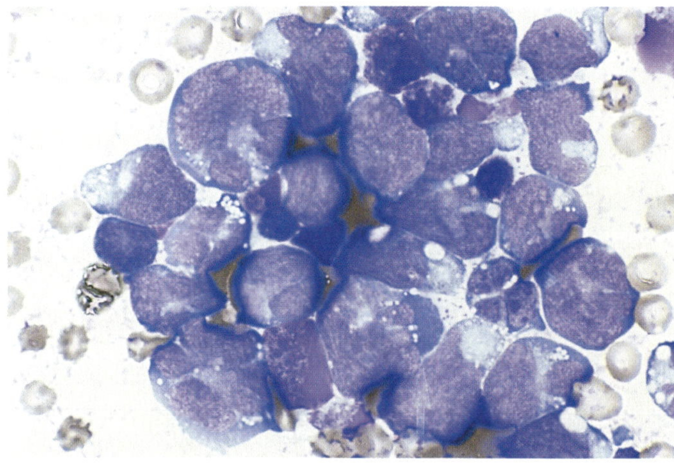

B

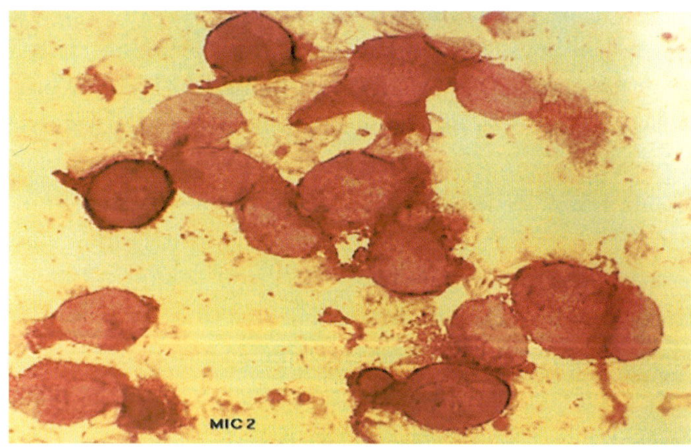

C

Figure 2.68 Peripheral neuroectodermal tumour (PNET). A 25-year-old patient presented with swelling in the neck, possibly salivary gland. **A.** FNAC reveals numerous aggregates and single small blue cells (MGG ×400). **B.** High-power view of one of the aggregates reveals blast-type cells with cytoplasmic vacuolation. However, unlike lymphoid blasts, these cells seem to have definite arrangement in clusters and rosettes (MGG ×1000). **C.** CD56 positivity confirms PNET (APAAP anti-MYC 2 ×1000).

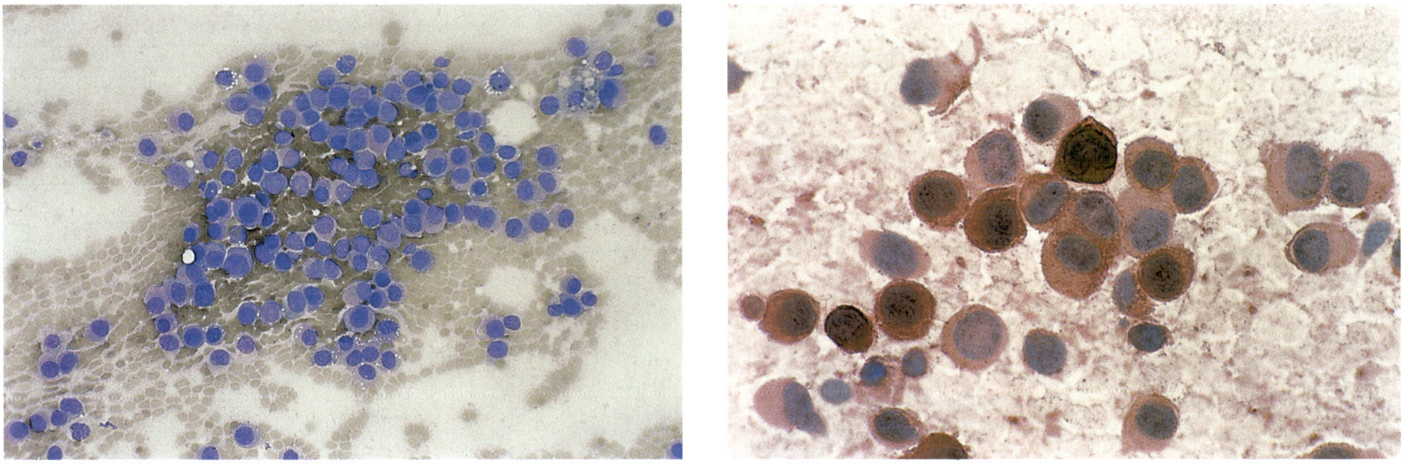

A B

Figure 2.69 Metastatic melanoma. **A.** FNAC of parotid in a patient with no known history reveals numerous single malignant cells with eccentric nuclei, well-outlined cytoplasm and prominent nucleoli. No pigment was seen (MGG ×400). **B.** S-100 positivity in melanoma cells (APAAP anti S100 ×600).

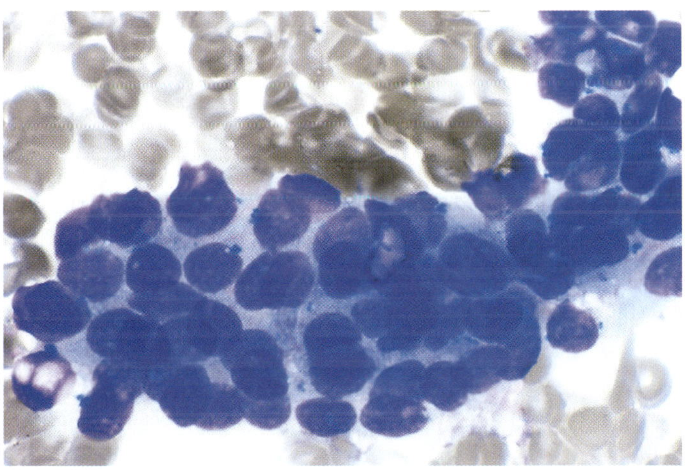

Figure 2.70 Basal cell carcinoma. Local spread of a known basal cell carcinoma helped the diagnosis in this case where aggregates of malignant cells showed no obvious pallisading or any other evidence of cell of origin.

also Chapter 5, Fig. 5.14). Numerous intact single cells with fragile cytoplasm, finely granular chromatin and inconspicuous nucleoli are present together with single nuclei in the background.[218]

Metastatic tumours

Salivary glands are a not infrequent site of metastases. Metastases or secondary deposits account for 16% of the malignant neoplasms involving the major salivary glands. A correct diagnosis of a secondary neoplasm is important for appropriate management to avoid unnecessary radical surgery and to guide further therapy. FNAC is a non-invasive diagnostic tool for evaluating metastatic lesions. Zhang et al[210] reviewed 36 metastatic tumours in the salivary glands and found a mixture of adenocarcinomas, squamous cell carcinomas, undifferentiated carcinomas, cutaneous basal cell carcinomas, cutaneous melanomas, osteosarcomas, non-Hodgkin's lymphomas and multiple myelomas (Figs 2.69 and 2.70).[219] FNAC is a reliable tool to differentiate haematological malignant neoplasms and melanomas from other salivary gland neoplasms. Knowledge of clinical history, review of previous pathological materials and, in some instances, the use of ancillary studies are crucial for recognising malignant neoplasms secondarily involving the salivary glands.

In their review of 20 cases of metastatic carcinoma Malata et al[220] found that most tumours originated from the head and neck region, the two main types being squamous cell carcinoma and malignant melanoma. All 20 presented with a parotid mass and 11 of the 20 had associated lymphadenopathy. Patients underwent superficial, total or radical parotidectomy, neck dissection and adjuvant postoperative radiotherapy. The cumulative 5-year survival rate was 51%.[220] Superficial parotidectomy is usually an adequate treatment for secondary parotid tumours (when disease is clinically limited to the superficial lobe). Patients in whom metastatic disease of the parotid gland is suspected do not require neck dissection if they have no palpable lymph nodes and MRI shows no evidence of spread. There seems to be no survival advantage in radical over modified neck dissection. Small cell lung carcinoma adenocarcinoma from upper airways and digestive tracts and renal cell carcinoma have been described as occurring in the parotid.[221–223]

REFERENCES

1. Orell SR. Diagnostic difficulties in the interpretation of fine needle aspirates of salivary gland lesions: the problem revisited. *Cytopathology* 1995; 6(5): 285–300.
2. Young JA. *Fine Needle Aspiration Cytopathology*: London: Blackwell, 1993.
3. Chan MK, McGuire LJ, King W, Li AK, Lee JC. Cytodiagnosis of 112 salivary gland lesions. Correlation with histologic and frozen section diagnosis. *Acta Cytol* 1992; 36(3): 353–63.
4. Al-Khafaji BM, Nestok BR, Katz RL. Fine-needle aspiration of 154 parotid masses with histologic correlation: ten-year experience at the University of Texas M. D. Anderson Cancer Center. *Cancer* 1998; 84(3): 153–9.
5. Cristallini EG, Ascani S, Farabi R et al. Fine needle aspiration biopsy of salivary gland, 1985–1995. *Acta Cytol* 1997; 41(5): 1421–5.
6. Candel A, Gattuso P, Reddy V, Matz G, Castelli M. Is fine needle aspiration biopsy of salivary gland masses really necessary? *Ear Nose Throat J* 1993; 72(7): 485–9.
7. Cajulis RS, Gokaslan ST, Yu GH, Frias-Hidvegi D. Fine needle aspiration biopsy of the salivary glands. A five-year experience with emphasis on diagnostic pitfalls. *Acta Cytol* 1997; 41(5): 1412–20.
8. Frable MA, Frable WJ. Fine-needle aspiration biopsy of salivary glands. *Laryngoscope* 1991; 101(3): 245–9.
9. Kocjan G, Nayagam M, Harris M. Fine needle aspiration cytology of salivary gland lesions: advantages and pitfalls. *Cytopathology* 1990; 1(5): 269–75.
10. Stewart CJ, MacKenzie K, McGarry GW, Mowat A. Fine-needle aspiration cytology of salivary gland: a review of 341 cases. *Diagn Cytopathol* 2000; 22(3): 139–46.

10a. Goh YH, Sethi DS. Submandibular gland excision: a five year review. *J Laryngol Otol* 1998; 112(3): 269–73.

11. Shintani S, Matsuura H, Hasegawa Y. Fine needle aspiration of salivary gland tumors. *Int J Oral Maxillofac Surg* 1997; 26(4): 284–6.
12. Murthy P, Laing MR, Palmer TJ. Fine needle aspiration cytology of head and neck lesions: an early experience. *J R Coll Surg Edinb* 1997; 42(5): 341–6.
13. Young JA, Smallman LA, Thompson H, Proops DW, Johnson AP. Fine needle aspiration cytology of salivary gland lesions. *Cytopathology* 1990; 1(1): 25–33.

13a. Jayaram G, Verma AK, Sood N, Khurana N. Fine needle aspiraton cytology of salivary gland lesions. *J Oral Pathol Med* 1994; 23(6): 256–61.

14. Choi DS, Na DG, Byun HS et al. Salivary gland tumors: evaluation with two-phase helical CT. *Radiology* 2000; 214(1): 231–6.
15. Takashima S, Takayama F, Wang Q, Kurozumi M, Sekiyama Y, Sone S. Parotid gland lesions: diagnosis of malignancy with MRI and flow cytometric DNA analysis and cytology in fine-needle aspiration biopsy. *Head Neck* 1999; 21(1): 43–51.
16. Shaha AR, Webber C, DiMaio T, Jaffe BM. Needle aspiration biopsy in salivary gland lesions. *Am J Surg* 1990; 160(4): 373–6.
17. Heller KS, Dubner S, Chess Q, Attie JN. Value of fine needle aspiration biopsy of salivary gland masses in clinical decision-making. *Am J Surg* 1992; 164(6): 667–70.
18. Raab SS, Sigman JD, Hoffman HT. The utility of parotid gland and level I and II neck fine-needle aspiration. *Arch Pathol Lab Med* 1998; 122(9): 823–7.
19. Zajicek J. 1. Introduction to aspiration biopsy. *Monogr Clin Cytol* 1974; 4(0): 1–211.
20. Seifert G, Sobin LH. The World Health Organization's Histological Classification of Salivary Gland Tumors. A commentary on the second edition. *Cancer* 1992; 70(2): 379–85.
21. Orell SR, Nettle NJ. Fine needle aspiration biopsy of salivary gland tumours. Problems and pitfalls. Pathology 1988; 20: 332–7.
22. Young JA. Diagnostic problems in fine needle aspiration cytopathology of the salivary glands. *J Clin Pathol* 1994; 47(3): 193–8.
23. Gray W. *Diagnostic Cytopathology*: Edinburgh: Churchill Livingstone, 1995.
24. Layfield LJ, Glasgow BJ. Aspiration cytology of clear-cell lesions of the parotid gland: morphologic features and differential diagnosis. *Diagn Cytopathol* 1993; 9(6): 705–11, discussion 711–2.
25. Layfield LJ, Glasgow BJ. Diagnosis of salivary gland tumors by fine-needle aspiration cytology: a review of clinical utility and pitfalls. *Diagn Cytopathol* 1991; 7(3): 267–72.
26. MacLeod CB, Frable WJ. Fine-needle aspiration biopsy of the salivary gland: problem cases. *Diagn Cytopathol* 1993; 9(2): 216–24, discussion 224–5.
27. Boccato P, Altavilla G, Blandamura S. Fine needle aspiration biopsy of salivary gland lesions. A reappraisal of pitfalls and problems. *Acta Cytol* 1998; 42(4): 888–98.
28. Carvalho MB, Soares JM, Rapoport A et al. Perioperative frozen section examination in parotid gland tumors. *Sao Paulo Med J* 1999; 117(6): 233–7.
29. Layfield LJ, Tan P, Glasgow BJ. Fine-needle aspiration of salivary gland lesions. Comparison with frozen sections and histologic findings. *Arch Pathol Lab Med* 1987; 111(4): 346–53.
30. Zakowski MF. Fine-needle aspiration cytology of tumors: diagnostic accuracy and potential pitfalls. *Cancer Invest* 1994; 12(5): 505–15.
31. Rimm DL, Stastny JF, Rimm EB, Ayer S, Frable WJ. Comparison of the costs of fine-needle aspiration and open surgical biopsy as methods for obtaining a pathologic diagnosis. *Cancer* 1997; 81(1): 51–6.
32. Roland NJ, Caslin AW, Smith PA, Turnbull LS, Panarese A, Jones AS. Fine needle aspiration cytology of salivary gland lesions reported immediately in a head and neck clinic. *J Laryngol Otol* 1993; 107(11): 1025–8.

33. Dey P, Ray R. Comparison of fine needle sampling by capillary action and fine needle aspiration. *Cytopathology* 1993; 4(5): 299–303.

34. Hamaker RA, Moriarty AT, Hamaker RC. Fine-needle biopsy techniques of aspiration versus capillary in head and neck masses. *Laryngoscope* 1995; 105(12 pt 1): 1311–4.

35. Mair S, Dunbar F, Becker PJ, Du Plessis W. Fine needle cytology – is aspiration suction necessary? A study of 100 masses in various sites [see comments]. *Acta Cytol* 1989; 33(6): 809–13.

36. Santos JE, Leiman G. Nonaspiration fine needle cytology. Application of a new technique to nodular thyroid disease [see comments]. *Acta Cytol* 1988; 32(3): 353–6.

37. Yue XH, Zheng SF. Cytologic diagnosis by transthoracic fine needle sampling without aspiration. *Acta Cytol* 1989; 33(6): 805–8.

38. Rajasekhar A, Sundaram C, Chowdhary T, Charanpal M, Ratnakar KS. Diagnostic utility of fine-needle sampling without aspiration: a prospective study. *Diagn Cytopathol* 1991; 7(5): 473–6.

39. Di Palma S, Simpson RH, Skalova A, Michal M. Metaplastic (infarcted) Warthin's tumour of the parotid gland: a possible consequence of fine needle aspiration biopsy. *Histopathology* 1999; 35(5): 432–8.

40. Lee SS, Cho KJ, Jang JJ, Ham EK. Differential diagnosis of adenoid cystic carcinoma from pleomorphic adenoma of the salivary gland on fine needle aspiration cytology. *Acta Cytol* 1996; 40(6): 1246–52.

41. Pinkston JA, Cole P. Incidence rates of salivary gland tumors: results from a population-based study. *Otolaryngol Head Neck Surg* 1999; 120(6): 834–40.

42. Saleh HA, Ram B, Harmse JL, Michie BA, Blair RL. Lipomatosis of the minor salivary glands. *J Laryngol Otol* 1998; 112(9): 895–7.

43. Coleman H, Altini M, Nayler S, Richards A. Sialadenosis: a presenting sign in bulimia [see comments]. *Head Neck* 1998; 20(8): 758–62.

44. Kim D, Uy C, Mandel L. Sialosis of unknown origin. *N Y State Dent J* 1998; 64(7): 38–40.

45. Ascoli V, Albedi FM, De Blasiis R, Nardi F. Sialadenosis of the parotid gland: report of four cases diagnosed by fine-needle aspiration cytology. *Diagn Cytopathol* 1993; 9(2): 151–5.

46. Mandel L, Hamele-Bena D. Alcoholic parotid sialadenosis. *J Am Dent Assoc* 1997; 128(10). 1411 5.

47. Gupta S, Sodhani P. Sialadenosis of parotid gland: a cytomorphologic and morphometric study of four cases. *Anal Quant Cytol Histol* 1998; 20(3): 225–8.

48. Mooney EE, Dodd LG, Layfield LJ. Squamous cells in fine-needle aspiration biopsies of salivary gland lesions: potential pitfalls in cyto logic diagnosis. *Diagn Cytopathol* 1996; 15(5): 447–52.

49. Jayaram G, Pathmanathan R, Khanijow V. Cystic lesion of the parotid gland with squamous metaplasia mistaken for squamous cell carcinoma. A case report. *Acta Cytol* 1998; 42(6): 1468–72.

50. Maiorano E, Favia G, Viale G. Lymphoepithelial cysts of salivary glands: an immunohistochemical study of HIV-related and HIV-unrelated lesions. *Hum Pathol* 1998; 29(3): 260–5.

51. Vicandi B, Jimenez-Heffernan JA, Lopez-Ferrer P et al. HIV-1 (p24)-positive multinucleated giant cells in HIV-associated lymphoepithelial lesion of the parotid gland. A report of two cases. *Acta Cytol* 1999; 43(2): 247–51.

52. Lopez-Rios F, Ballestin C, Martinez-Gonzalez MA, Serrano R, de Agustin PP. Lymphoepithelial cyst with crystalloid formation. Cytologic features of two cases. *Acta Cytol* 1999; 43(2): 277–80.

53. Kavishwar VS, Rege JD, Naik LP. Fine needle aspiration diagnosis of lymphoepithelial cyst of the parotid gland [letter]. *Acta Cytol* 1999; 43(5): 972–4.

54. Chhieng DC, Argosino R, McKenna BJ, Cangiarella JF, Cohen JM. Utility of fine-needle aspiration in the diagnosis of salivary gland lesions in patients infected with human immunodeficiency virus. *Diagn Cytopathol* 1999; 21(4)· 260–4.

55. Chaushu G, Buchner A, David R. Multiple oncocytic cysts with tyrosine-crystalloids in the parotid gland [see comments]. *Hum Pathol* 1999; 30(2): 237–9.

56. Moody AB, Avery CM, Harrison JD. Dermoid cyst of the parotid gland. *Int J Oral Maxillofac Surg* 1998; 27(6): 461–2.

57. Righi PD, Wells WA, Wagner JD, Kim SA, Anderson MW, Longardner NR. Odontogenic keratocyst of the mandible: an unusual cause of a parotid mass. *Ann Plast Surg* 1998; 41(1): 89–93.

58. Bhatty MA, Piggot TA, Soames JV, McLean NR. Chronic non-specific parotid sialadenitis. *Br J Plast Surg* 1998; 51(7). 517 21.

59. Hogg RP, Ayshford C, Watkinson JC. Parotid duct carcinoma arising in bilateral chronic sialadenitis. *J Laryngol Otol* 1999; 113(7): 686–8.

60. Boutonnat J, Ducros V, Pinel C et al. Identification of amylase crystalloids in cystic lesions of the parotid gland. *Acta* Cytol 2000; 44(1): 51–6.

61. Gupta RK, Green C, Fauck R, Lallu S, Naran S. Fine needle aspiration cytodiagnosis of sialadenitis with crystalloids. *Acta Cytol* 1999; 43(3): 390–2.

62. Nasuti JF, Gupta PK, Fleisher SR, LiVolsi VA. Nontyrosine crystalloids in salivary gland lesions: report of seven cases with fine-needle aspiration cytology and follow-up surgical pathology. *Diagn Cytopathol* 2000; 22(3): 167–71.

63. Granter SR, Renshaw AA, Cibas ES. Nontyrosine crystalloids in fine-needle aspiration specimens of the parotid gland: a report of two cases and review of the literature. *Diagn Cytopathol* 1999; 20(1): 11–6.

64. Batsakis JG. Granulomatous sialadenitis. *Ann Otol Rhinol Laryngol* 1991; 100(2): 166–9.

65. Van der Walt JD, Leake J. Granulomatous sialadenitis of the major salivary glands. A clinicopathological study of 57 cases. *Histopathology* 1987; 11(2): 131–44.

66. Mair S, Leiman G, Levinsohn D. Fine needle aspiration cytology of parotid sarcoidosis. *Acta Cytol* 1989; 33(2): 169–72.

67. Santiago K, Rivera A, Cabaniss D, Dhurhar N, Moroz K. Fine-needle aspiration of cytomegalovirus sialadenitis in a patient with acquired immunodeficiency syndrome: pitfalls of diff-quik staining. *Diagn Cytopathol* 2000; 22(2): 101–3.

68. Raab SS, Thomas PA, Cohen MB. Fine-needle aspiration biopsy of salivary gland mycoses. *Diagn Cytopathol* 1994; 11(3): 286–90.

68a. Patton LL, McKaig R, Strauss R, Rogers D, Eron JJ Jr. Changing prevalence of oral manifestations of human immumodeficiency virus in the era of protease inhibitor therapy. *Oral Surg Oral Med Oral Pathol Oral Radiol Endod* 2000; 89: 299–304.

68b. Langford RJ, Whear NM. Serology should be a routine investigation when presented with a major salivary gland lump. *Br J Oral Maxillofac Surg* 2000; 38: 158–9.

69. Ussmuller J, Donath K. [Histopathogenesis of chronic sialectatic parotitis as precursor of myoepithelial sialadenitis lesion (Sjogren syndrome)]. *Laryngorhinootologie* 1998; 77(12): 723–7.

70. Haddad J, Deny P, Munz-Gotheil C et al. Lymphocytic sialadenitis of Sjogren's syndrome associated with chronic hepatitis C virus liver disease [see comments]. *Lancet* 1992; 339(8789): 321–3.

71. Jordan J, Babinski D, Sova J. [Adenolymphoma (Warthin's tumor) of the larynx: coexistence with the bilateral laryngocele. Contribution to differential diagnosis with oncocytic papillary cystadenoma]. *Otolaryngol Pol* 1999; 53(2): 213–6.

72. Isaacson PG. Mucosa-associated lymphoid tissue lymphoma. *Semin Hematol* 1999; 36(2): 139–47.

73. Isaacson PG. Gastrointestinal lymphomas of T- and B-cell types. *Mod Pathol* 1999; 12(2): 151–8.

74. Harris NL, Isaacson PG. What are the criteria for distinguishing MALT from non-MALT lymphoma at extranodal sites? *Am J Clin Pathol* 1999; 111(1 suppl 1): S126–32.

75. Banks PM, Isaacson PG. MALT lymphomas in 1997. Where do we stand? *Am J Clin Pathol* 1999; 111(1 suppl 1): S75–83.

76. Du MQ, Isaacson PG. Recent advances in our understanding of the biology and pathogenesis of gastric mucosa-associated lymphoid tissue (malt) lymphoma. *Forum (Genova)* 1998; 8(2): 162–73.

77. Lasota J, Miettinen MM. Coexistence of different B-cell clones in consecutive lesions of low-grade MALT lymphoma of the salivary gland in Sjogren's disease. *Mod Pathol* 1997; 10(9): 872–8.

77a. Nishimura M, Miyajima S, Okada N. Salivary gland MALT lymphoma associated with Helicobacter pylori infection in patients with Sjogren's syndrome. *J Dermatol* 2000; 27: 450–2.

78. Harris NL. Lymphoid proliferations of the salivary glands. *Am J Clin Pathol* 1999; 111(1 suppl 1): S94–103.

79. Aiello A, Du MQ, Diss TC et al. Simultaneous phenotypically distinct but clonally identical mucosa-associated lymphoid tissue and follicular lymphoma in a patient with Sjogren's syndrome. *Blood* 1999; 94(7): 2247–51.

80. Quintana PG, Kapadia SB, Bahler DW, Johnson JT, Swerdlow SH. Salivary gland lymphoid infiltrates associated with lymphoepithelial lesions: a clinicopathologic, immunophenotypic, and genotypic study [see comments]. *Hum Pathol* 1997; 28(7): 850–61.

81. Klussmann JP, Guntinas-Lichius O, Heilig B, Wagner M, Jungehulsing M, Michel O. [Sjogren syndrome and bilateral MALT lymphoma of the parotid gland]. *HNO* 1999; 47(7): 637–41.

82. Ruschenburg I, Korabiowska M, Schlott T, Kubitz A, Droese M. The value of PCR technique in fine needle aspiration biopsy of salivary gland for diagnosis of low-grade B-cell lymphoma. *Int J Mol Med* 1998; 2(3): 339–341.

83. MacCallum PL, Lampe HB, Cramer H, Matthews TW. Fine-needle aspiration cytology of lymphoid lesions of the salivary gland: a review of 35 cases. *J Otolaryngol* 1996; 25(5): 300–4.

84. Joshi VV, Gagnon GA, Chadwick EG et al. The spectrum of mucosa-associated lymphoid tissue lesions in pediatric patients infected with HIV: A clinicopathologic study of six cases. *Am J Clin Pathol* 1997; 107(5): 592–600.

85. Cha I, Long SR, Ljung BM, Miller TR. Low-grade lymphoma of mucosa-associated tissue in the parotid gland: a case report of fine-needle aspiration cytology diagnosis using flow cytometric immunophenotyping. *Diagn Cytopathol* 1997; 16(4): 345–9.

86. Burke JS. Are there site-specific differences among the MALT lymphomas – morphologic, clinical? *Am J Clin Pathol* 1999; 111(1 suppl 1): S133–43.

87. Christensen NR, Charabi S, Sorensen WT, Dethloff T, Balle VH, Tos M. [Benign neoplasms in the parotid gland in the county of Copenhagen 1986–1995]. *Ugeskr Laeger* 1998; 160(42): 6066–9.

88. Buenting JE, Smith TL, Holmes DK. Giant pleomorphic adenoma of the parotid gland: case report and review of the literature. *Ear Nose Throat J* 1998; 77(8): 634, 637–8, 640.

89. Ahn MS, Hayashi GM, Hilsinger RL Jr, Lalwani AK. Familial mixed tumors of the parotid gland. *Head Neck* 1999; 21(8): 772–5.

90. Klijanienko J, El-Naggar AK, Vielh P. Fine-needle sampling findings in 26 carcinoma ex pleomorphic adenomas: diagnostic pitfalls and clinical considerations. *Diagn Cytopathol* 1999; 21(3): 163–6.

91. Viguer JM, Vicandi B, Jimenez-Heffernan JA, Lopez-Ferrer P, Limeres MA. Fine needle aspiration cytology of pleomorphic adenoma. An analysis of 212 cases. *Acta Cytol* 1997; 41(3): 786–94.

92. Klijanienko J, Vielh P. Fine-needle sampling of salivary gland lesions. I. Cytology and histology correlation of 412 cases of pleomorphic adenoma. *Diagn Cytopathol* 1996; 14(3): 195–200.

93. Laskawi R, Schott T, Schroder M. Recurrent pleomorphic adenomas of the parotid gland: clinical evaluation and long-term follow-up. *Br J Oral Maxillofac Surg* 1998; 36(1): 48–51.

94. Kapadia SB, Dusenbery D, Dekker A. Fine needle aspiration of pleomorphic adenoma and adenoid cystic carcinoma of salivary gland origin. *Acta Cytol* 1997; 41(2): 487–92.

95. Elsheikh TM, Bernacki EG. Fine needle aspiration cytology of cellular pleomorphic adenoma. *Acta Cytol* 1996; 40(6): 1165–75.

96. Domanski HA. Intravenous pyogenic granuloma mimicking pleomorphic adenoma in a fine needle aspirate. A case report. *Acta Cytol* 1999; 43(3): 439–41.

97. Auclair PL, Ellis GL. Atypical features in salivary gland mixed tumors: their relationship to malignant transformation. *Mod Pathol* 1996; 9(6): 652–7.

98. Di Palma S, Guzzo M. Myoepithelial carcinoma with predominance of plasmacytoid cells arising in a pleomorphic adenoma of the parotid gland [letter, comment]. *Histopathology* 1998; 33(5): 485.

99. Pitman MB, Thor AD, Goodman ML, Rosenberg AE. Benign metastasizing pleomorphic adenoma of salivary gland: diagnosis of bone lesions by fine-needle aspiration biopsy. *Diagn Cytopathol* 1992; 8(4): 384–7.

100. Klijanienko J, El-Naggar AK, Servois V, Rodriguez J, Validire P, Vielh P. Clinically aggressive metastasizing pleomorphic adenoma: report of two cases. *Head Neck* 1997; 19(7): 629–33.

101. Bottles K, Lowhagen T, Miller TR. Mast cells in the aspiration cytology differential diagnosis of adenolymphoma. *Acta Cytol* 1985; 29(4): 513–5.

102. Kobayashi TK, Ueda M, Nishino T, Kushima R, Nakajima S, Kaneko C. Association of mast cells with Warthin's tumor in fine needle aspirates of the salivary gland. *Acta Cytol* 1999; 43(6): 1052–8.

103. Klijanienko J, Vielh P. Fine-needle sampling of salivary gland lesions. II. Cytology and histology correlation of 71 cases of Warthin's tumor (adenolymphoma). *Diagn Cytopathol* 1997; 16(3): 221–5.

104. Ballo MS, Shin HJ, Sneige N. Sources of diagnostic error in the fine-needle aspiration diagnosis of Warthin's tumor and clues to a correct diagnosis. *Diagn Cytopathol* 1997; 17(3): 230–4.

105. Ryska A, Seifert G. Adenolymphoma (Warthin's tumor) with multiple sarcoid-like granulomas. *Pathol Res Pract* 1999; 195(12): 835–9.

106. Hürthle K. Beitrage zur Kenntnis de Sekretions-vorganges in der Schilddruse. *Arch F D Ges Physiol* 1894; 56: 1–44.

107. Jahan-Parwar B, Huberman RM, Donovan DT, Schwartz MR, Ostrowski ML. Oncocytic mucoepidermoid carcinoma of the salivary glands. *Am J Surg Pathol* 1999; 23(5): 523–9.

108. Shick PC, Brannon RB. Oncocytoid artifact of the parotid gland: a newly reported artifact. *Oral Surg Oral Med Oral Pathol Oral Radiol Endod* 1998; 86(6): 720–2.

109. Strassburger S, Hyckel P, Kosmehl H. Multifocal oncocytic adenomatous hyperplasia of the parotid gland. A case report. *Int J Oral Maxillofac Surg* 1999; 28(6): 457–8.

110. Park CK, Manning JT Jr, Battifora H, Medeiros LJ. Follicle center lymphoma and Warthin tumor involving the same anatomic site. Report of two cases and review of the literature. *Am J Clin Pathol* 2000; 113(1): 113–9.

111. Nagao T, Sugano I, Ishida Y, Tajima Y, et al. Mucoepidermoid carcinoma arising in Warthin's tumour of the parotid gland: report of two cases with histopathological, ultrastructural and immunohistochemical studies. *Histopathology* 1998; 33(4): 379–86.

112. Seifert G. [Carcinoma in pre-existing Warthin tumors (cystadenolymphoma) of the parotid gland. Classification, pathogenesis and differential diagnosis]. *Pathologe* 1997; 18(5): 359–67.

113. Patterson JW, Wright ED, Camden S. Extraparotid Warthin's tumor. *J Am Acad Dermatol* 1999; 40(3): 468–70.

114. Layfield LJ. Fine needle aspiration cytology of a trabecular adenoma of the parotid gland. *Acta Cytol* 1985; 29(6): 999–1002.

115. Klijanienko J, el-Naggar AK, Vielh P. Comparative cytologic and histologic study of fifteen salivary basal-cell tumors: differential diagnostic considerations. *Diagn Cytopathol* 1999; 21(1): 30–4.

116. Stanley MW, Horwitz CA, Rollins SD et al. Basal cell (monomorphic) and minimally pleomorphic adenomas of the salivary glands. Distinction from the solid (anaplastic) type of adenoid cystic carcinoma in fine-needle aspiration. *Am J Clin Pathol* 1996; 106(1): 35–41.

117. Thompson LD, Wenig BM, Ellis GL. Oncocytomas of the submandibular gland. A series of 22 cases and a review of the literature. *Cancer* 1996; 78(11): 2281–7.

118. Skalova A, Starek I, Michal M, Leivo I. Malignancy-simulating change in parotid gland oncocytoma following fine needle aspiration. Report of 3 cases. *Pathol Res Pract* 1999; 195(6): 399–405.

119. Rajan PB, Wadehra V, Hemming JD, Hawkesford JE. Fine needle aspiration cytology of malignant oncocytoma of the parotid gland – a case report [see comments]. *Cytopathology* 1994; 5(2): 110–3.

120. Vo-Ngoc H, Dellagi K, Marandas P, Micheau C. [Myoepithelioma (or myoepithelial cell adenoma). Report of a case]. *Ann Pathol* 1994; 14(2): 112–5.

121. Tanimura A, Nakamura Y, Nagayama K, Tanaka S, Hachisuka H. Myoepithelioma of the parotid gland. Report of two cases with immunohistochemical technique for S-100 protein and electron microscopic observation. *Acta Pathol Jpn* 1985; 35(2): 409–17.

122. Dodd LG, Caraway NP, Luna MA, Byers RM. Myoepithelioma of the parotid. Report of a case initially examined by fine needle aspiration biopsy. *Acta Cytol* 1994; 38(3): 417–21.

123. Alos L, Cardesa A, Bombi JA, Mallofre C, Cuchi A, Traserra J. Myoepithelial tumors of salivary glands: a clinicopathologic, immunohistochemical, ultrastructural, and flow-cytometric study. *Semin Diagn Pathol* 1996; 13(2): 138–47.

124. Sironi M, Taccagni G, Assi A. A cytologic, immunocytochemical and ultrastructural study of a malignant parotid gland myoepithelioma. *Cytopathology* 1997; 8(1): 53–62.

125. Orell SR, Nettle WJ. Fine needle aspiration biopsy of salivary gland tumours. Problems and pitfalls. *Pathology* 1988; 20(4): 332–7.

126. King PH, Hill J. Intraduct papilloma of parotid gland. *J Clin Pathol* 1993; 46(2): 175–6.

127. Soofer SB, Tabbara S. Intraductal papilloma of the salivary gland. A report of two cases with diagnosis by fine needle aspiration biopsy. *Acta Cytol* 1999; 43(6): 1142–6.

128. Nagao T, Sugano I, Matsuzaki O, Hara H, Kondo Y, Nagao K. Intraductal papillary tumors of the major salivary glands [in process citation]. *Arch Pathol Lab Med* 2000; 124(2): 291–5.

129. Derias NW, Chong WH, Pambakian H. Sebaceous adenoma of parotid gland – a rare tumour diagnosed by fine needle aspiration cytology. *Cytopathology* 1994; 5(6): 392–5.

130. Mahler V, Schell H. Papillary cystadenoma: a rare tumor of the minor salivary glands. *Eur J Dermatol* 1999; 9(5): 387–9.

131. Graham CT, Roberts AH, Padel AF. Pleomorphic lipoma of the parotid gland. *J Laryngol Otol* 1998; 112(2): 202–3.

132. Ide F, Shimoyama T, Horie N, Tanaka H. Collagenous fibroma (desmoplastic fibroblastoma) presenting as a parotid mass. *J Oral Pathol Med* 1999; 28(10): 465–8.

133. Carr MM, Fraser RB, Clarke KD. Nodular fasciitis in the parotid region of a child. *Head Neck* 1998; 20(7): 645–8.

134. Malata CM, Camilleri IG, McLean NR et al. Malignant tumours of the parotid gland: a 12-year review. *Br J Plast Surg* 1997; 50(8): 600–8.

135. Calearo C, Pastore A, Storchi OF, Polli G. Parotid gland carcinoma: analysis of prognostic factors. *Ann Otol Rhinol Laryngol* 1998; 107(11 Pt 1): 969–73.

136. Leverstein H, van der Wal JE, Tiwari RM et al. Malignant epithelial parotid gland tumours: analysis and results in 65 previously untreated patients. *Br J Surg* 1998; 85(9): 1267–72.

137. Nordkvist A, Roijer E, Bang G et al. Expression and mutation patterns of p53 in benign and malignant salivary gland tumors. *Int J Oncol* 2000; 16(3): 477–83.

138. Zhu Q, Tipoe GL, White FH. Proliferative activity as detected by immunostaining with Ki-67 and proliferating cell nuclear antigen in benign and malignant epithelial lesions of the human parotid gland. *Anal Quant Cytol Histol* 1999; 21(4): 336–42.

139. Pinto AE, Fonseca I, Soares J. The clinical relevance of ploidy and S-phase fraction determination in salivary gland tumors: a flow cytometric study of 97 cases. *Cancer* 1999; 85(2): 273–81.

140. Betkowski A, Cyran-Rymarz A, Domka W. [Bilateral acinar cell carcinoma of the parotid gland]. *Otolaryngol Pol* 1998; 52(1): 101–4.

141. Depowski PL, Setzen G, Chui A, Koltai PJ, Dollar J, Ross JS. Familial occurrence of acinic cell carcinoma of the parotid gland. *Arch Pathol Lab Med* 1999; 123(11): 1118–20.

142. Angeles-Angeles A, Caballero-Mendoza E, Tapia-Rangel B, Cortes-Gonzalez R, Larriva-Sahd J. [Giant acinic cell parotid gland adenocarcinoma of the papillary-cystic type]. *Rev Invest Clin* 1998; 50(3): 245–8.

143. Laskawi R, Rodel R, Zirk A, Arglebe C. Retrospective analysis of 35 patients with acinic cell carcinoma of the parotid gland. *J Oral Maxillofac Surg* 1998; 56(4): 440–3.

144. Klijanienko J, Vielh P. Fine-needle sample of salivary gland lesions. V: Cytology of 22 cases of acinic cell carcinoma with histologic correlation. *Diagn Cytopathol* 1997; 17(5): 347–52.

145. Hoffman HT, Karnell LH, Robinson RA, Pinkston JA, Menck HR. National Cancer Data Base report on cancer of the head and neck: acinic cell carcinoma. *Head Neck* 1999; 21(4): 297–309.

146. Nagel H, Laskawi R, Buter JJ, Schroder M, Chilla R, Droese M. Cytologic diagnosis of acinic-cell carcinoma of salivary glands. *Diagn Cytopathol* 1997; 16(5): 402–12.

147. Plambeck K, Friedrich RE, Schmelzle R. Mucoepidermoid carcinoma of salivary gland origin: classification, clinical-pathological correlation, treatment results and long-term follow-up in 55 patients. *J Craniomaxillofac Surg* 1996; 24(3): 133–9.

148. Cohen MB, Fisher PE, Holly EA, Ljung BM, Lowhagen T, Bottles K. Fine needle aspiration biopsy diagnosis of mucoepidermoid carcinoma. Statistical analysis. *Acta Cytol* 1990; 34(1): 43–9.

149. Klijanienko J, Vielh P. Fine-needle sampling of salivary gland lesions. IV. Review of 50 cases of mucoepidermoid carcinoma with histologic correlation. *Diagn Cytopathol* 1997; 17(2): 92–8.

150. Hamed G, Shmookler BM, Ellis GL, Punja U, Feldman D. Oncocytic mucoepidermoid carcinoma of the parotid gland. *Arch Pathol Lab Med* 1994; 118(3): 313–4.

151. Klijanienko J, El-Naggar AK, Servois V, Rodriguez J, Validire P, Vielh P. Mucoepidermoid carcinoma ex pleomorphic adenoma: nonspecific preoperative cytologic findings in six cases. *Cancer* 1998; 84(4): 231–4.

152. Jacobs JC. Low grade mucoepidermoid carcinoma ex pleomorphic adenoma. A diagnostic problem in fine needle aspiration biopsy. *Acta Cytol* 1994; 38(1): 93–7.

153. Frankenthaler RA, el-Naggar AK, Ordonez NG, Miller TS, Batsakis JG. High correlation with survival of proliferating cell nuclear antigen expression in mucoepidermoid carcinoma of the parotid gland. *Otolaryngol Head Neck Surg* 1994; 111(4): 460–6.

154. Klijanienko J, Vielh P. Fine-needle sampling of salivary gland lesions. III. Cytologic and histologic correlation of 75 cases of adenoid cystic carcinoma: review and experience at the Institut Curie with emphasis on cytologic pitfalls. *Diagn Cytopathol* 1997; 17(1): 36–41.

155. Orell SR S, Walters MN et al. *Manual and Atlas of Fine Needle Aspiration Cytology*. Edinburgh: Churchill Livingstone, 1992.

156. Nagel H, Hotze HJ, Laskawi R, Chilla R, Droese M. Cytologic diagnosis of adenoid cystic carcinoma of salivary glands. *Diagn Cytopathol* 1999; 20(6): 358–66.

157. Grenko RT, Abendroth CS, Davis AT, Levin RJ, Dardick I. Hybrid tumors or salivary gland tumors sharing common differentiation pathways? Reexamining adenoid cystic and epithelial-myoepithelial carcinomas. *Oral Surg Oral Med Oral Pathol Oral Radiol Endod* 1998; 86(2): 188–95.

158. Prasad AR, Savera AT, Gown AM, Zarbo RJ. The myoepithelial immunophenotype in 135 benign and malignant salivary gland tumors other than pleomorphic adenoma. *Arch Pathol Lab Med* 1999; 123(9): 801–6.

159. Puxeddu R, Puxeddu P, Parodo G, Faa G. Polymorphous low-grade adenocarcinoma of the parotid gland. *Eur J Morphol* 1998; 36(suppl): 262–6.

160. Barak AP, Grobbel MA, Rabaja DR. Polymorphous low-grade adenocarcinoma of the parotid gland. *Am J Otolaryngol* 1998; 19(5): 322–4.

161. Vincent SD, Hammond HL, Finkelstein MW. Clinical and therapeutic features of polymorphous low-grade adenocarcinoma. *Oral Surg Oral Med Oral Pathol* 1994; 77(1): 41–7.

162. Simpson RH, Clarke TJ, Sarsfield PT, Gluckman PG, Babajews AV. Polymorphous low-grade adenocarcinoma of the salivary glands: a clinicopathological comparison with adenoid cystic carcinoma [see comments]. *Histopathology* 1991; 19(2): 121–9.

163. Gibbons D, Saboorian MH, Vuitch F, Gokaslan ST, Ashfaq R. Fine-needle aspiration findings in patients with polymorphous low grade adenocarcinoma of the salivary glands. *Cancer* 1999; 87(1): 31–6.

164. Frierson HF Jr, Covell JL, Mills SE. Fine-needle aspiration cytology of terminal duct carcinoma of minor salivary gland. *Diagn Cytopathol* 1987; 3(2): 159–62.

165. Klijanienko J, Vielh P. Salivary carcinomas with papillae: cytology and histology analysis of polymorphous low-grade adenocarcinoma and papillary cystadenocarcinoma. *Diagn Cytopathol* 1998; 19(4): 244–9.

166. Cleveland DB, Cosgrove MM, Martin SE. Tyrosine-rich crystalloids in a fine needle aspirate of a polymorphous low grade adenocarcinoma of a minor salivary gland. A case report. *Acta Cytol* 1994; 38(2): 247–51.

167. Watanabe K, Ono N, Saito K, Saito A, Suzuki T. Fine-needle aspiration cytology of polymorphous low-grade adenocarcinoma of the tongue. *Diagn Cytopathol* 1999; 20(3): 167–9.

168. Thiebault S, Mogras A, Brun I et al. [Epithelial-myoepithelial carcinoma of the salivary glands: report of a case]. *Ann Pathol* 1999; 19(1): 30–2.

169. Kasper HU, Mellin W, Kriegsmann J, Cheremet E, Lippert H, Roessner A. Epithelial-myoepithelial carcinoma of the salivary gland – a low grade malignant neoplasm? Report of two cases and review of the literature. *Pathol Res Pract* 1999; 195(3): 189–92.

170. Batsakis JG, el-Naggar AK, Luna MA. Epithelial-myoepithelial carcinoma of salivary glands. *Ann Otol Rhinol Laryngol* 1992; 101(6): 540–2.

171. Brocheriou C, Auriol M, de Roquancourt A, Gaulard P, Fornes P. [Epithelial-myoepithelial carcinoma of the salivary glands. Study of 15 cases and review of the literature]. *Ann Pathol* 1991; 11(5–6): 316–25.

172. Ng WK, Choy C, Ip P, Shek WH, Collins RJ. Fine needle aspiration cytology of epithelial-myoepithelial carcinoma of salivary glands. A report of three cases. *Acta Cytol* 1999; 43(4): 675–80.

173. Carrillo R, Poblet E, Rocamora A, Rodriguez-Peralto JL. Epithelial-myoepithelial carcinoma of the salivary gland. Fine needle aspiration cytologic findings. *Acta Cytol* 1990; 34(2): 243–7.

174. Yang GC, Soslow RA. Epithelial-myoepithelial carcinoma of the parotid. A case of ductal-predominant presentation with cytologic, histologic and ultrastructural correlations. *Acta Cytol* 1999; 43(6): 1113–8.

175. Kocjan G, Milroy C, Fisher EW, Eveson JW. Cytological features of epithelial-myoepithelial carcinoma of salivary gland: potential pitfalls in diagnosis. *Cytopathology* 1993; 4(3): 173–80.

176. Plath T, Dallenbach F. [Basal cell adenocarcinoma of the minor salivary glands of the palate. Case report and review of the literature]. *Mund Kiefer Gesichtschir* 1998; 2(5): 275–8.

177. Pisharodi LR. Basal cell adenocarcinoma of the salivary gland. Diagnosis by fine-needle aspiration cytology. *Am J Clin Pathol* 1995; 103(5): 603–8.

178. Moroz K, Ferreira C, Dhurandhar N. Fine needle aspiration of basal cell adenocarcinoma of the parotid gland. Report of a case with assessment of DNA ploidy in aspirates and tissue sections by image analysis. *Acta Cytol* 1996; 40(4): 773–8.

179. Foss RD, Ellis GL, Auclair PL. Salivary gland cystadenocarcinomas. A clinicopathologic study of 57 cases. *Am J Surg Pathol* 1996; 20(12): 1440–7.

180. Tambouret RH, Yantiss RK, Kirby R, Eichhorn JH. Mucinous adenocarcinoma of the parotid gland. Report of a case with fine needle aspiration findings and histologic correlation. *Acta Cytol* 1999; 43(5): 842–6.

181. Ardekian L, Manor R, Peled M, Laufer D. Malignant oncocytoma of the parotid gland: case report and analysis of the literature. *J Oral Maxillofac Surg* 1999; 57(3): 325–8.

182. Nakada M, Nishizaki K, Akagi H, Masuda Y, Yoshino T. Oncocytic carcinoma of the submandibular gland: a case report and literature review. *J Oral Pathol Med* 1998; 27(5): 225–8.

183. Gray SR, Cornog JL Jr, Seo IS. Oncocytic neoplasms of salivary glands: a report of fifteen cases including two malignant oncocytomas. *Cancer* 1976; 38(3): 1306–17.

184. Brandwein MS, Jagirdar J, Patil J, Biller H, Kaneko M. Salivary duct carcinoma (cribriform salivary carcinoma of excretory ducts). A clinicopathologic and immunohistochemical study of 12 cases. *Cancer* 1990; 65(10): 2307–14.

185. Fyrat P, Cramer H, Feczko JD et al. Fine-needle aspiration biopsy of salivary duct carcinoma: report of five cases. *Diagn Cytopathol* 1997; 16(6): 526–30.

186. Gilcrease MZ, Guzman-Paz M, Froberg K, Pambuccian S. Salivary duct carcinoma. Is a specific diagnosis possible by fine needle aspiration cytology? *Acta Cytol* 1998; 42(6): 1389–96.

187. Dee S, Masood S, Issacs JH Jr, Hardy NM. Cytomorphologic features of salivary duct carcinoma on fine needle aspiration biopsy. A case report. *Acta Cytol* 1993; 37(4): 539–42.

188. Klijanienko J, Vielh P. Cytologic characteristics and histomorphologic correlations of 21 salivary duct carcinomas. *Diagn Cytopathol* 1998; 19(5): 333–7.

189. Garcia-Bonafe M, Catala I, Tarragona J, Tallada N. Cytologic diagnosis of salivary duct carcinoma: a review of seven cases. *Diagn Cytopathol* 1998; 19(2): 120–3.

190. Ersoz C, Cetik F, Aydin O, Cosar EF, Talas DU. Salivary duct carcinoma ex pleomorphic adenoma: analysis of the findings in fine-needle aspiration cytology and histology. *Diagn Cytopathol* 1998; 19(3): 201–4.

191. Lewis JE, McKinney BC, Weiland LH, Ferreiro JA, Olsen KD. Salivary duct carcinoma. Clinicopathologic and immunohistochemical review of 26 cases. *Cancer* 1996; 77(2): 223–30.

192. Colecchia M, Frigo B, Leopardi OM. Salivary duct carcinoma of the parotid gland. Report of a case with cytologic and immunocytochemical findings on fine needle aspiration biopsy. *Acta Cytol* 1997; 41(2): 593–7.

193. Cerilli LA, Swartzbaugh JR, Saadut R et al. Analysis of chromosome 9p21 deletion and p16 gene mutation in salivary gland carcinomas. *Hum Pathol* 1999; 30(10): 1242–6.

194. Felix A, El-Naggar AK, Press MF, Ordonez NG, Fonseca I, Tucker SL, et al. Prognostic significance of biomarkers (c-erbB-2, p53, proliferating cell nuclear antigen, and DNA content) in salivary duct carcinoma. *Hum Pathol* 1996; 27(6): 561–6.

195. Klijanienko J, Vielh P. Reply: cytology of salivary duct carcinoma. *Diagn Cytopathol* 2000; 22(2): 135.

196. Kim T, Yoon GS, Kim O, Gong G. Fine needle aspiration diagnosis of malignant mixed tumor (carcinosarcoma) arising in pleomorphic adenoma of the salivary gland. A case report. *Acta Cytol* 1998; 42(4): 1027–31.

197. Flynn MB, Maguire S, Martinez S, Tesmer T. Primary squamous cell carcinoma of the parotid gland: the importance of correct histological diagnosis. *Ann Surg Oncol* 1999; 6(8): 768–70.

198. Seifert G, Donath K. [Differential diagnosis of squamous epithelial carcinoma of the salivary glands]. *Pathologe* 1998; 19(3): 201–8.

199. Klijanienko J, Vielh P. Fine-needle sampling of salivary gland lesions. VI. Cytological review of 44 cases of primary salivary squamous-cell carcinoma with histological correlation. *Diagn Cytopathol* 1998; 18(3): 174–8.

200. Franzen A, Schmid S, Pfaltz M. [Primary small cell carcinomas and metastatic disease in the head and neck]. *HNO* 1999; 47(10): 912–7.

201. Vural C, Dogan O, Yavuz E, Ozcelik HS, Senvar A. Small cell neuroendocrine carcinoma of the parotid gland. *Otolaryngol Head Neck Surg* 2000; 122(1): 151–2.

202. Mair S, Phillips JI, Cohen R. Small cell undifferentiated carcinoma of the parotid gland. Cytologic, histologic, immunohistochemical and ultrastructural features of a neuroendocrine variant. *Acta Cytol* 1989; 33(2): 164–8.

203. Moore JG, Bocklage T. Fine-needle aspiration biopsy of large-cell undifferentiated carcinoma of the salivary glands: presentation of two cases, literature review, and differential cytodiagnosis of high-grade salivary gland malignancies. *Diagn Cytopathol* 1998; 19(1): 44–50.

204. Batsakis JG, Luna MA. Undifferentiated carcinomas of salivary glands. *Ann Otol Rhinol Laryngol* 1991; 100(1): 82–4.

205. Gunhan O, Celasun B, Safali M et al. Fine needle aspiration cytology of malignant lymphoepithelial lesion of the salivary gland. A report of two cases. *Acta Cytol* 1994; 38(5): 751–4.

206. Safneck JR, Ravinsky E, Yazdi HM, Nason RW, Dort JC, Anderson BJ. Fine needle aspiration biopsy findings in lymphoepithelial carcinoma of salivary gland. *Acta Cytol* 1997; 41(4): 1023–30.

207. Kuczkowski J, Jagielski J. [A case of schwannoma in the parotid gland]. *Otolaryngol Pol* 1997; 51(3): 324–7.

208. Mair S, Leiman G. Benign neurilemoma (schwannoma) masquerading as a pleomorphic adenoma of the submandibular salivary gland. *Acta Cytol* 1989; 33(6): 907–10.

209. Gil-Benso R, Carda-Batalla C, Navarro-Fos S, Pellin-Perez A, Llombart-Bosch A. Cytogenetic study of a spindle-cell rhabdomyosarcoma of the parotid gland. *Cancer Genet Cytogenet* 1999; 109(2): 150–3.

210. Grayson W, Nayler SJ, Jena GP. Synovial sarcoma of the parotid gland. A case report with clinicopathological analysis and review of the literature. *S Afr J Surg* 1998; 36(1): 32–4, discussion 34–5.

211. Shimizu K, Ogura S, Kobayashi TK et al. Fine-needle aspiration cytology of malignant hemangiopericytoma of the salivary gland: A case report. *Diagn Cytopathol* 1999; 21(6): 398–401.

212. Perez del Rio MJ, Garcia-Garcia J, Diaz-Iglesias JM, Fresno MF. Radiation-associated angiosarcoma involving the parotid gland [letter]. *Histopathology* 1998; 33(6): 586–7.

213. Kang J, Levinson JA, Hitti IF. Leiomyosarcoma of the parotid gland: a case report and review of the literature. *Head Neck* 1999; 21(2): 168–71.

214. Gutierrez Triguero M, Escamilla Carpintero Y, Martinez Guirado T, Bodoque Cano M, Scola Yurrita B, Fernandez-Vega M. [Granulocytic sarcoma. A case with an unusual location]. *Acta Otorrinolaringol Esp* 1998; 49(8): 667–70.

215. Orvidas LJ, Kasperbauer JL, Lewis JE, Olsen KD, Lesnick TG. Pediatric parotid masses. *Arch Otolaryngol Head Neck Surg* 2000; 126(2): 177–84.

216. Roebuck DJ, Ahuja AT. Hemangioendothelioma of the parotid gland in infants: sonography and correlative MR imaging. *AJNR Am J Neuroradiol* 2000; 21(1): 219–23.

217. Deb RA, Desai SB, Amonkar PP, Aiyer PM, Borges AM. Primary primitive neuroectodermal tumour of the parotid gland [see comments]. *Histopathology* 1998; 33(4): 375–8.

218. Helsel JC, Mrak RE, Hanna E, Parham DH, Bardales RH. Peripheral primitive neuroectodermal tumor of the parotid gland region: report of a case with fine-needle aspiration findings. *Diagn Cytopathol* 2000; 22(3): 161–6.

219. Zhang C, Cohen JM, Cangiarella JF, Waisman J, McKenna BJ, Chhieng DC. Fine-needle aspiration of secondary neoplasms involving the salivary glands. A report of 36 cases. *Am J Clin Pathol* 2000; 113(1): 21–8.

220. Malata CM, Camilleri IG, McLean NR, Piggott TA, Soames JV. Metastatic tumours of the parotid gland. *Br J Oral Maxillofac Surg* 1998; 36(3): 190–5.

221. Pisani P, Krengli M, Ramponi A, Guglielmetti R, Pia F. Metastases to parotid gland from cancers of the upper airway and digestive tract. *Br J Oral Maxillofac Surg* 1998; 36(1): 54–7.

222. Gangopadhyay K, Abuzeid MO, Martin JM, Saleem M. Metastatic renal cell carcinoma of the parotid gland presenting as a neck mass. *Int J Clin Pract* 1998; 52(3): 196–8.

223. Takatsugi K, Komuta K, Hosen N, Kitada S, Iida S, Nishihara K, et al. [Metastasis of small cell lung cancer to the parotid gland as the initial clinical manifestation, followed by metastases to the pituitary gland and lumber spinal cord]. *Nihon Kokyuki Gakkai Zasshi* 1998; 36(3): 246–50.

3

Thyroid

Introduction
Non-neoplastic and inflammatory conditions
Neoplasms
Metastatic tumours in thyroid

INTRODUCTION

Thyroid nodules are extremely common, affecting from 4% to 7% of the population. Since most of these lesions are benign, indications for surgical removal should be as narrow as possible. Fine needle aspiration cytology is the most accurate and cost-effective technique for nodule diagnosis. It is simple, safe, and should be the first test used in patient investigations.[1–23]

FNAC procedure

FNAC of the thyroid gland is simple but requires skill and practice; this is particularly important since, being an endocrine organ, much emphasis is put on the cellularity and the cell:colloid ratio rather than the detailed cell morphology. Excess of blood, so often produced by the inexperienced aspirators, has the cells trapped in the strands of fibrin giving a false impression of focal hypercellularity with very little possibility of studying the cell detail due to their artifactual crowding, poor fixation and/or poor penetration of stain. These smears are the ones most commonly reported as 'indeterminate', giving no useful information for clinical management. Given the relatively small number of thyroid nodules in the non-endemic areas, ideally, there should be a dedicated team of aspirators, who also interpret material, or have a continuous feedback from the microscopists as to the adequacy of the material they are collecting. In our experience, cytopathologists are in a good position to evaluate the adequacy of the material during and after the procedure, prepare the material in the optimal way, and interpret the findings against the known clinical background. Even more so than any other branch of medicine, endocrine pathology diagnostic work-up is possible only as a concerted team effort. To that end, cytopathologists are members of a team and should see FNAC as being part of the framework of other clinical and laboratory investigations. Cytopathologists examining the patients and reporting the FNAC smears should have the results of other investigations available and, if necessary, refer to them in the report. Similarly, if following microscopic examination diagnosis is unclear and could be elucidated by further investigations, this should be clearly stated in the report. This approach, although requiring a lot of coordination, discipline and mutual understanding, will produce meaningful results and will not alienate the continuing use of FNAC as a key investigation of solitary thyroid lumps.

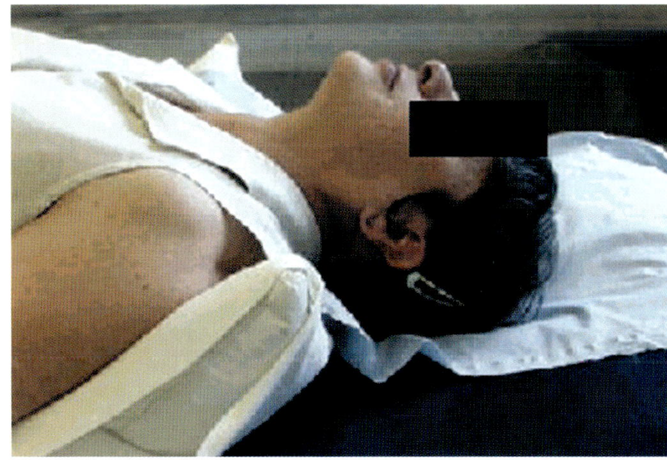

Figure 3.1 FNAC of the thyroid. The procedure is performed with the patient in a supine position with the neck extended.

FNAC is performed with the patient in a supine position with the neck extended over the cushion (Fig. 3.1). The FNAC test is explained to the patient, and he or she is requested not to swallow or speak during the procedure. After this, the thyroid is palpated while the patient is asked to swallow (Fig. 3.2). The enlarged nodule is fixed between the fingers of the non-dominant hand. Thyroid enlargements are usually situated in the groove between the trachea and the anterior edge of the sternocleidomastoid muscle. After cleaning the skin, the patient is reminded not to swallow or speak during the procedure. A 23G or smaller needle without the attached syringe is passed vertically into

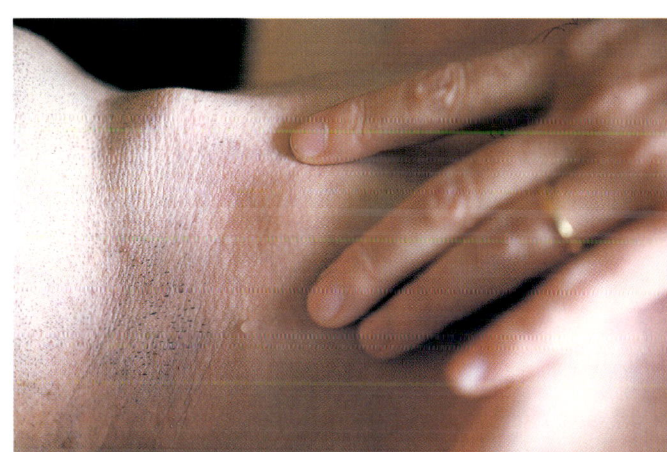

Figure 3.2 FNAC of the thyroid. The thyroid is palpated while the patient is asked to swallow. The enlarged nodule is fixed between the fingers of the non-dominant hand. Thyroid enlargements are usually situated in the groove between the trachea and the anterior edge of the sternocleidomastoid muscle.

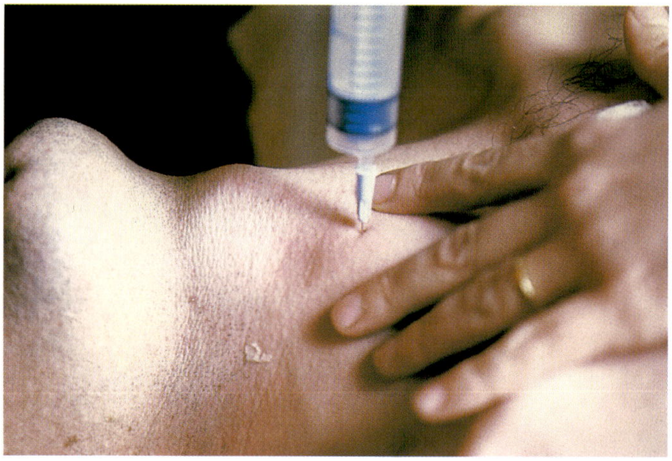

A

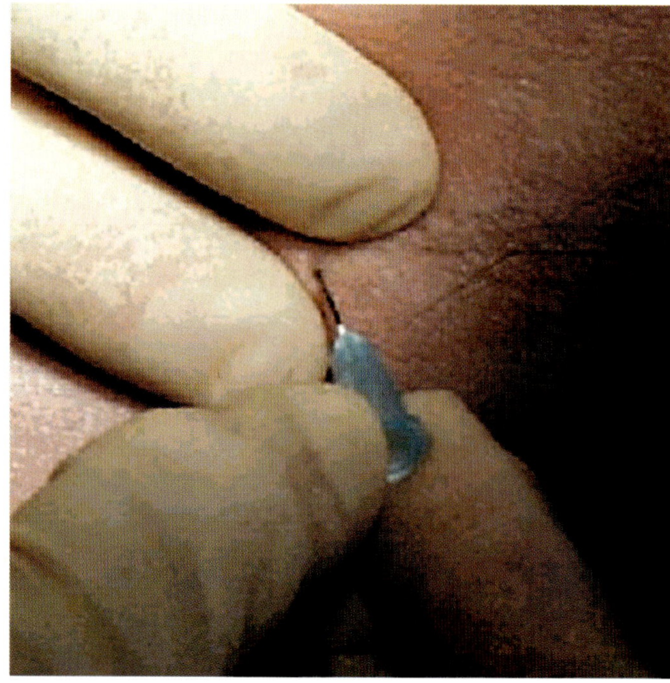

B

Figure 3.3 FNAC of the thyroid. A 23G or smaller needle **A.** with or **B.** without the attached syringe is passed vertically into the nodule. The direction of the needle remains vertical, tangential to the trachea throughout the procedure. Once in the nodule, several fast passes, pushing and withdrawing the needle from the lesion, are made. The procedure lasts only a few seconds.

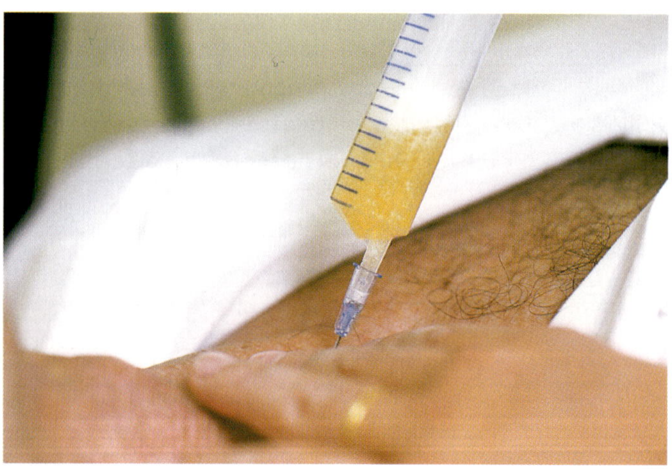

A

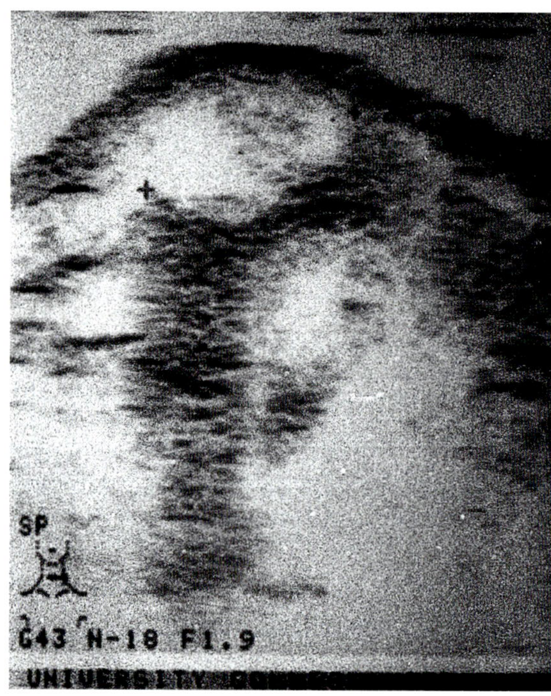

B

Figure 3.4 FNAC of thyroid cysts. **A.** Cystic fluid is drained as much as possible without changing the direction of the needle. Repeat aspirates are not advised since they usually produce bleeding into the cystic space and refilling of the cyst. **B.** Complex cystic lesions may be aspirated under ultrasound guidance. Ultrasound appearances of a 29-year-old woman show a growth within the cystic space. FNAC showed papillary carcinoma (see Fig. 3.24).

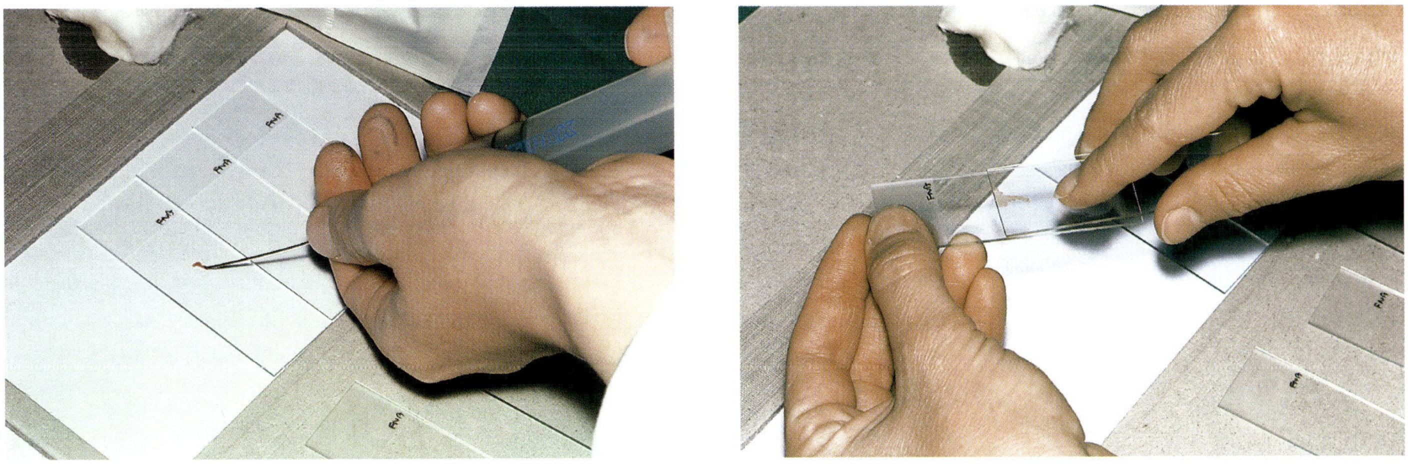

A B

Figure 3.5 FNAC of the thyroid. Material is **A.** expelled on the centre of glass slide and **B.** spread with the help of another slide positioned flat against the test slide, sliding over it in parallel, avoiding edges which push cells to one side and account for ridge-like effects.

the nodule. The direction of the needle should remain vertical, tangential to the trachea, throughout the procedure. Once in the nodule, several fast passes, pushing and withdrawing the needle, are made. The procedure lasts only a few seconds (Fig. 3.3). After withdrawing the needle, the patient is placed in a comfortable position and allowed to swallow and speak. Occasionally, the procedure is repeated, except when cysts are drained. If anticipating a cystic lesion, a 20 ml syringe and Cameco syringe holder are used (Fig. 3.4). Otherwise, capillary action of the needle is usually sufficient to obtain ample diagnostic material. The material is either spread on the glass slides or expelled into a container (Fig. 3.5). Alcohol fixation and air drying are both used in interpretation of thyroid aspirates so that the method of fixation will vary according to the local preference. More recently, with the introduction of the thin layer preparations, there are studies comparing the conventional smear preparation with that from a thin layer. Their findings are mixed, with the general conclusion that there is no significant differences between thin layer and direct smears[4].

If examination fails to reveal thyroid enlargement, the patient is repositioned with a further attempt at extending the neck. If the lesion is still impalpable, it is advisable not to proceed with the procedure 'blind' but to refer the patient for ultrasound-guided FNAC. Ultrasound-guided FNAC of the thyroid is performed in approximately 12% of cases of thyroid enlargements.[4] Apart from impalpable nodules, the indications for an ultrasound-guided FNAC are multiple nodules, complex nodules (Fig. 3.4b), prior failed FNAC, thyroid bed abnormalities post-thyroidectomy, difficult access and investigation of a recurrent tumour in a residual thyroid lobe. Ultrasound-guided FNAC provides additional information in 60% of those patients in whom conventional FNAC with palpation has failed to obtain material. Sensitivity (96%), specificity (91%), accuracy (94%), and positive (96%) and negative predictive values (91%) of ultrasound-guided FNAC for malignancy are not significantly different from those of palpation-guided FNAC (88%, 90%, 88%, 95% and 75%, respectively) for those nodules where an adequate FNAC is obtained.[5] Intraoperative touch-imprint cytological diagnosis has been used successfully as an adjunct to frozen sections in equivocal cases.[6–8]

Diagnostic accuracy

The rates of sensitivity and specificity of FNAC for the diagnosis of thyroid malignancy differ among various reported series. The values differ depending on whether only clearly positive and negative results are considered or whether 'positives' include 'suspicious for malignancy'; whether adenomas are considered neoplasms in the same category as carcinomas and whether only histologically proven cases are taken into calculation without regard for benign cases on clinical follow-up.[9]

When calculating diagnostic accuracy, most commonly four cytological diagnostic categories are used. Rates for these categories, based on data pooled from recent series, were as follows: benign, 69%; suspicious, 10%; malignant, 4%; and non-diagnostic, 17%. Analysis of recent data suggests sensitivity of 94% and a specificity of 96%, with positive predictive value of 93%[2, 11–23]. Diagnostic accuracy can be further improved when clinical data are considered e.g. risk of malignancy in "follicular lesion" are higher in men and in solitary nodules greater than 4 cm.

Diagnostic pitfalls

Limitations of fine-needle aspiration are mainly related to two major areas: the adequacy of material i.e. skill of the aspirator and the overlapping morphological features[24–26]. The latter relates to one or more of the following: hyperplasia vs neoplasia, oncocytic change, cystic change, giant cells, papillary change, spindle cells, lymphoid infiltrate and primary vs secondary tumours.

The following appearances, often in combination, may lead to overdiagnosis: cellularity; little colloid (e.g. in cellular adenoma); pseudopapillary changes due to regression of follicular epithelial cells in a multinodular goitre; cellular atypia of follicular epithelium; thick colloid simulating a psammoma body but without the characteristic lamellar appearance; papillary hyperplasia in Hashimoto's thyroiditis; cellular atypia of follicular epithelium in Hashimoto's disease; treatment with radioactive iodine; thyroid gland inhibitory or stimulatory drugs and chemotherapy or radiotherapy to the neck.

Material adequacy depends on the uniformity of collection and preparation of FNAC material by skilled staff and is essential for correct interpretation. Cell/colloid ratio in FNAC smears from thyroid is often more important than cell morphology and may be affected by poor sampling. As mentioned earlier, "too much" bloodstained material is not desirable.

Morphological features that overlap are common in thyroid FNAC. One of the commonest problems encountered is the distinction between hyperplasia and neoplasia. Cellularity, the amount of colloid, cell morphology and additional features all contribute to the correct diagnosis. Oncocytic change may be seen in several conditions e.g. lymphocytic thyroiditis, colloid goitre, oncocytic neoplasms as well as in papillary carcinoma. Cystic change may be seen in cystic goitre as well as in papillary carcinoma. Multinucleate giant cells may be present in subacute thyroiditis, lymphocytic thyroiditis, papillary carcinoma, anaplastic carcinoma as well as in palpation granuloma. Papillary change may be seen in papillary carcinoma and its variants (cystic hypocellular, oncocytic, clear cell, tall cell, dedifferentiated) in papillary hyperplasia in goitre, in metastatic renal cell carcinoma and hyalinising trabecular adenoma. Spindle cells may be seen in cysts, anaplastic carcinoma as well as in mesenchymal tumours. Lymphocytic infiltrate may be seen in lymphocytic thyroiditis, hyperthyroidism, specific infections, post transplant lymphoproliferative syndrome and in lymphoma. Distinction between primary and metastatic tumours may sometimes be difficult.

Role in clinical management

The introduction of FNAC has had a substantial effect on the management of patients with thyroid nodules, the critical question being whether to excise the lobe or not (Table 3.1). Current European practice regarding the investigation of thyroid nodules means that FNAC of the thyroid is performed in 95% of patients with a finding of a dominant "cold" area[27]. When analysing the most frequently utilised diagnostic modalities in detection of 5583 cases of thyroid carcinoma (USA cohort study), FNAC thyroid was used in 53% of cases, compared to scintigrafy in 38% and ultrasound in 39%[10a]. Current views on the role of FNAC in the management of thyroid nodules are that the FNAC is the "gold standard" for diagnosis[28] and that the "FNAC is the best modality available for the workup of thyroid nodules and is widely utilised in endocrine centres worldwide"[29].

The conventional criteria for requesting thyroid FNAC have traditionally been: a recently enlarged single nodule in an otherwise euthyroid patient, found by ultrasound to be solid with a scintigraphy showing a low radioiodine uptake ("cold"). Thyroid FNAC helps select patients appropriate for thyroid surgery. By using the FNAC, the percentage of patients undergoing thyroidectomy has decreased by 25%, and the yield of carcinoma in patients who undergo surgery has increased from 15% to at least 30%. Fine needle aspiration has decreased the cost of care by 25%[2]. Repeated FNAC is not useful in management of patients with benign thyroid nodular disease. With repeated FNAC there is no

Table 3.1 Clinical management of a thyroid nodule*

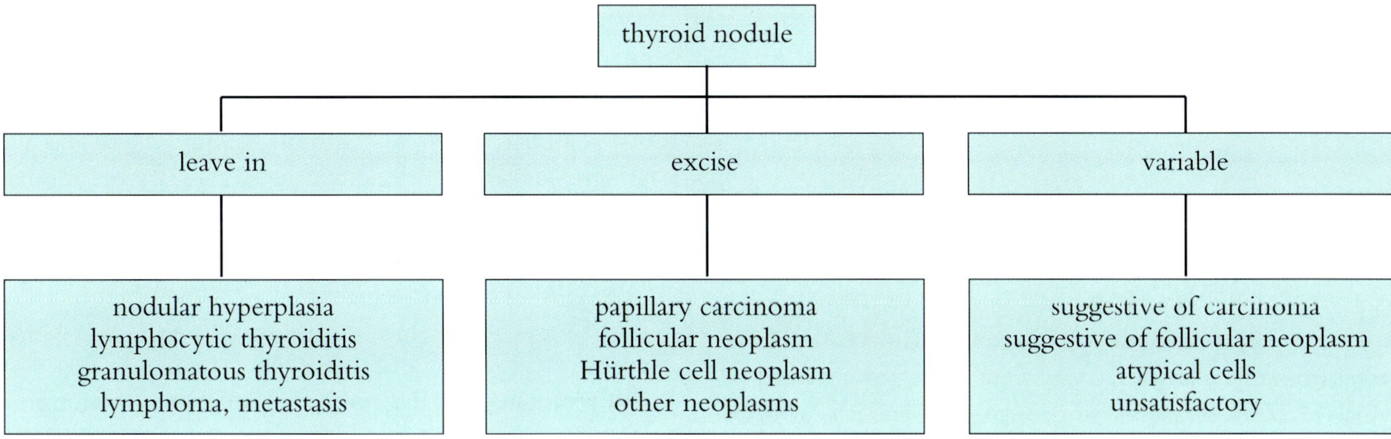

*Rab SS, *Am J Clin Pathol* 2000; 113: 765–768

additional detection of malignancy and the clinical factors may hold precedence over FNAC in surgical management[30].

In our own institution, we compared clinical diagnoses based on non-invasive diagnostic investigations (ultrasound scan, isotope scan, immunoassays and hormonal assays) with FNAC. FNAC represents no improvement on the diagnosis of benign colloid/cystic goitre (55% vs 54% respectively). It represents an improvement on the diagnosis of thyroiditis (9% vs 17% respectively). It decreases clinically suspicious lesions from 37% to 15%. FNAC has an essential role in the diagnosis and management of 23% of our patients, a confirmatory role in 61% of patients, a non-contributory role in 13% when specimens are inadequate, and is misleading in 3% where results are false negative. The positive identification of thyroiditis and neoplasia stands on its own as a justification for FNAC.[26] FNAC is the single most important procedure for differentiating benign from malignant thyroid nodules, and its role in evaluation and management of nodular thyroid disease cannot be overemphasised.[27]

The majority of invasive cancers (82%) are found in patients whose lesions are suspicious for papillary carcinoma or in patients aged 50 years or older with follicular or Hürthle cell neoplasms. The risk of carcinoma in these combined subgroups (60%) warrants early surgical intervention.[28] Since the introduction of aspiration cytology, 21–25% fewer operations for isolated thyroid swellings have been performed.[25–29] The method is cost-effective and should be available to primary care.[30]

The majority of paediatric thyroid nodules are benign. The prevalence of malignancy in paediatric patients with thyroid nodules in one series was 24.6%. High diagnostic accuracy of thyroid FNAC improves selection of paediatric patients requiring surgery.[31]

The place of FNAC as the first step in the diagnostic management of thyroid nodules seems justified. It has decreased costs substantially because it enables selection of patients who need surgery. Introduction of FNAC reduces the cost of thyroid operations by 25% and doubles the yield of carcinoma.[29,32,33] The limitations of cytological examination, non-diagnostic results and cellular follicular neoplasms should be borne in mind but need not prevent continued use of FNAC. Negative (benign) and positive (malignant) cytological results are conclusive; careful clinical follow-up of benign nodules and surgical excision of malignant nodules is recommended. Non-diagnostic results are inconclusive; further evaluation by repeated FNAC, ultrasound-guided biopsy or radioisotope scanning is necessary. Suspicious cytological results are also inconclusive and are associated with a 20% chance of malignant involvement; surgical treatment is necessary for clarification.[34] Clinical characteristics (larger diameter, fixation of the mass, and younger age of the patient) may be used for more accurate assessment of the risk of the presence of a malignant lesion when FNAC of a thyroid nodule is reported as suspicious for follicular neoplasm.[35]

Comparison of FNAC with frozen section histology

Fine needle aspiration cytology is widely used in the diagnosis and management of solitary thyroid nodules. It is the most accurate tool available and decreases the need for ultrasonography and thyroid scanning. FNAC is used to assist in planning surgical strategy for differentiated thyroid cancer mainly by determining the likely extent of contralateral lobe resection and nodal dissection required.[36] Frozen section, which usually serves as the surgeon's guide, and FNAC both have varying accuracy rates.[37–39] In a series of Kopald et al[40] carcinoma was diagnosed by frozen section in 69% of cases of true positive carcinomas. Frozen section analysis was incorrect in 5–31% of cases of carcinoma diagnosed on FNAC and confirmed on definitive histology.[40,41] Frozen section examination is therefore indicated for intraoperative decision making in patients with a 'suspicious', 'cellular' or 'indeterminate' FNAC diagnosis but is unnecessary when the FNAC diagnosis is either benign or malignant.[41–45] If the fine needle aspiration is suspicious for papillary carcinoma of the thyroid, the incidence of cancer is 54%, and patients with these conditions should undergo surgery with frozen section. When either gross findings or frozen sections suggest malignancy, definitive thyroidectomy can be performed because 90% of such cases will be cancer.[46]

FNAC is at least as accurate as frozen section analysis with less morbidity and expense. When papillary carcinoma of the thyroid or follicular-variant papillary carcinoma of the thyroid is definitively diagnosed on FNAC, the surgeon can perform definitive thyroidectomy without frozen section because of the high specificity for cancer.[40,46,47] If the frozen section is not diagnostic of malignancy, a thyroid lobectomy/isthmusectomy is recommended because 71% have a benign lesion. This systematic approach to papillary carcinoma of the thyroid will obviate unnecessary frozen sections while maintaining excellent diagnostic specificity.

Ancillary techniques

Immunocytochemistry: Immunodetection of galectin-3 and CD44v6

Immunocytochemical staining of thyroid FNAC specimens for CD44v6, a marker for the detection of the deregulated cell growth and galectin-3, a marker for thyreocytes that have undergone malignant transformation appear to distinguish between carcinomas and benign lesions of the thyroid, irrespective of histological type[53]. CD44v6 shows positivity in 88% classic, surgically confirmed, papillary thyroid carcinomas on FNAC with no staining of benign aspirates. The authors conclude that most papillary carcinomas of the thyroid express the cell adhesion molecule CD44, which may be of clinical value in confirming the diagnosis on borderline fine-needle aspiration specimens[54].

Thyroid peroxidase (TPO) is another recently used marker which promises to be diagnostically useful by distinguishing benign from malignant nodules and therefore may help in selecting patients for surgery[55].

The monoclonal antibody HBME-1, generated against the microvillous surface of mesothelial cells, has been shown to have significant reactivity in histological sections of follicular-derived thyroid malignancies. Sack et al[49] examined the diagnostic utility of HBME-1 in thyroid FNACs. Authors conclude that a positive immunostaining for HBME-1 on a thyroid FNAC is supportive evidence that the lesion is a carcinoma, that a negative result for HBME-1 does not preclude the diagnosis of thyroid carcinoma, and that HBME-1 can be effectively applied to thyroid FNAC specimens and can be a valuable adjunct in the cytological diagnosis of thyroid malignancies (Fig. 3.25b).[49] Cyclin-dependent Kinase Inhibitor p27Kip1 expression can also be detected in FNAC thyroid. P27Kip1 is an inhibitor of cell cycle progression present in quiescent and differentiated cells and not present in cell division. Loss of p27 has been found in poorly differentiated tumours. A high p27 expression is found in goitre and low in neoplasms[57].

The ribonucleoprotein telomerase has been noted to be activated in a wide variety of carcinomas. Saji et al[50] examined 30 papillary carcinomas for telomerase activity to determine whether this would be a useful adjunct to FNAC in the diagnosis. Telomerase activity was documented in 67% of the papillary carcinomas, 0 of 3 benign nodules and 0 of 10 normal thyroids. The telomerase assay appears useful in the distinction between benign and malignant thyroid lesions that have FNAC suspicious for but not diagnostic of papillary carcinoma.[50] Microsatellite instability (MSI) appears also to have a potential use in the pathology of thyroid. MSI is a molecular landmark of mutations in DNA mismatch repair genes.

Impaired DNA repair mechanism promotes carcinogenesis. Recent research shows that there are more MSI and LOH in papillary carcinoma than in multinodular hyperplasia[59].

Complications of FNAC

A single case is reported in the literature of a slow-growing papillary carcinoma of the thyroid that caused clinically apparent implantation along the tract of a FNAC. This appears to be the first report of a cutaneous needle tract metastasis from a papillary thyroid carcinoma. It represents a highly unusual complication of a FNAC of an indolent, slow-growing tumour.[51]

A puzzling artefact caused by previous fine needle aspiration of the thyroid has been reported.[52] Histological changes following aspiration cytology in the thyroid can be varied and should always be kept in mind in order to avoid misdiagnoses. Infarction of thyroid neoplasms following FNAC has been reported.[53] Potential problems in such cases include: (1) post-FNAC infarction may obscure the nature of a cytologically diagnosed neoplasm, making histological confirmation difficult; and (2) with fine needle aspiration of an infarcted nodule there may be difficulties in obtaining diagnostic material, potentially resulting in a false-negative diagnosis. A review of the literature on thyroid infarction shows this to be a rare event, with most reported cases occurring after FNAC of a neoplasm. The finding of necrosis and fibrosis in an aspirate or surgical specimen should thus suggest the presence of a neoplasm.

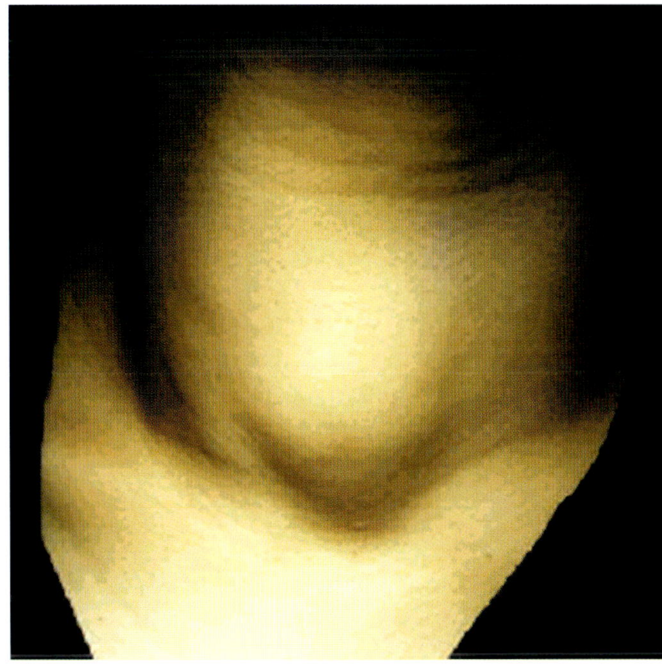

Figure 3.6 Multinodular non-toxic goitre. This used to be the commonest form of thyroid gland enlargement; this is an example of a young patient from an endemic area.

NON-NEOPLASTIC AND INFLAMMATORY CONDITIONS

Thyroid hyperplasia, goitre

Colloid goitre (non-toxic goitre, adenomatous hyperplasia, multinodular goitre)

Multinodular non-toxic goitre used to be the commonest form of thyroid gland enlargement; it was an endemic abnormality in areas where iodine deficiency was prevalent, which is now extremely uncommon due to the addition of iodine to table salt (Fig. 3.6). Sporadic forms are encountered in clinical practice by primary care doctors, endocrinologists, surgeons and otolaryngologists. Epidemiological data suggest that in the non-endemic areas (e.g. the USA), the incidence of such goitres is approximately 0.1–1.5% per year, translating into 250 000 new nodules annually. Nodular goitre is more common in women than in men, with advancing age, and after exposure to external irradiation. These goitres may be asymptomatic, with normal TSH levels (non-toxic), or may be associated with systemic thyrotoxic symptoms (toxic multinodular goitre or Plummer's disease).

Diagnostic evaluation of patients with nodular goitres consists of clinical evaluation, biochemical testing, FNAC and imaging studies. The serum TSH level is a sensitive and reliable index of thyroid function. FNAC results are pivotal to assess cancer risk in patient management for prominent palpable and suspicious nodules. Chest radiography, high-resolution ultrasonography and CT help to delineate the size and extent of goitre in evaluating compression symptoms. Indications for treatment in patients with multinodular goitre include: hyperthyroidism, local compression symptoms attributed to the goitre, cosmesis and concern about malignancy based on FNAC results. Management of toxic multinodular goitre by surgery is well established. Radioiodine is also effective therapy for many of these patients. When treatment is necessary for non-toxic multinodular goitre, surgical excision is preferred. The management policy, for patients who have small non-toxic multinodular goitres that are clinically asymptomatic, who are biochemically euthyroid according to serum TSH levels, and who have prominent palpable or suspicious nodules benign by FNAC, is yearly evaluation with serum TSH determinations and thyroid palpation. For large non-toxic multinodular goitres with local compression symptoms, the preferred treatment is surgery.[54] Routine performance of repeated FNAC in the follow-up of females with benign nodular thyroid disease, without any clinical changes, is of limited usefulness.[55]

Histologically, multinodular goitre is composed of variably sized, partly encapsulated nodules composed of follicles, which also vary in size. There are usually extensive regressive changes (oedema, infarction, haemorrhage, fibrosis, calcification and occasional bone formation) The follicular epithelium is often oncocytic and sometimes shows clear cell metaplasia. The gland may show diffuse nodularity, focal nodularity or solitary hyperplastic nodules.

The distinction between an adenoma and a solitary, hyperplastic, adenomatous nodule is arbitrary. The term 'adenoma' is usually used to describe solitary lesions with a microscopically complete capsule; the thyroid gland parenchyma in an adenoma differs in that in the surrounding thyroid gland, the follicles are compressed by the extensive growth of the adenoma. Also in adenoma, extensive regressive changes may be seen. It is not certain if all solitary nodules are true adenomata (neoplasms) or if some of them represent hyperplastic (physiological) lesions.

Cytological features. Cytological features of multinodular goitre are variable.[56] Aspirates from adenomatous areas are cellular with little colloid; aspirates from a multinodular goitre contain abundant thin colloid (pale blue on MGG staining) with sparse follicular epithelium (Fig. 3.7). Cells are uniform, arranged in loose aggregates or flat sheets lying within the colloid. Individual cells have oval or round pyknotic nuclei, inconspicuous nucleoli and poorly defined cytoplasm. They are regular in size and monotonous in appearance. They may be difficult to differentiate from lymphocytes. Minor variations in size of the nuclei are common. Microfollicles may be present. Occasionally, there is oncocytic change: sharply circumscribed cell borders, abundant finely granular grey/blue cytoplasm, anysonucleosis and occasionally prominent nucleoli (Fig. 3.8). In heavily bloodstained aspirates, the concentration of cells along the strands of fibrin may give an impression of hypercellularity. However, a lack of consistency of this finding throughout the sample is important. Macrophages are often seen, even in a predominantly colloid goitre. Fragments of hyaline stroma may be seen in generously sampled aspirates. Calcium oxalate crystals showing birefringence may be seen. Although they can be seen in all, they are more commonly seen in nodular goitres than in

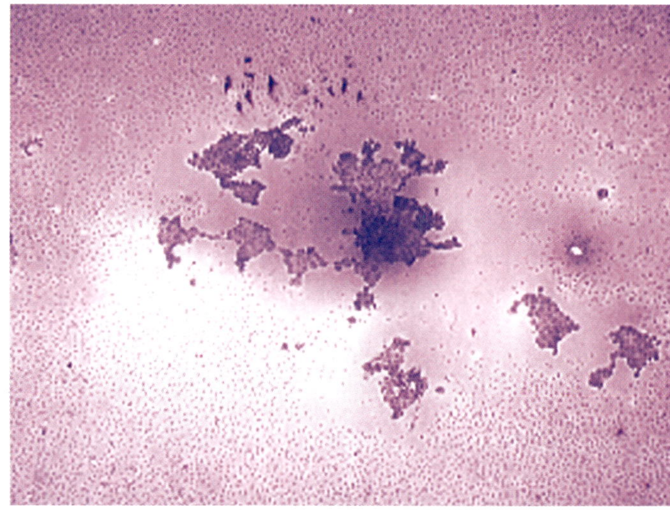

A

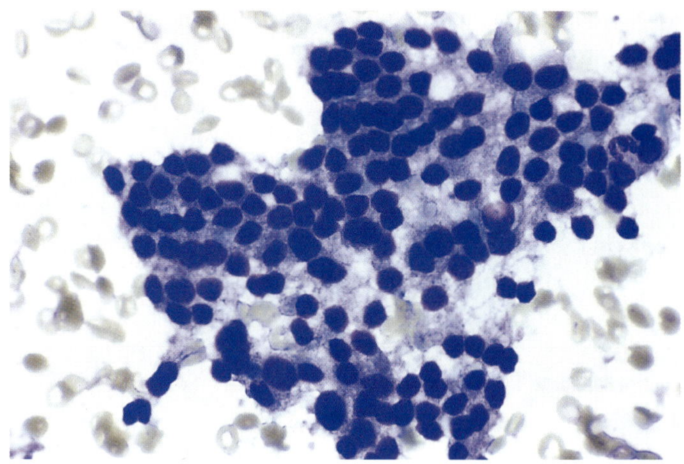

B

Figure 3.7 Multinodular goitre. Cytological features of multinodular goitre are variable. **A.** Aspirates from a multinodular goitre contain abundant thin colloid (pale blue on MGG staining) with sparse follicular epithelium. Cells are uniform, arranged in loose aggregates or flat sheets lying within the colloid (MGG ×100). **B.** Individual cells have oval or round pyknotic nuclei, inconspicuous nucleoli and poorly defined cytoplasm. They are regular in size and monotonous in appearance (MGG ×600 oil immersion).

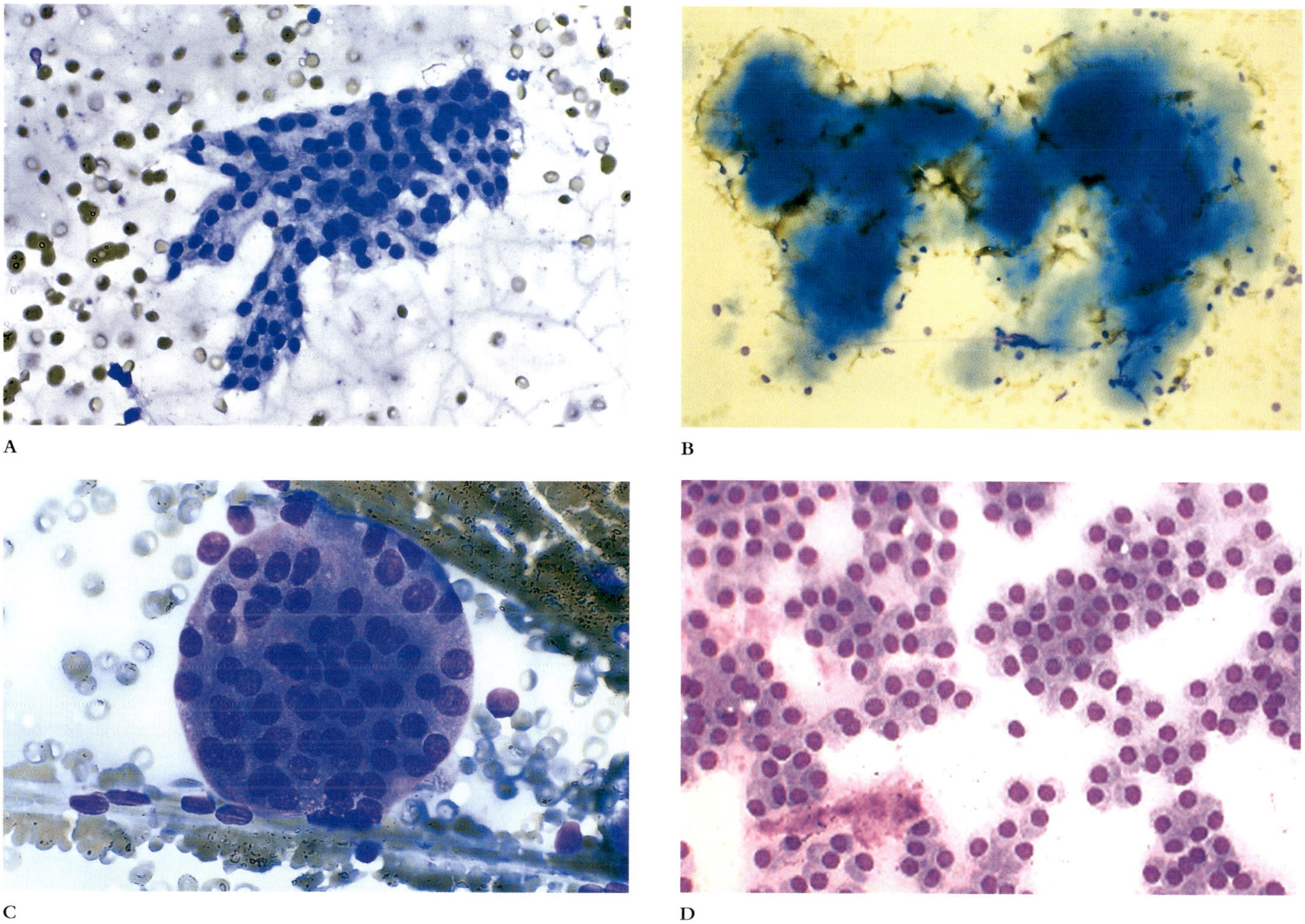

Figure 3.8 Multinodular goitre. **A.** Thin and **B.** thick colloid may be seen. Minor variations in size of the nuclei are common (MGG ×600). **C.** Microfollicles may be present (MGG ×600 oil). **D.** Occasionally there is oncocytic change: sharply circumscribed cell borders, abundant finely granular grey/blue cytoplasm, anysonucleosis and occasionally prominent nucleoli (MGG ×600 oil).

adenomas or carcinomas. Psammoma bodies may be seen (Fig. 3.9). Psammoma bodies are not pathognomonic of papillary carcinoma, and their presence, in the absence of other cytological criteria for malignancy, should not necessarily lead to diagnosis of carcinoma.[57] However, the presence of psammoma bodies in a FNAC smear cytologically consistent with a colloid goitre should raise the possibility of coexistent papillary hyperplasia or neoplasia. Because of the strong statistical association of psammoma bodies with malignant thyroid neoplasms, histological confirmation is mandatory in such cases.[58] Occasionally, multicentric papillary hyperplasia presents with cytological features suggestive of thyroid papillary carcinoma. While the cytological criteria for papillary thyroid carcinoma are well defined, occasional diagnostic difficulties can arise. Cytologically, the presence of focal papillary aggregates, the presence of a psammoma body within a background of copious colloid and scattered follicular cells may lead to diagnostic errors.[59]

Follicular epithelium may show *degenerative changes*; foamy cytoplasm containing granules makes epithelium indistinguishable from macrophages (Fig. 3.10). Sometimes the follicular epithelium may be spindle shaped, particularly in the wall of the cystic goitre, and have prominent nucleoli resembling repair epithelium (Fig. 3.11). Large, bare nuclei with structureless chromatin may be seen in hypothyroidism. Antithyroid drug treatment, Hashimoto's disease, chemotherapy and radiotherapy can all produce marked degenerative changes that may be source of diagnostic errors (Fig. 3.12).

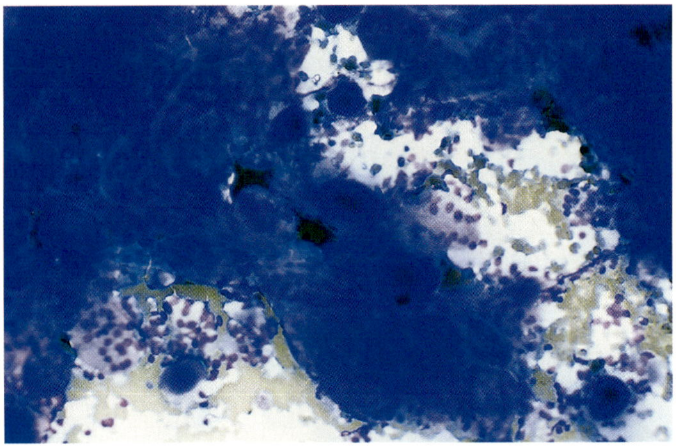

A

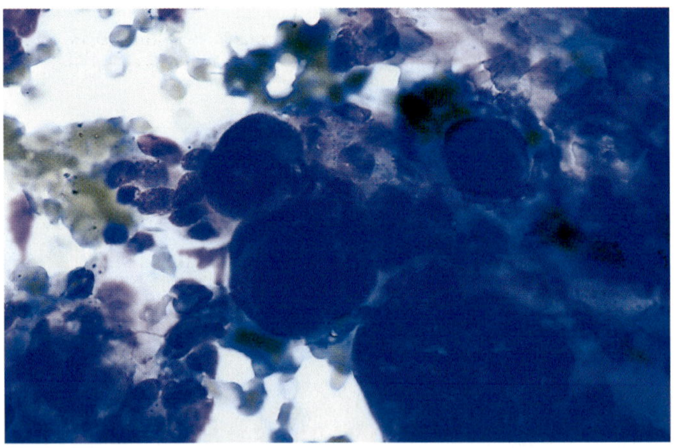

B

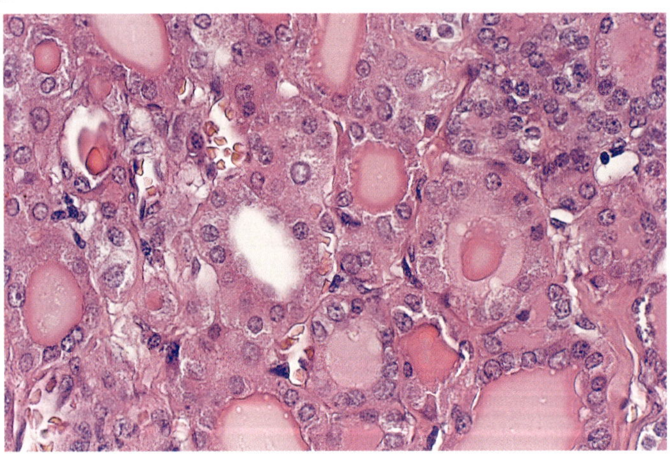

C

Figure 3.9 Multinodular goitre. **A.** Aspirates from adenomatous areas are cellular with little colloid. Psammoma bodies may be seen. **B.** High-power view shows psammoma bodies. Apart from papillary carcinoma, psammoma bodies may be present in colloid goitre. Their presence, in the absence of other cytological criteria for malignancy, should not necessarily lead to diagnosis of carcinoma. However, the presence of psammoma bodies in a FNAC smear cytologically consistent with a colloid goitre should raise the possibility of coexistent papillary hyperplasia or neoplasia. Because of the strong statistical association of psammoma bodies with malignant thyroid neoplasms, histological confirmation is mandatory in such cases. **C.** Histological section shows colloid goitre with psammoma bodies within the follicles (H&E).

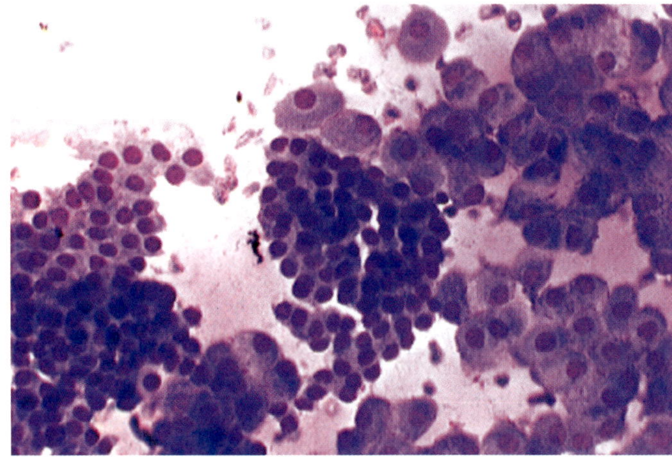

A

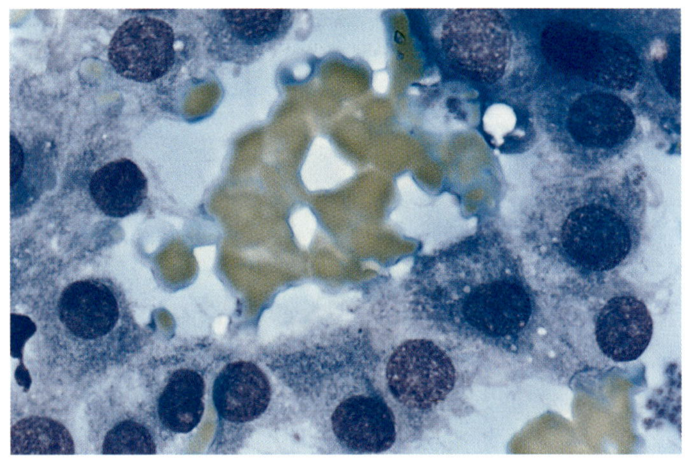

B

Figure 3.10 Degenerative changes. **A.** Foamy cytoplasm containing granules makes epithelium indistinguishable from macrophages (MGG ×600 oil immersion). **B.** Higher power view shows cytoplasmic granules (MGG ×1000).

Cysts

In multinodular goitre with cyst formation, macrophages are often seen. They may be multinucleated and sometimes contain haemosiderin. Epithelial cells with degenerative changes may be seen; anisonucleosis and anisocytosis may be present although the N:C ratio remains normal (Figs 3.13 and 3.14).

Hyperactive goitre (toxic goitre, thyrotoxicosis, primary hyperthyroidism, Grave's disease)

FNAC smears from hyperactive goitre usually show little colloid (Fig. 3.15) Follicular epithelium may be hypercellular, arranged in microfollicles or acini. Obvious

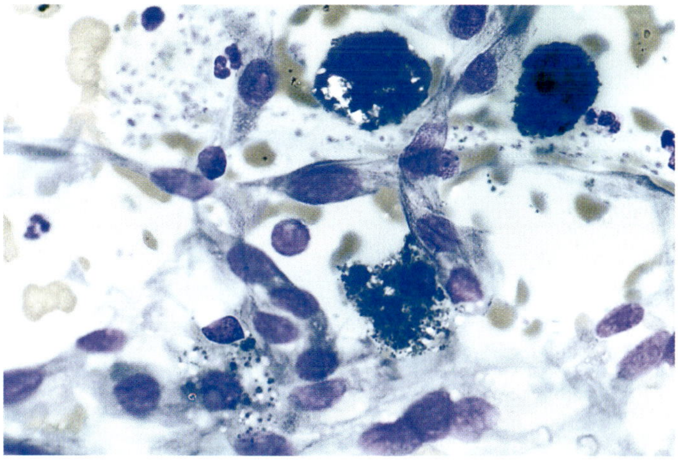

A

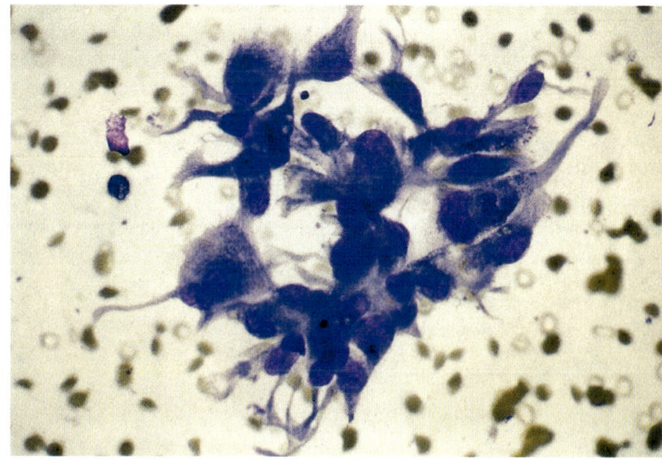

B

Figure 3.11 Regenerative changes. **A.** Spindle-shaped follicular epithelium and macrophages (MGG ×600 oil immersion). **B.** Spindle epithelial cells from the wall of the cystic goitre have prominent nucleoli resembling repair epithelium. This may be misleading into diagnosis of a mesenchymal lesion (MGG ×600 oil).

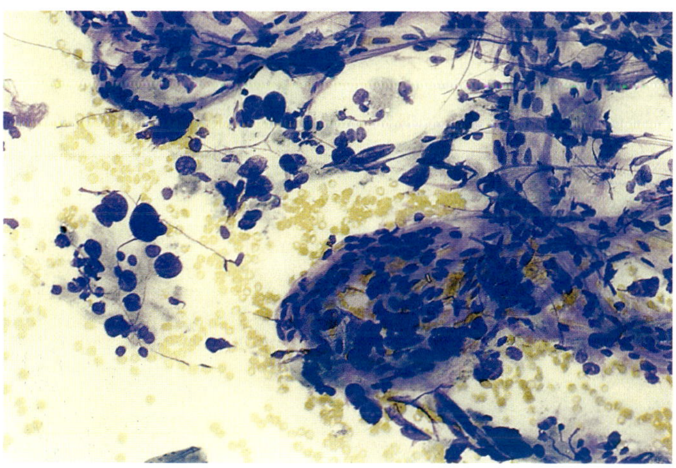

A

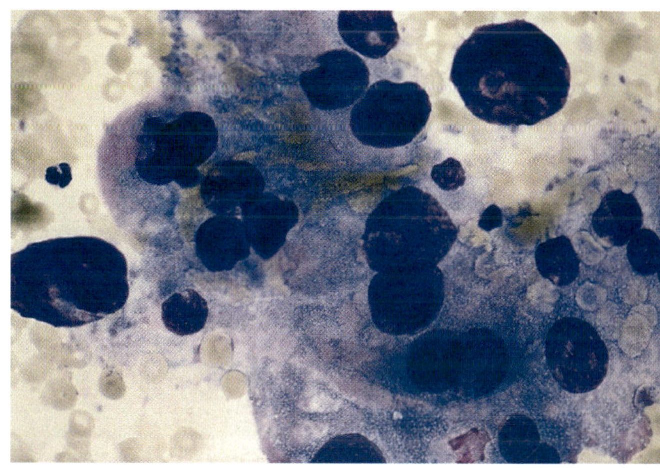

B

Figure 3.12 Degenerative changes. Radioiodine effect on follicular epithelium 30 years after the patient had treatment. **A.** Fragments of fibrous stroma with large bare nuclei (MGG ×400). **B.** Bare nuclei with structureless chromatin but prominent anisonucleosis and alarming pleomorphism (MGG ×1000 oil immersion).

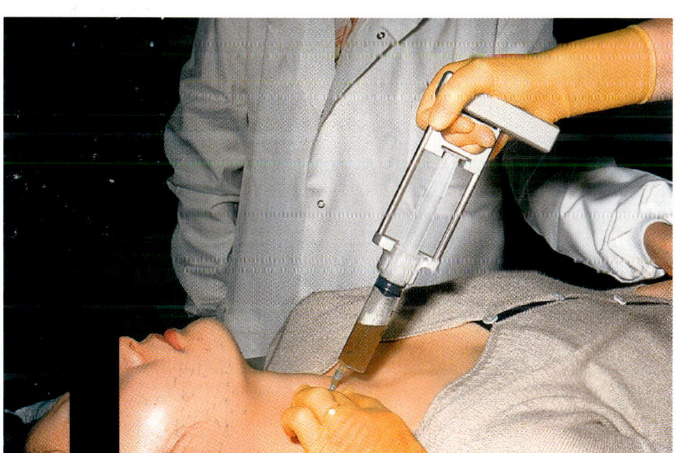

Figure 3.13 FNAC evacuation of the fluid from thyroid cyst. Patient is being reminded not to swallow or speak during the procedure to avoid trauma.

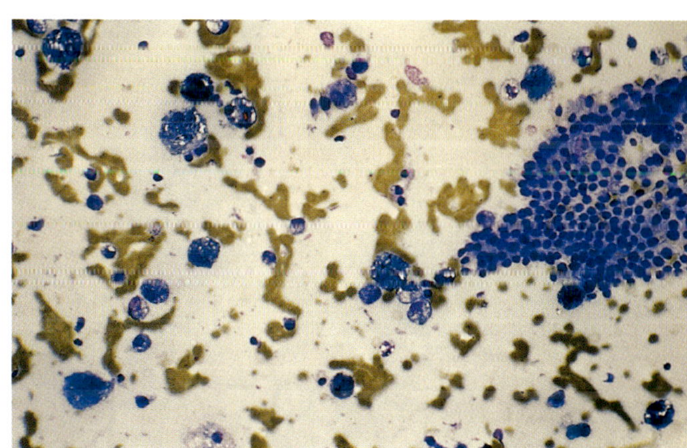

A

Figure 3.14 Thyroid cyst. **A.** A low-power view typical of a benign thyroid cyst. Sparse follicular epithelium and macrophages (MGG ×200).

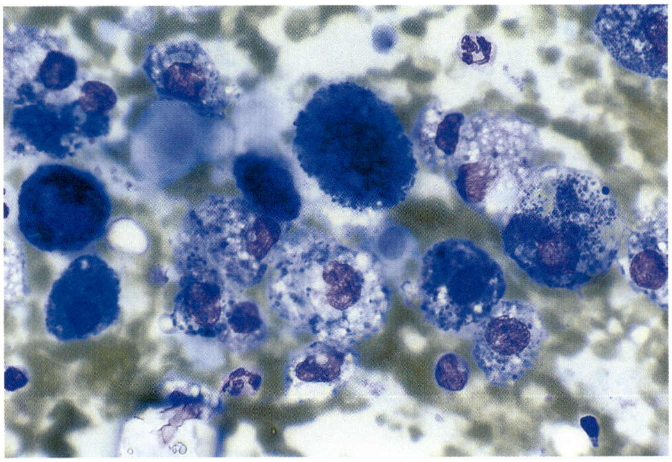

B

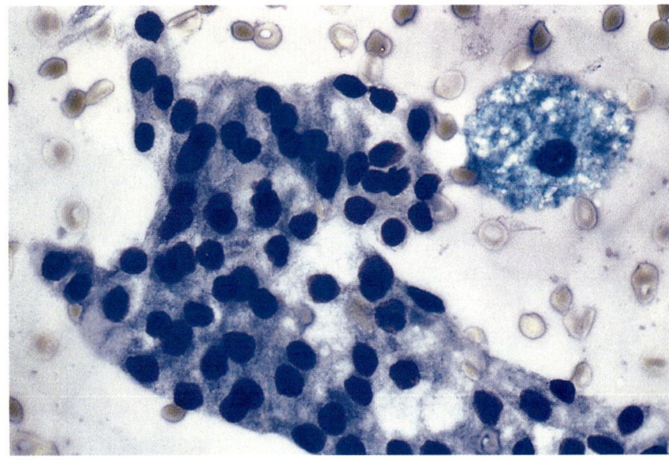

C

Figure 3.14 (*continued*) **B.** Epithelium shows degenerative changes. Macrophages are filled with haemosiderin (MGG ×400). **C.** Foamy macrophages and colloid (MGG ×600 oil immersion).

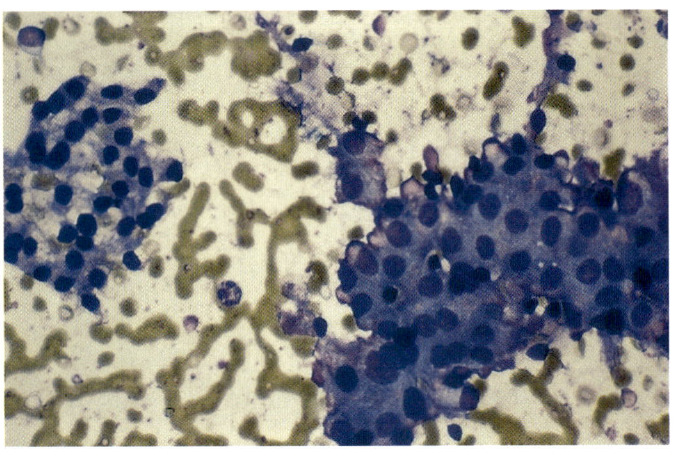

A

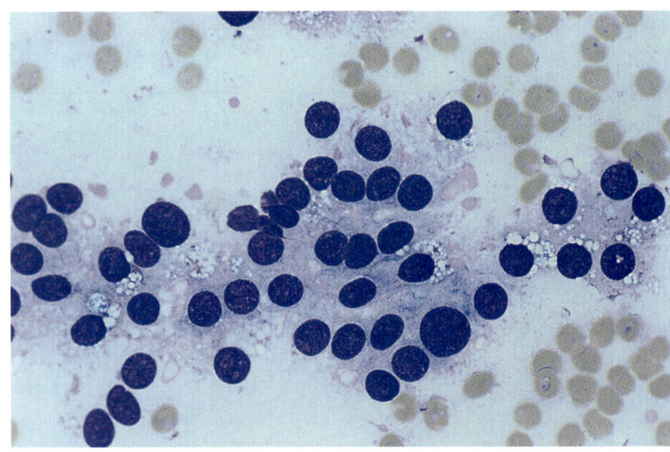

B

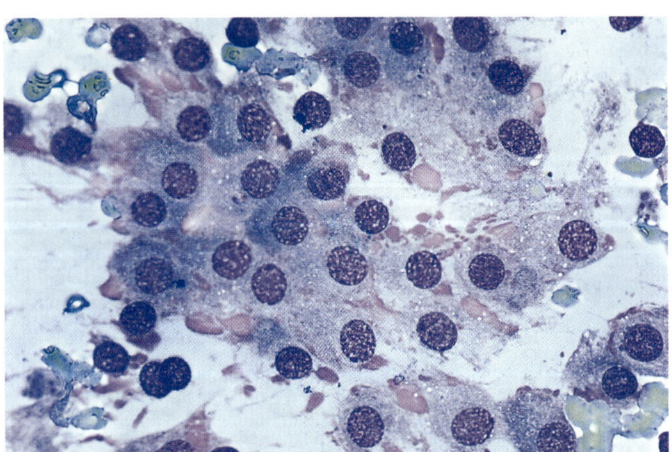

C

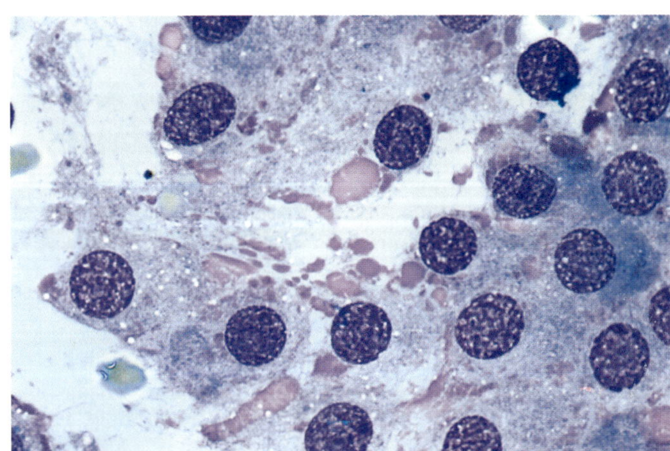

D

Figure 3.15 Hyperactive toxic goitre. **A.** FNAC smears from hyperactive goitre usually show little colloid. Follicular epithelium may be hypercellular, arranged in microfollicles or acini. **B.** Obvious anisonucleosis is seen (MGG ×600 oil immersion). **C,D.** Marginal vacuoles (fire-flare cells) and fine red granulation are present in the cytoplasm (MGG ×600, ×1000 oil immersion).

anisonucleosis is seen. Marginal vacuoles (fire-flare cells) and fine red granulation are present in the cytoplasm (Fig. 3.16). Apart from the hyperactive (thyrotoxic goitre) in which marginal vacuoles are seen in 100% of cases, they are also seen in 42.6% of hyperplastic nodules, 5.2% of colloid goitre and 13.3% of neoplasms. Marginal vacuoles are limited to neoplasms with a follicular component, which includes 15% of follicular neoplasms and 50% of follicular variant of papillary carcinoma. A multiparameter study of FNAC from toxic goitre showed that a fire-flare appearance of the follicular cells and a good cellularity of the smears were the features most frequently observed in these cases.[60] Hürthle cell changes were present in 47% of the cases and small numbers of lymphocytes were seen in smears from 41% of the cases. Epithelioid cell granulomata and multinucleated giant cells were observed in less than one-quarter of the cases. About half of the cases showed some degree of pleomorphism of the follicular cells.

Fine needle aspiration of the thyroid has a limited value in differentiating hyperplastic nodular goitres from true follicular neoplasms (Fig. 3.17) and in separating follicular adenomas from follicular carcinomas. Only two of the cellular patterns (honeycomb and single dispersed) and the average maximum nuclear diameter show trends in differentiating these lesions.[61]

The cytological differential diagnosis of colloid nodule and the follicular variant of papillary carcinoma are difficult with common morphologic features. The follicular variant of papillary carcinoma can be differentiated from colloid nodule based on nuclear changes, which include a larger size, higher N:C ratio, and presence of pseudoinclusions.

Thyroiditis

Acute (purulent) thyroiditis

Acute thyroiditis is rarely seen. The cause is bacteria, fungi or parasites. Differential diagnosis includes anaplastic carcinoma, which can be associated with a background with numerous granulocytes. Granulocytes may also be seen in subacute thyroiditis.

Subacute thyroiditis (granulomatous thyroiditis, De Quervain's thyroiditis)

Subacute thyroiditis presents usually in young women, frequently after viral respiratory infection. There is painful asymmetric thyroid gland enlargement. Clinically, there is a raised ESR, occasionally fever and mild hypothyroidism. Patients complain of pain in the thyroid typically irradiating into the ear. The illness lasts several weeks to several months and usually ends in complete recovery. Histologically there is destruction of follicular epithelium with a granulomatous reaction to colloid. There is variably dense lymphocytic infiltrate and variable fibrosis. The cause is unknown and is assumed to be viral.

Cytological features. Granulomatous thyroiditis has a variably cellular appearance with multinucleated giant cells, sometimes of Langerhans' type with fragments of colloid, epithelioid cells, macrophages, lymphocytes, fibroblasts and frequently small epithelial cells with degenerative changes (Fig. 3.18). Hürthle cells may be seen. Stromal cells with large pleomorphic nuclei may be present.

Apart from in subacute thyroiditis, *multinucleate giant cells* may be seen in papillary carcinoma and Hashimoto's thyroiditis, thyroid granuloma, adenomatous goitre and Hürthle cell adenoma.[62] Anaplastic carcinoma of the thyroid may cause painful swelling of the gland with inflammatory cells, spindled cells and osteoclast-like giant cells.

Lymphocytic thyroiditis (Hashimoto's thyroiditis)

Lymphocytic thyroiditis occurs most often in females above the age of 40 and causes a symmetric diffuse thyroid gland enlargement (Fig. 3.19). Initially there is often mild hyperthyroidism; eventually the patient is clinically hypothyroid. Histologically, there is intralobular fibrosis, a dense lymphoplasmacytic infiltrate with lymphoid follicle formation, extension of the infiltrate around atrophic follicles and extensive oncocytic metaplasia of the follicular epithelium. The epithelium often shows nuclear enlargement, nuclear overlap and occasionally clearing of the nuclear structure to produce appearances similar to those of papillary carcinoma. Squamous cell metaplasia may be seen. The cause is autoimmune; high levels of different antibodies, including antibodies to thyroglobulin, are found in serum.

Cytological features. Hashimoto's thyroiditis is the commonest thyroiditis encountered by cytopathologists. Smears are cellular with lymphocytes and lymphoid follicle centre cells, centrocytes, centroblasts and plasma cells (Fig. 3.20). Oncocytic epithelial cells are seen. They may have prominent anisonucleosis and anisocytosis with prominent

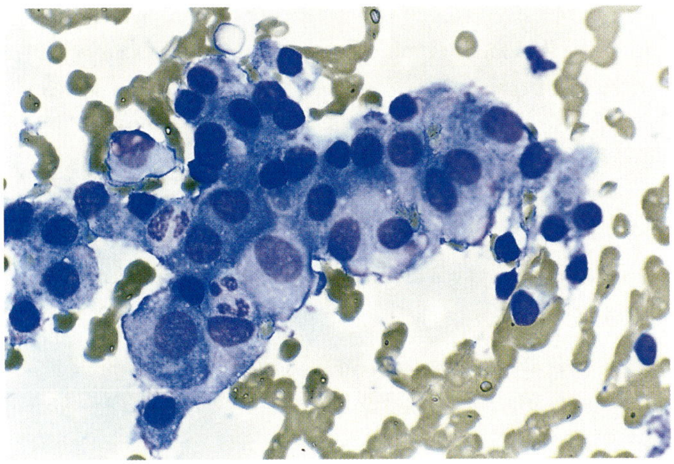

Figure 3.16 Hyperactive goitre. Although not pathognomonic of hyperactive nodules, fire-flare appearance of the follicular cells and a good cellularity of the smears are the features most frequently observed in these cases. Appearances of a well-outlined cytoplasm of oncocytic type with scalloped edges may be misleading (see Fig. 3.24) (MGG ×600).

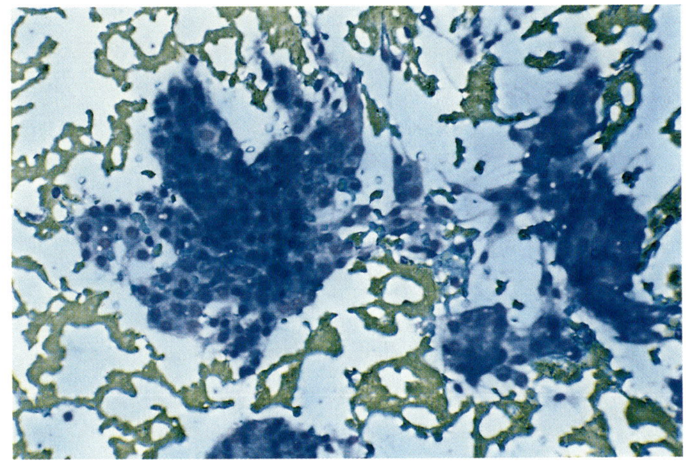

Figure 3.17 Adenomatous goitre vs follicular adenoma. Fine needle aspiration of the thyroid is limited in differentiating hyperplastic nodular goitres from true follicular neoplasms. This is an aspirate from an adenomatous colloid goitre. Note plenty of thin colloid in the background (MGG ×400).

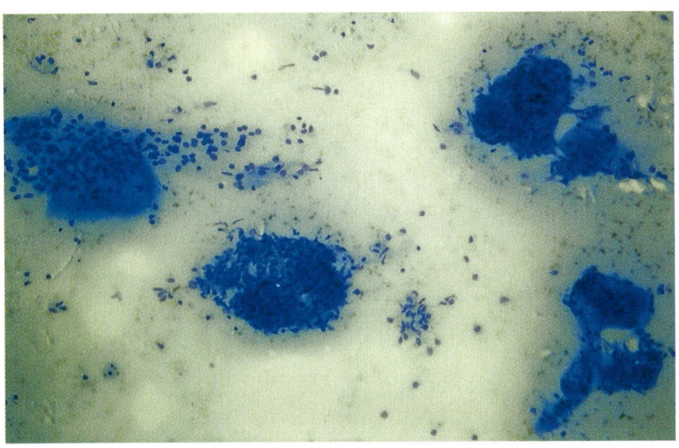

A

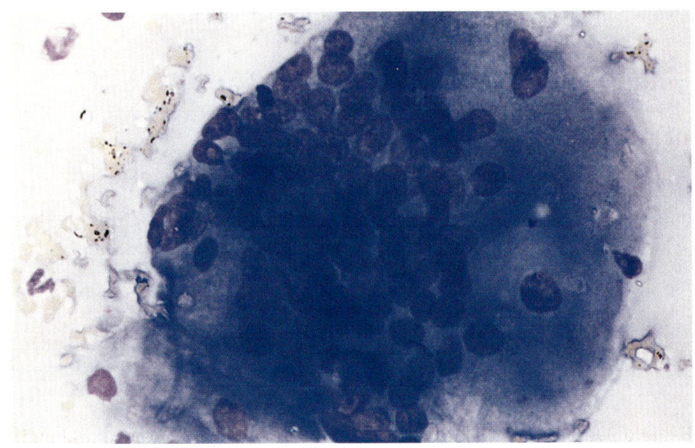

B

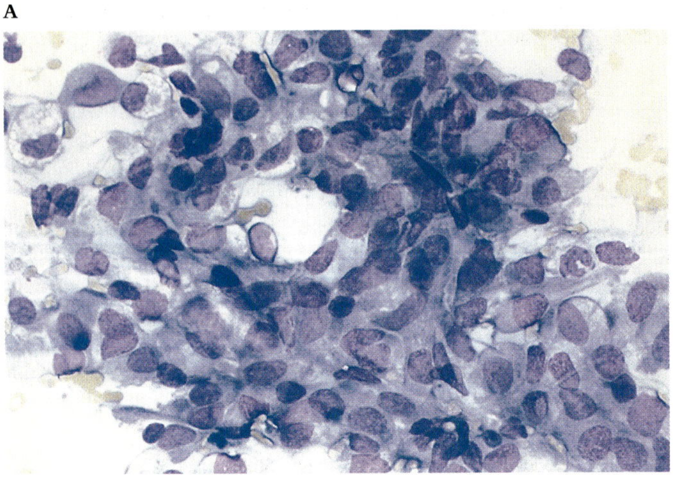

C

Figure 3.18 Granulomatous thyroiditis. **A.** A low-power view shows variably cellular appearance with multinucleated giant cells with fragments of colloid, epithelioid cells and macrophages (MGG ×100). **B.** Multinucleate giant cells may be of Langerhans' type (MGG ×600 oil immersion). **C.** Epithelioid cells forming granulomas often replace any thyroid epithelium in aspirates (MGG ×600 oil immersion).

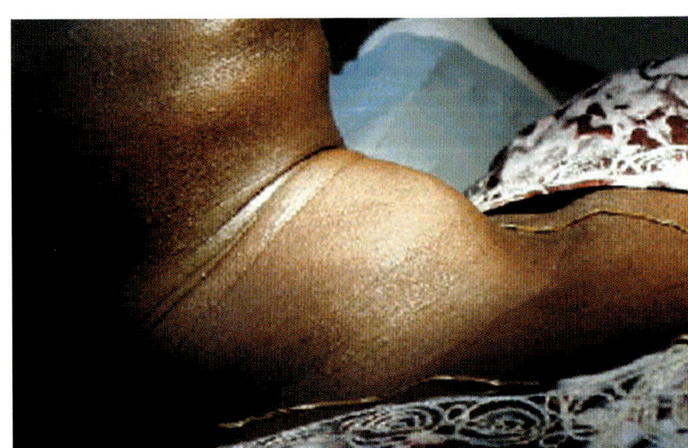

Figure 3.19 Lymphocytic thyroiditis occurs most often in females above the age of 40 and causes a symmetric diffuse thyroid gland enlargement.

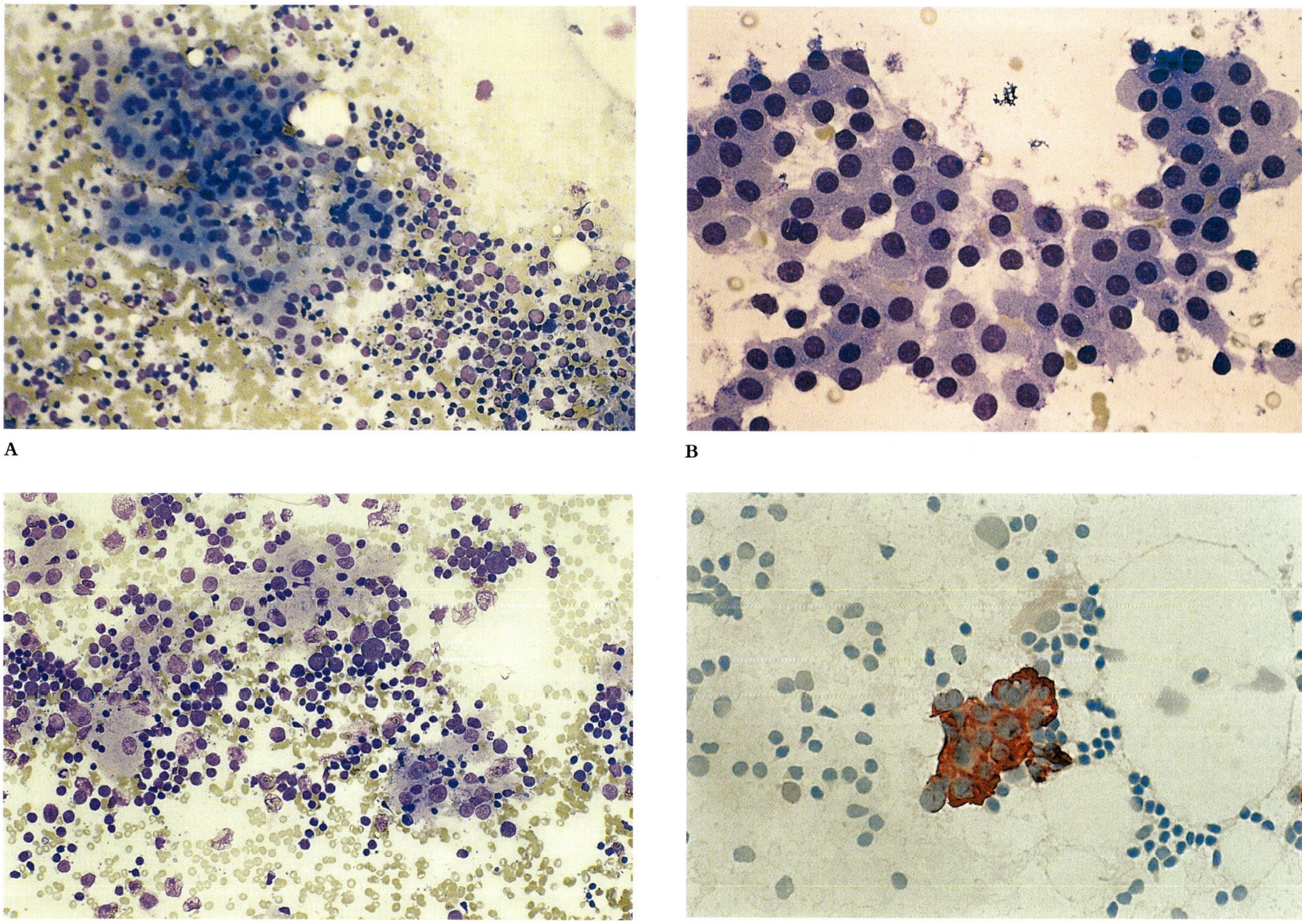

A B C D

Figure 3.20 Lymphocytic thyroiditis. **A.** Smears are cellular with lymphocytes and lymphoid follicle centre cells, centrocytes, centroblasts, plasma cells and oncocytic epithelial cells (MGG ×400). **B.** Oncocytic epithelial cells (×600 oil immersion). **C.** Residual follicle centre fragments are often indistinguishable from epithelium (MGG ×400). **D.** Cytokeratin marker confirms epithelial islands within the lymphoid background (CAM 5.2, APAAP ×600 oil immersion).

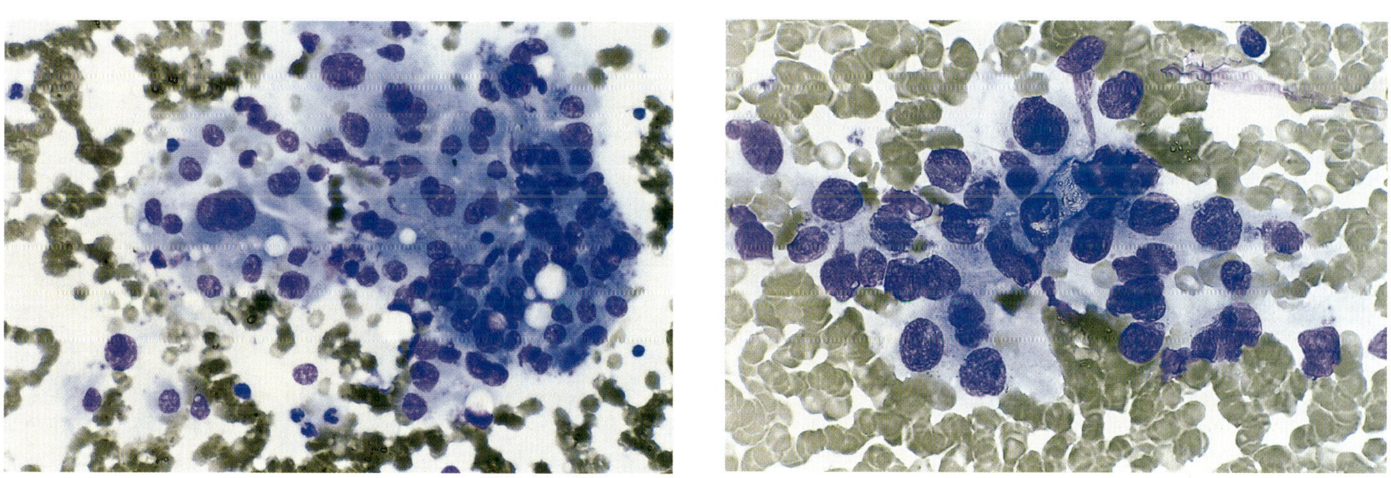

A B

Figure 3.21 Lymphocytic thyroiditis. **A.** Oncocytic epithelial atypia, which occurs in longstanding lymphocytic thyroiditis, may be interpreted as malignancy, particularly if associated with multinucleated giant cells as in papillary carcinoma (MGG ×600). **B.** Same case (MGG×1000).

nucleoli. Multinucleated giant cell histiocytes may also be seen.[63] FNAC is highly sensitive in diagnosing Hashimoto's thyroiditis, with a diagnostic accuracy rate of 92%.[64]

Potential pitfalls in diagnosis relate to both lymphoid and epithelial components.[65] Epithelial atypia may be interpreted as malignancy, particularly if associated with multinucleated giant cells as in papillary carcinoma (Fig. 3.21). On the other hand, pleomorphic Hürthle cells may be present in aspirates from Hürthle cell neoplasms and underdiagnosed as Hashimoto's thyroiditis, especially when they are associated with a few lymphocytes.[66] Papillary carcinomas and anaplastic carcinomas may have lymphocytic infiltrates. Non-Hodgkin's lymphoma of the thyroid arises against a background of lymphocytic thyroiditis (Fig. 3.32). False-positive diagnoses may be possible on the basis of epithelial atypia or suspicion of a lymphoma. False-negative results may be due to lymphocytic infiltrates in tumours with thyroiditis component. Differential diagnosis of Hashimoto's thyroiditis includes subacute thyroiditis, oncocytic hyperplasia, oncocytic tumours, follicular tumours, papillary carcinoma and malignant lymphoma.

Riedel's thyroiditis

This is the rarest form of thyroiditis. A poorly cellular aspirate usually contains occasional fibroblasts.

NEOPLASMS

FNAC is a diagnostic tool useful as a guide to patient management. Oertel & Oertel[67] believe that its role in solving the diagnostic dilemmas presented by thyroid nodules is still underappreciated. Current constraints in health care might bring about a wider use of this simple technique to select patients for surgery. Care in sampling a mass is essential to obtain aspirates that are representative of the lesion and adequate in quantity for interpretation. Several aspirates are needed from all but the smallest masses. Most thyroid carcinomas are well differentiated with a low grade of malignancy. The majority of these are papillary carcinomas, which are easily diagnosed from good cytological smears. With FNAC, the goal is to diagnose a follicular neoplasm and to separate it from the adenomatoid nodule. The follicular neoplasm then can be classified as adenoma or carcinoma on the histological sections. The minimally invasive carcinoma still can be challenging to recognise.[67]

Follicular adenoma

This is a solitary encapsulated lesion composed of a proliferation of follicular epithelium. Patients usually have normal thyroid gland function and present with a palpable lesion which by immunoscintigraphy is usually 'cold' (non-hormonally active).

Histologically the lesion is usually 'round, encapsulated, and has an expansive growth pattern with compression of the surrounding thyroid gland tissue. The growth pattern may vary with macrofollicles (colloid adenoma), microfollicles (foetal adenoma), trabeculae and solid areas (embryonal adenoma). The cell type may vary among Hürthle cell, clear cell and signet ring cell. These microscopic variations have no clinical significance. The distinction between follicular adenoma and follicular carcinoma may be difficult due to pseudoinfiltrative growth in the capsule and the often extremely close relationship between the follicular epithelium and thin-walled blood vessels. Pseudopapillary hyperplastic structures, cellular atypia and nuclear pleomorphism (especially in Hürthle cell tumours) may also cause diagnostic difficulty.[68] A rare variant is hyalinising trabecular adenoma, a tumour with a large cell type that may be confused microscopically with a medullary or papillary carcinoma. The term 'atypical adenoma' is used for encapsulated lesions with cytological atypia, mitoses and necrosis. Follow-up studies have shown that these lesions are benign.

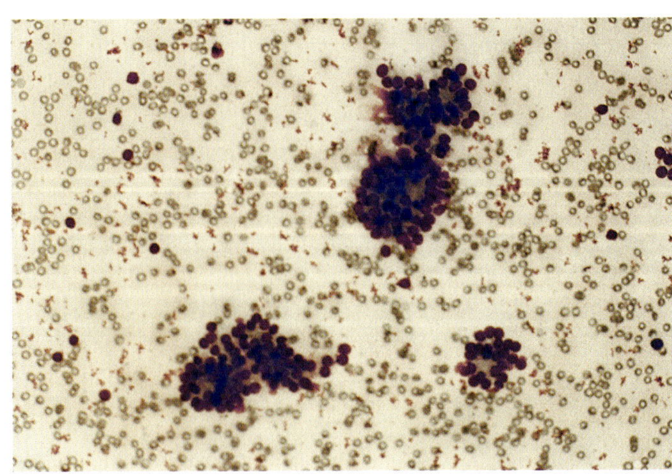

A

Figure 3.22 Follicular adenoma. **A.** In microfollicular adenoma the aspirate is cellular with cells arranged in follicular structures (MGG ×200). ***(continued)***

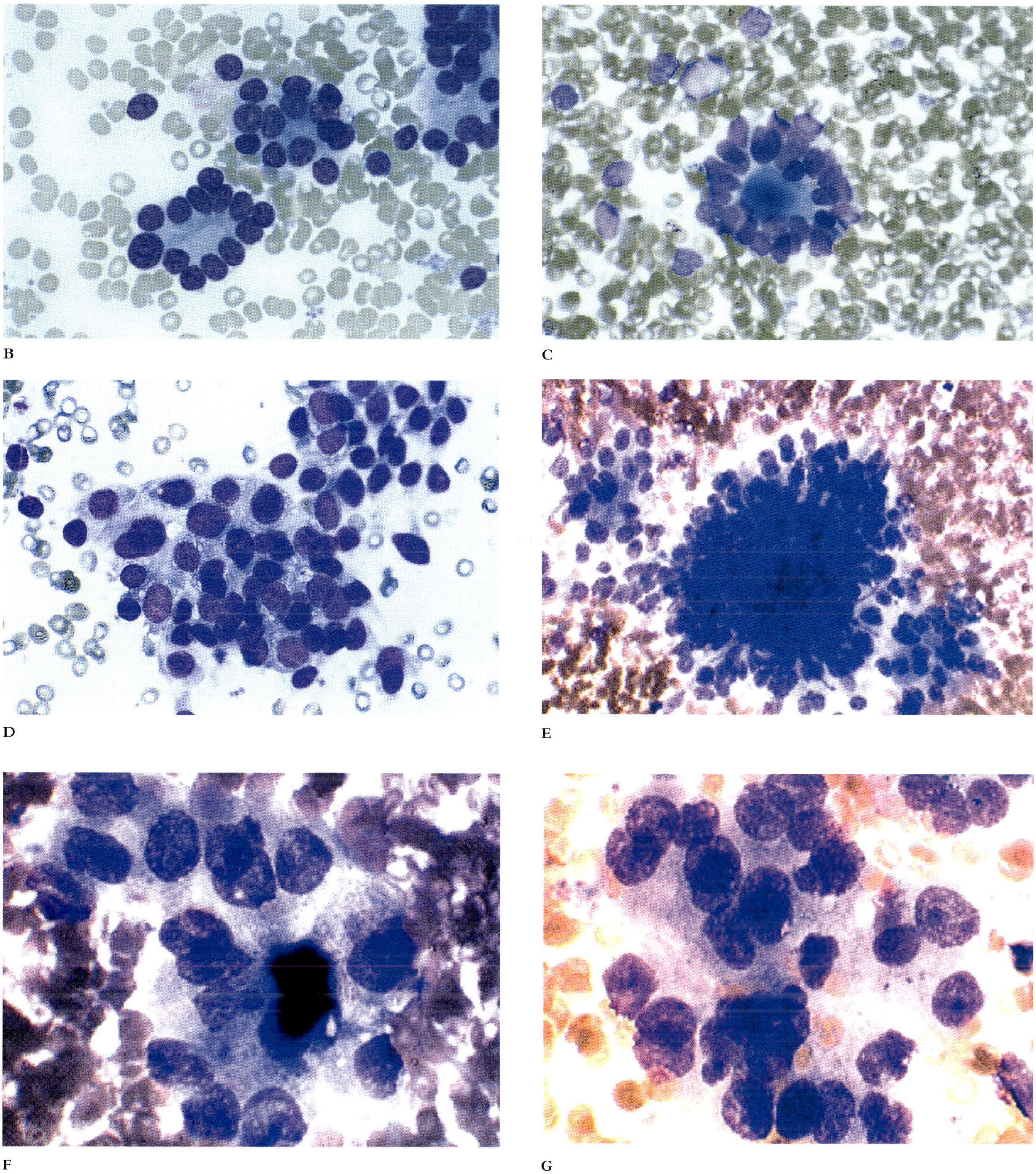

Figure 3.22 Follicular adenoma. ***(continued)*** **B.** These are arranged in the form of rings or rosettes with cytoplasm centrally and without obvious cytoplasmic borders. **C.** There is little or no colloid present (MGG ×600 oil immersion). **D, E, F.** Occasionally, pleomorphism may lead to a diagnosis of follicular proliferation as follicular carcinoma. This was erroneous in this case; after excision the lesion was diagnosed as follicular adenoma. (MGG ×500, ×1000, oil immersion). **G** Same case as 3.22D, E, F. Cellular atypia in follicular adenoma should not be overinterpreted (MGG ×1000).

Cytological features. FNAC of follicular adenoma is not possible to distinguish from follicular carcinoma. In microfollicular adenoma, the aspirate is cellular, with cells arranged in follicular structures in the form of rings or rosettes with cytoplasm centrally and without obvious cytoplasmic borders. There is little or no colloid present. When present, it is seen in particles in microfollicles (Fig. 3.22). There is usually little pleomorphism and nucleoli are small. In macrofollicular adenomata there is usually abundant colloid and the appearance may be similar to that of nodular goitre. In adenomata, anisonucleosis is common.

Hürthle cell tumours

FNACs from Hürthle cell adenomas are predominantly composed of large, monomorphic Hürthle cells with oval nuclei, prominent nucleoli and abundant, well-defined, granular cytoplasm, present singly, in acinar arrangement and in monolayered sheets of variable sizes. Nuclear pleomorphism is noted (Fig. 3.23). Occasional small syncytial tumour cell clusters and a few naked tumour cell nuclei are observed.[69] The FNACs from Hürthle cell carcinomas are hypercellular; tumour cells are relatively small and show monomorphic or pleomorphic nuclei, prominent nucleoli and ill-defined cytoplasm. Syncytial tumour cell clusters are present in abundance, and numerous naked tumour cell nuclei are noted. The presence of small tumour cells with ill-defined cytoplasm and prominent nucleoli in syncytial clusters and abundant naked tumour cell nuclei in the FNAC of a thyroid nodule should alert the observer about the strong possibility of a Hürthle cell carcinoma.[69]

Cellular thyroid aspirates with follicular groups and little or no colloid are seen in microfollicular adenomas, well-differentiated carcinoma, follicular-variant papillary carcinoma, nodular hyperplasia, proliferations following antithyroid drugs, parathyroid gland adenomata and glomus tumours. In all these cases the cytological conclusion should be 'follicular proliferation' and the management advice should be for a histological examination. In the classification of follicular lesions of the thyroid by fine needle aspiration, adherence to strict cytological criteria helps to identify those patients who will benefit most from surgery.[70]

When trying to develop clinical criteria capable of predicting malignancy in patients with a FNAC diagnosis of follicular neoplasm, Tuttle et al[71] analysed the data and showed that after a FNAC showing a follicular neoplasm, the risk of malignancy in males with large nodules was nearly 80%, compared with a rate of only 3% in females with small nodules. These results suggest that clinical features including gender, nodule size, and character of the gland by palpation can be systematically integrated into the decision analysis, thereby improving the selection of patients for surgical referral.[71]

Hyalinising trabecular adenoma

Hyalinising trabecular adenoma is a recently described benign thyroid tumour almost exclusively occurring in

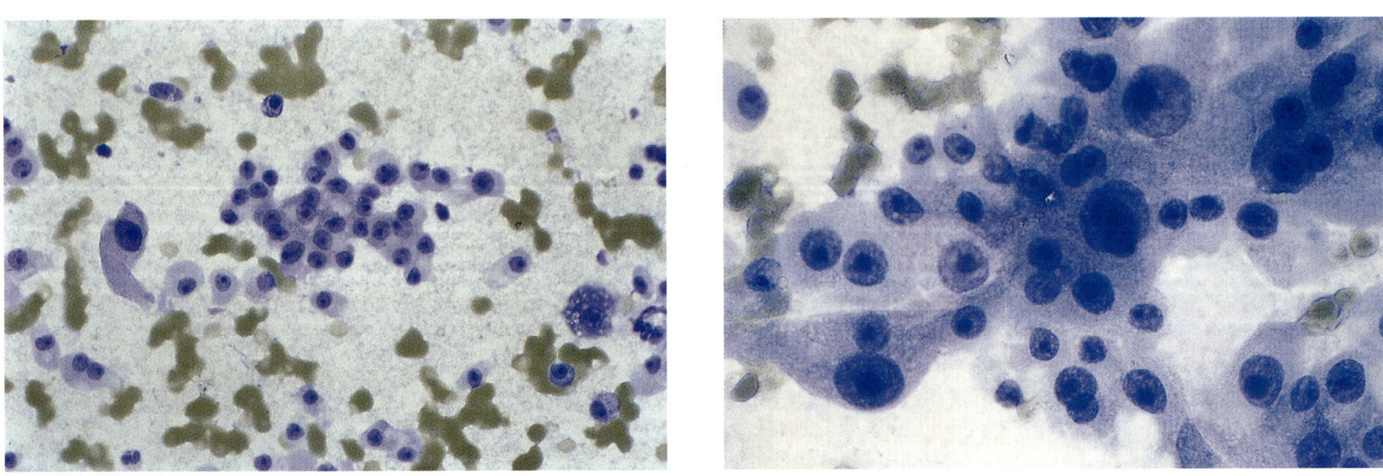

A B

Figure 3.23 Hürthle cell adenoma. **A.** FNACs from Hürthle cell adenomas are predominantly composed of large monomorphic Hürthle cells with oval nuclei, prominent nucleoli and abundant, well-defined, granular cytoplasm present singly, in acinar arrangement and in monolayered sheets of variable sizes (MGG ×400). **B.** Anisonucleosis and prominent nucleoli may mislead into diagnosis of malignancy (MGG ×600 oil immersion).

women.[72] The morphological features of this entity overlap with both papillary and medullary carcinoma to varying extents. This in turn creates a situation of potential diagnostic error, particularly for a false- positive diagnosis of papillary carcinoma in FNAC. False consideration of medullary carcinoma is also possible by the unwary, especially if staining for congo red and/or immunostaining for calcitonin is not resorted to.

Cytological features. Hyalinising trabecular adenomas contain cells with mild nuclear atypia, nuclear grooves and nuclear pseudoinclusions but lack psammoma bodies, high cellularity and papillary structures. Collections of an amorphous colloid-like material are noted, surrounded by follicular cells. The purplish red stromal deposits corresponding to accumulations of basement membrane material helps to prevent cytological overdiagnosis of malignancy in this rare, benign tumour.[73,74] Inflammatory cells in the background may suggest the possibility of a thyroiditis.[75] Immunohistochemistry using anticalcitonin and antithyroglobulin antibodies is helpful in distinguishing these tumours from medullary carcinoma. The low Ki-67 (nuclear) index and absence of p53 immunostaining are consistent with the benign behaviour of this tumour.[76] Tumour cells of hyalinising trabecular adenoma reveal an intense cytoplasmic immunopositivity for MIB1. In contrast, cytoplasmic immunostaining for MIB1 has been found to be negative in all other thyroid tumours and non-neoplastic lesions. Positive cytoplasmic immunostaining for MIB1 is a characteristic finding of hyalinising trabecular adenoma and is useful in differentiating it from other thyroid tumours.[77]

All of the cases in a series by Goellner et al[78] initially had been interpreted as either suspicious or positive for malignancy. On retrospective review, many of the cytological features did mimic those of other lesions, particularly papillary carcinoma. The smears tended to hypercellularity and nuclei were often slightly enlarged with pale chromatin, intranuclear holes and longitudinal grooving of the nuclear membrane. On the other hand, some cytological features were more suggestive of medullary carcinoma: poor cohesion of cells with elongated and spindle cell forms and hyaline acellular areas. The authors suggest awareness of the histological and cytological features of hyalinising trabecular adenoma which may enable cytopathologists to avoid false-positive diagnoses of papillary carcinoma or medullary carcinoma, although they consider it unrealistic to expect a definitive diagnosis of hyalinising trabecular adenoma on FNAC.[73,77–84]

Papillary carcinoma

Approximately 95% of malignant thyroid gland tumours arise from the follicular epithelium and the remainder from C-cells. The commonest carcinomas are papillary, follicular, anaplastic and medullary.

Papillary carcinoma is the commonest type of thyroid carcinoma. It is more common in females than in males, and presents in all age groups. Histologically, papillary carcinoma is characterised by characteristic cytological features and papillary structures. Papillae are complex with a variable amount of stroma and lined by a single layer of epithelium. Occasionally the entire tumour may be follicular without papillary structures. The biological behaviour of both the classical and follicular types is similar. Tumours may become cystic, particularly in lymph node metastases. Psammoma bodies in the stroma are characteristic for papillary carcinoma but may be seen in other conditions (Fig. 3.9). Papillary carcinoma tends to spread via the lymphatics. Distant metastases are infrequent. Prognosis is good (20-year survival is 90%). Unfavourable prognostic features are old age at presentation, extension of the tumour outside the thyroid gland and the presence of poorly differentiated areas.

Variants of papillary carcinoma – oncocytic, diffuse sclerosing, tall and columnar cell – have a poorer prognosis. They are associated with aggressive behaviour, early visceral metastasis and a rapidly fatal course. Cases of papillary carcinoma merging with squamous carcinoma, mucoepidermoid carcinoma, insular carcinoma, columnar cell carcinoma, poorly differentiated carcinoma, anaplastic carcinoma and medullary carcinoma have been reported.[85]

Can papillary carcinoma be managed on the basis of FNAC report?

When papillary carcinoma of the thyroid or follicular variant of papillary carcinoma of the thyroid is definitively diagnosed on FNAC, the surgeon can perform definitive thyroidectomy without frozen section because of the high specificity for cancer. If the FNAC is suspicious for papillary

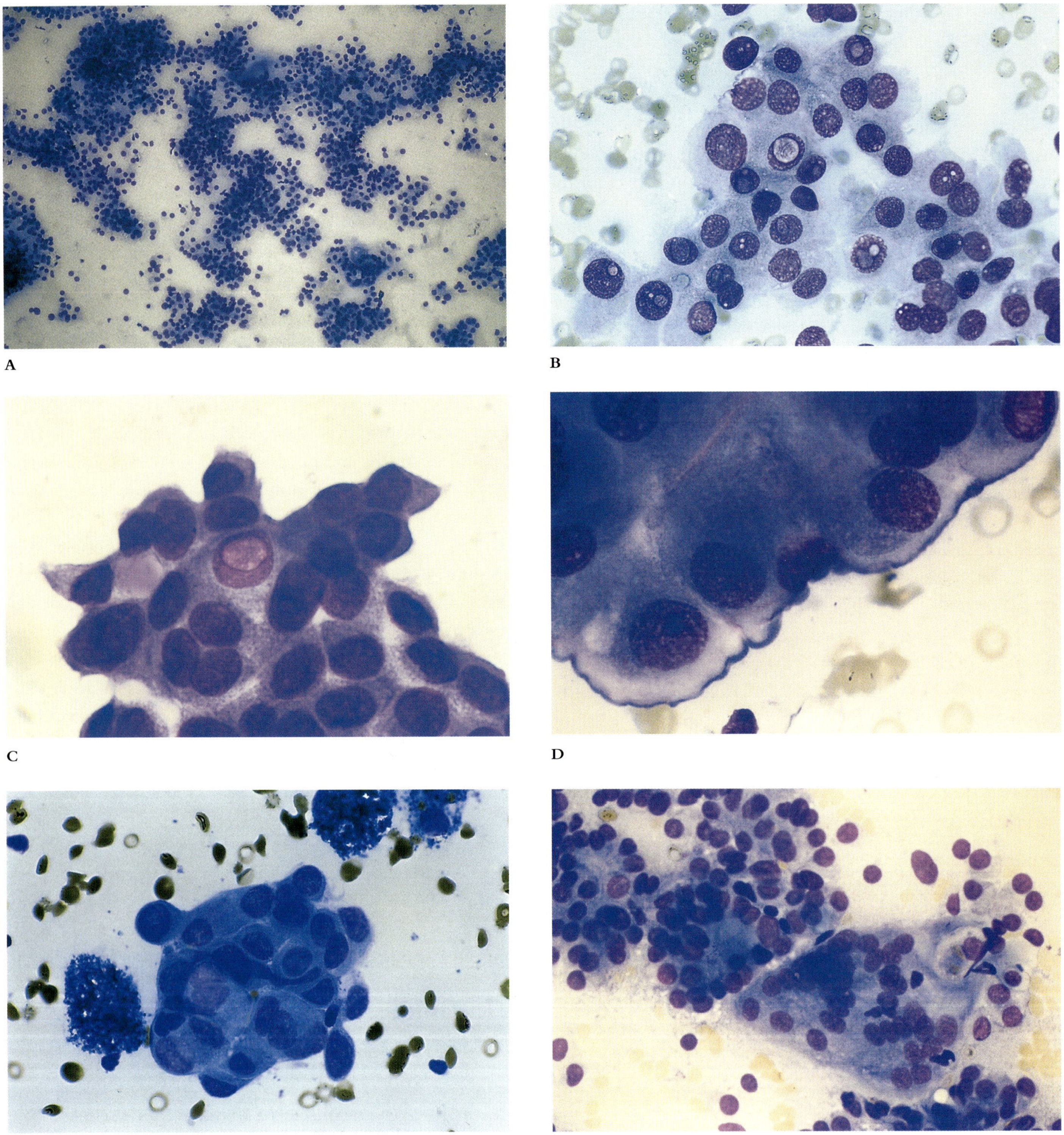

Figure 3.24 Papillary carcinoma. **A.** FNAC smears are cellular. Follicular cells with dense cytoplasm, well-defined cell margins and presence of papillary clusters are the most consistent features observed (MGG ×200). **B.** Intranuclear cytoplasmic inclusions, though characteristics, are found in 66.6% of cases (MGG x600 oil immersion). **C.** Nuclear grooves are also a useful criterion in the diagnosis of papillary thyroid carcinoma. 88% of papillary carcinomas have nuclear grooves in at least 20% of tumour cells. They are better appreciated on PAP-stained smears and H&E (MGG ×600 oil immersion). **D.** Well defined cytoplasmic borders with scalloping of the cytoplasm is often seen (MGG ×1000, oil immersion). **E.** Cystic change may be present (MGG×600, oil immersion). **F.** Multinucleate giant cells are frequemtly present in papillary carcinoma and follicula variant of papillary carcinoma (MGG×600, oil immersion).

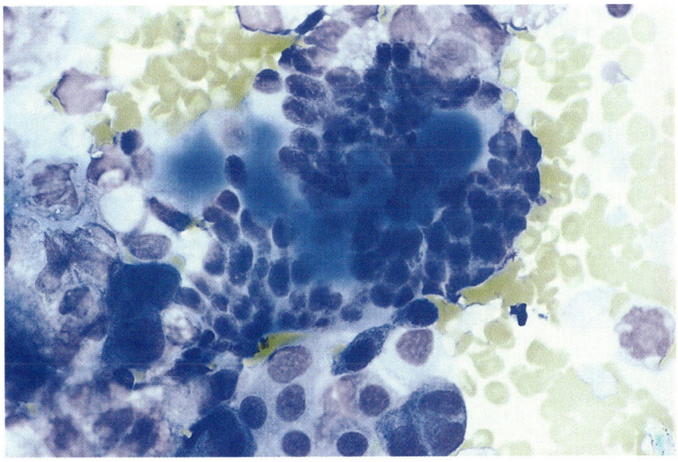

G

Figure 3.24 (*continued*) G. Colloid is sparse and tenaceous (MGG ×600 oil immersion).

carcinoma of the thyroid, the incidence of cancer is 54%, and patients with these conditions should undergo surgery with frozen section. When either gross findings or frozen sections suggest malignancy, definitive thyroidectomy can be performed because 90% of such cases will be carcinoma. If frozen section is not diagnostic of malignancy, a thyroid lobectomy/isthmusectomy is recommended because 71% have a benign lesion. This systematic approach to papillary carcinoma of the thyroid will obviate unnecessary frozen sections while maintaining excellent diagnostic specificity.[46,86] FNAC can detect a virtually harmless occult papillary carcinoma that will oblige patients to have surgery. This very occasional 'pitfall' of FNAC should not preclude this method from being used in the management of thyroid disease.[87]

Cytological features. Cytological features are characteristic enough to enable accurate tumour typing.[88] FNAC smears are cellular. Follicular cells with dense cytoplasm, well-defined cell margins, and presence of papillary clusters are the most consistent features observed (Fig. 3.24). Intranuclear cytoplasmic inclusions, though characteristic, are found in 66.6% of cases.[89] Psammoma bodies may be seen but are not pathognomonic for papillary carcinoma (Fig 3.9).[58] Isolated psammoma bodies are an unreliable predictor of papillary carcinoma in the absence of cytological features.[90] The presence of psammoma bodies, in the absence of other cytological criteria for malignancy, should not necessarily lead to immediate surgical exploration. If surgery is carried out, the approach should be limited and conservative, given the reduced likelihood of malignancy.[57] Nuclear grooves are also a useful criterion in the diagnosis of papillary thyroid carcinoma. Eighty-eight percent of papillary carcinomas have nuclear grooves in at least 20% of tumour cells, whereas none of the other thyroid diseases exceed this level.[91–93] Nuclear grooves are better seen in H&E and PAP-stained smears. However, in MGG-stained smears the number of cells with nuclear grooves is also significantly higher as com-

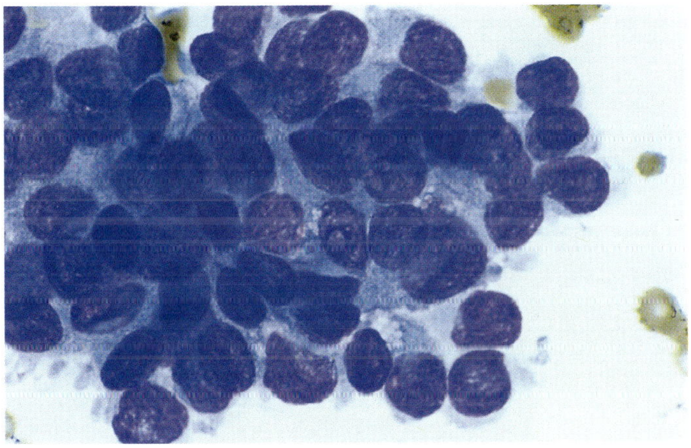

A

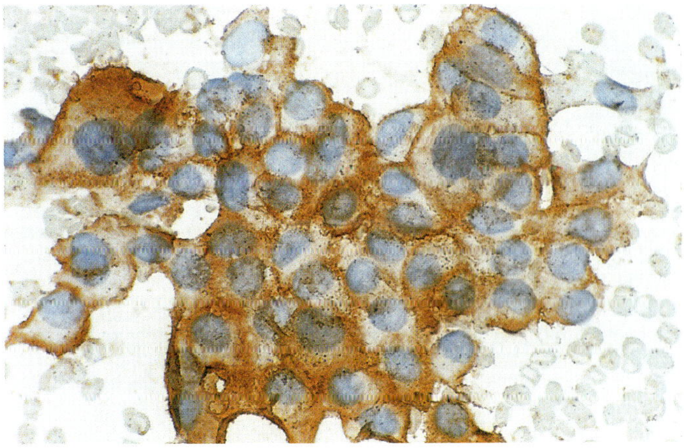

B

Figure 3.25 Papillary carcinoma, follicular variant. **A.** The smears of FVPTC reveal multi-layered microfollicles (rosettes), numerous nuclear grooves and inclusions in the follicular cells, very rare giant cells with absence of calcification and papillary clusters (MGG ×600 oil immersion). **B.** Positive immunostaining for HBME-1 on a thyroid FNAC is supportive evidence that the lesion is a carcinoma. A negative result for HBME-1 does not preclude the diagnosis of thyroid carcinoma. HBME-1 can be effectively applied to thyroid FNAC specimens and can be a valuable adjunct in the cytological diagnosis of thyroid malignancies.

pared to other thyroid disorders (multi-nodular goitre, follicular adenoma, Hürthle cell adenoma, pure thyroiditis, thyroiditis with nodular hyperplasia)[94]. Nuclear grooving, when seen in abundance, can be considered a reliable criterion for the diagnosis of papillary carcinoma. The presence of occasional grooves, however, should be regarded as a non-specific finding.[93] Grooved nuclei are somewhat difficult to recognise in the aspiration smears, although lobulated nuclei are identified easily. The latter are a significant feature in the diagnosis of papillary carcinoma. Ultrastructurally, grooved nuclei showed a deep, linear indentation of the nuclear membranes. Lobulated nuclei are characterised by multiple indentations that divide the nucleus into several lobules.[95] Cystic change may be present.[96] Multinucleate giant cells are frequently present in papillary carcinoma and follicular-variant papillary carcinoma. They are usually absent from follicular adenomas.[97]

Variants of papillary carcinoma

The *follicular variant* of papillary thyroid carcinoma presents significant diagnostic difficulty in FNAC.[98] Diagnoses by FNAC vary considerably and usually are categorised as 'follicular proliferations'[99] (Fig. 3.25). The smears of follicular-variant papillary thyroid carcinoma reveal numerous colloid balls in the background, multilayered microfollicles (rosettes), numerous nuclear grooves and inclusions in the monolayer sheets of follicular cells, very rare giant cells, absence of calcification and papillary clusters.[100] Nuclei are twice the size of red blood cells, have smooth contours, are hyperchromatic, and vary in shape but not much in size. Nuclear overlapping is common. Some nuclei have one small and almost pointed end, thereby resembling arrowheads. Although present, intranuclear inclusions, multinucleated histiocytes, and psammoma bodies are uncommon.[101,102] Marginal vacuoles may be seen in 50% of follicular-variant papillary carcinoma.[103] Cases of follicular adenoma, follicular carcinoma and adenomatous goitre share many of these features but notably lack inclusions and abundant nuclear grooves.[104] A careful microscopic search for nuclear grooves should be attempted in aspirates yielding a diagnosis of follicular neoplasia that could otherwise be indistinguishable from the follicular variant of papillary carcinoma of the thyroid.[105] Given the variable presence of characteristic nuclear features, in order to avoid a false-negative report, suspicion of a follicular-variant papillary thyroid carcinoma should be conveyed in the cytopathology report, which may prompt intraoperative assessment to avoid a second surgical intervention for completion thyroidectomy.[106] Follicular-variant, papillary carcinoma is a distinct cytological entity, different from other papillary carcinomas, in that it has a higher number of cases with acinar formation, tubular formation and marginal vacuoles and a lower number of cases with nuclear grooves. It also differs from follicular neoplasm with respect to papillary formation, tubular formation, intranuclear inclusions and nuclear grooves.[107]

The *macrofollicular variant* of papillary thyroid carcinoma is defined as a combination of numerous macrofollicles occupying 50% of the tumour and foci of the conventional follicular variant of papillary carcinoma.[108,109]

The *tall cell variant* of papillary carcinoma represents 8.5% of all papillary carcinomas. Tall cells are defined as cells with abundant eosinophilic, elongated cytoplasm; the height of these cells is at least twice their width and they have to constitute more than 30% of the tumour cell population (Fig. 3.26). They show round or oval tall columnar cells with basal nuclei with finely granular or stippled chromatin pattern (ground glass), pseudonuclear inclusions, small or inconspicuous nucleoli, nuclear grooves and abundant oxyphilic cytoplasm which can be vacuolated and has indistinct borders. Mitoses are seen. The identification of both tall cells and mitotic figures in the same smear is highly indicative of tall cell-variant of papillary carcinoma.[110] It is important to distinguish this tumour from the common thyroid papillary carcinoma because of its much more aggressive behaviour, from metastatic adenocarcinoma for obvious treatment considerations, medullary carcinoma and Hürthle cell papillary neoplasm of the thyroid.[111–118]

The *columnar cell variant* of papillary carcinoma thyroid is a rare and aggressive tumour composed of tall columnar cells that form papillae, glands and solid structures. FNAC smears show tall columnar cells in monolayered, three-dimensional, acinar and occasional papillary clusters. Nuclei are oval or elongated and monomorphic.[119] Nuclear pseudostratification, resembling that seen in respiratory epithelial cells, is present in some of the cell clusters.[117] Occasional cells show squamous or Hürthle cell metaplasia. Nuclear grooves and intranuclear cytoplasmic inclusions are not seen. Tall cell-variant papillary

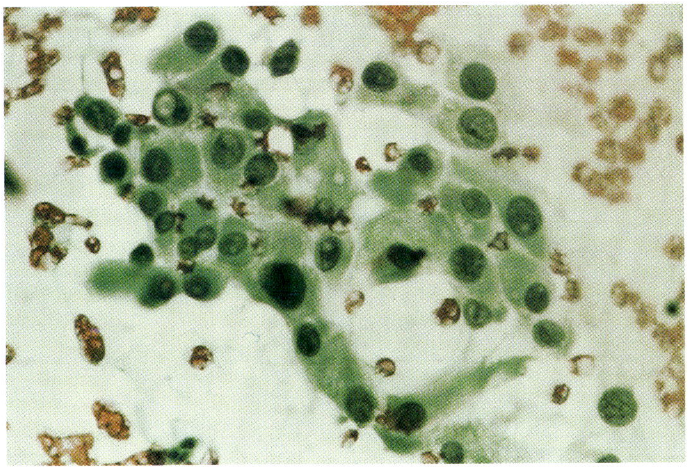

A

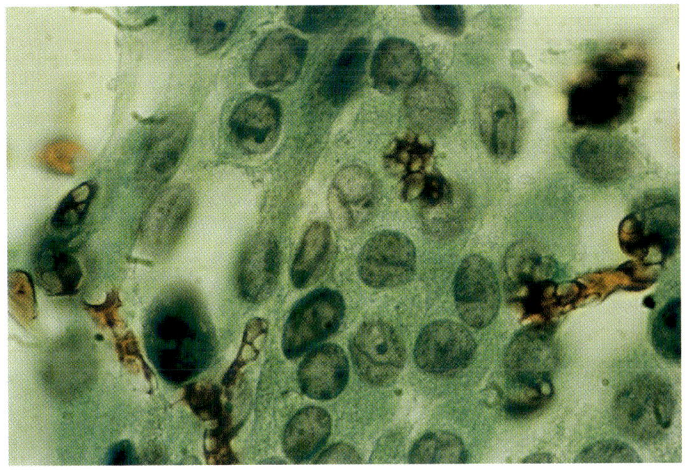

B

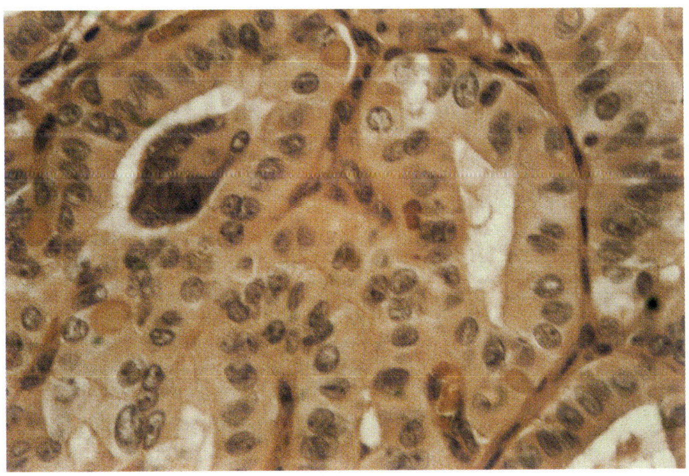

C

Figure 3.26 Papillary carcinoma, tall cell variant. **A.** 'Tall cells' are defined as cells with abundant eosinophilic, elongated cytoplasm; the height of these cells is twice their width or more, and they have to constitute more than 30% of the tumour cell population (PAP ×600 oil immersion.) **B.** They show round or oval tall columnar cells with basal nuclei with finely granular or stippled chromatin pattern (ground glass), pseudonuclear inclusions, small or inconspicuous nucleoli, nuclear grooves and abundant oxyphilic cytoplasm which can be vacuolated and has indistinct borders (PAP ×1000 oil immersion.) **C.** Histology of the tall cell variant of papillary carcinoma shows similar features to those seen in cytology (H&E ×400). (Courtesy of Dr R Dina)

carcinoma can be distinguished from the columnar cell variant by the oxyphilia of the tumour cells and the absence of nuclear pseudostratification. The differential diagnosis of the columnar cell variant includes medullary carcinoma of thyroid and metastatic adenocarcinoma (colorectal and endometrial adenocarcinomas).[117]

Only a few cases of the *oxyphil cell variant* of papillary thyroid carcinoma have been detailed cytologically.[120] Smears show scattered papillary groups and monolayered sheets. The large neoplastic cells have abundant granular cytoplasm and eccentrically placed nuclei (Fig. 3.27). Nuclear grooves and intranuclear inclusions are variably present. Psammoma bodies and colloid are not identified. Histologically, the tumours consist predominantly of oxyphilic cells arranged in papillary patterns and with nuclear features of usual papillary carcinoma. Oxyphil cell-variant papillary thyroid carcinoma can be diagnosed in smears composed predominantly of large oxyphilic cells but showing features associated with usual papillary carcinoma and can be cytologically distinguished from follicular oxyphilic tumours and usual papillary carcinoma.[120]

Papillary Hürthle cell carcinoma with lymphoplasmacytic stroma is a newly recognised variant of papillary carcinoma of the thyroid gland. FNAC findings yield cellular smears, mostly

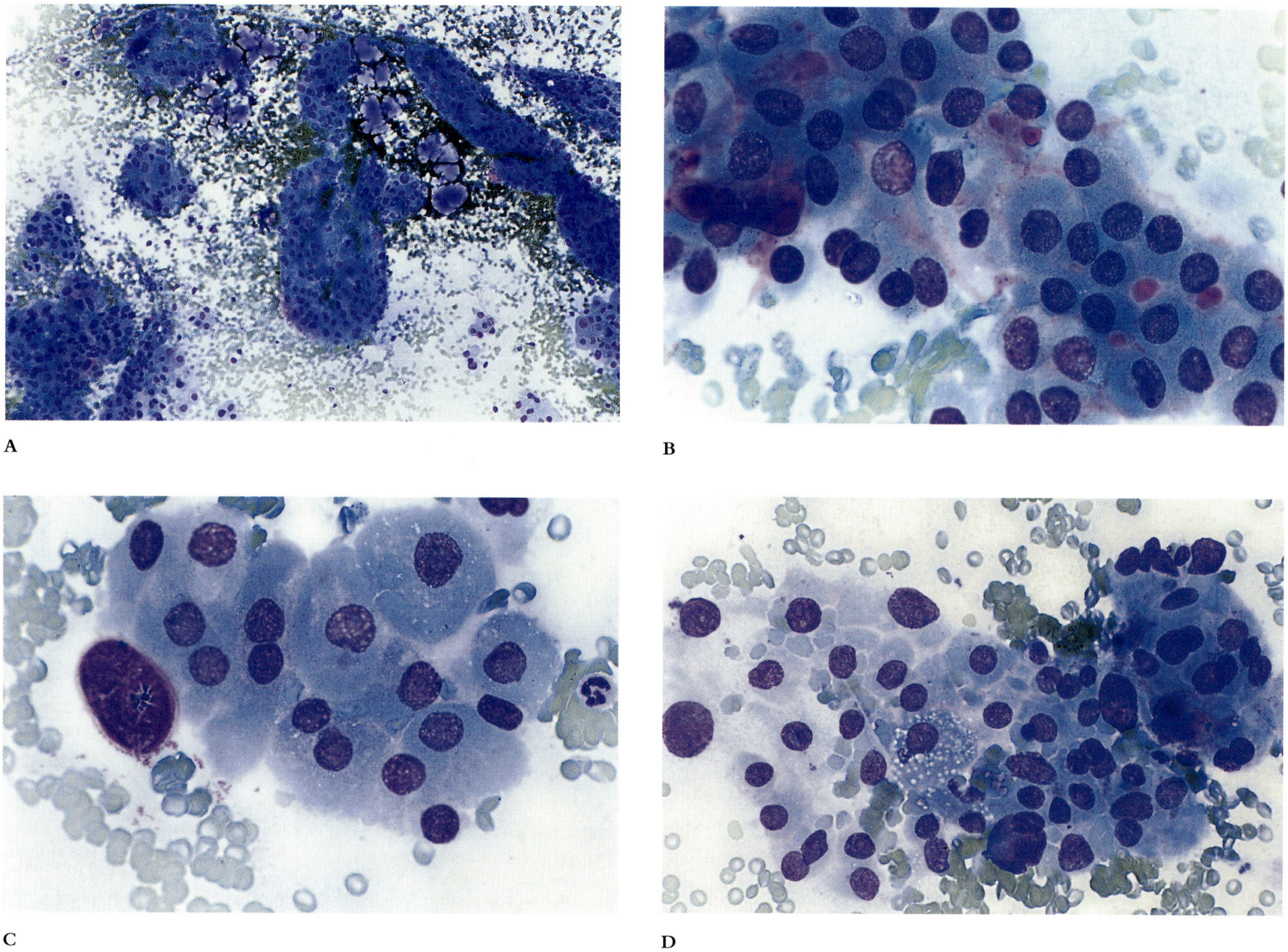

Figure 3.27 Papillary carcinoma, oxyphil cell variant. **A.** Smears show scattered papillary groups and monolayered sheets (MGG ×200). **B,C.** The large, neoplastic cells have abundant, granular cytoplasm and eccentrically placed nuclei. Intra- and extracellular eosinophillic granular material is present (MGG ×600, ×1000 oil immersion). **D.** Nuclear grooves and intranuclear inclusions are variably present. Psammoma bodies and colloid were not identified (MGG ×600 oil).

in large and small papillary clusters of Hürthle cells, with nuclear grooves and rare nuclear inclusions in a lymphoplasmacytic background. Isolated Hürthle cells and multinucleated giant cells are also seen. The presence of papillary clusters with nuclear features of papillary carcinoma and oxyphilic cytoplasm in a lymphoplasmacytic background should raise the diagnosis of Warthin-like tumour of the thyroid.[121,122]

The *diffuse sclerosing variant* of papillary carcinoma is characterised by diffuse involvement of one or both thyroid lobes showing histologically prominent sclerosis, an intense lymphocytic infiltrate, numerous psammoma bodies and squamous metaplasia together with the characteristic cytoarchitectural pattern of classical papillary carcinoma. A diagnosis of diffuse sclerosing-variant papillary carcinoma on FNAC should be considered when a combination of clinicocytological features consisting of numerous psammoma bodies, lymphocytes, squamous metaplasia and absence of stringy colloid are noted with otherwise typical cytoarchitectural features of papillary carcinoma obtained from diffusely nodular, firm thyroid enlargement.[123,124]

The presence of a prominent *nodular fasciitis-like stromal com-*

ponent may result in low-power microscopic appearances resembling fibroadenoma, phyllodes tumour, or fibrocystic disease of the breast. The carcinomatous component grows in the form of anastomosing narrow tubules, clustered glands and solid sheets with or without squamous differentiation and/or papillae, and exhibits the typical nuclear features of papillary thyroid carcinoma. The abundant stroma may have a nodular fasciitis-like quality and be composed of short fascicles of spindle cells separated by varying amounts of mucoid matrix, collagen and extravasated red blood cells; this is interpreted as an exuberant mesenchymal reaction to the carcinoma. The importance of recognising this variant of papillary thyroid carcinoma is that, when one encounters a fibroproliferative lesion of the thyroid, a diligent search should be made for papillary carcinoma. This variant also must be distinguished from the vastly more aggressive papillary carcinomas with anaplastic transformation and the so-called carcinosarcomas.[125–128] Epithelium of papillary carcinoma may occasionally assume spindle shape.[129]

When correlating cytological features and the different histological variants, Leung et al[130] noted that single cells, monolayers and papillary fragments were present in all the variants. The presence of follicles was not restricted to the follicular variant. Nuclear grooves and cytoplasmic pseudoinclusions were present in most of the cases, with nuclear grooves the most common finding in all the variants (92.3–100%). Psammoma bodies were an infrequent finding (0–25%) and were absent from the follicular variant. Colloid was present in all the variants and was a frequent finding in the follicular variant (84.6%). The findings suggest that the exact histological variant of papillary carcinoma cannot be predicted from the appearance of the fine needle aspirate.[130] The question of clinical relevance of histological subtypes of papillary carcinoma, in terms of prognosis, is still not resolved. At the moment, it would appear that histological grading (tumour size, nuclear atypia, necrosis, vascular invasion) , mitotic rate, S-phase and G(2) phase fractions are more important in determining prognosis than histological subtypes .

The molecular genetics of papillary carcinoma has grown in recent years. Flow cytometry has shown a correlation between the aneuploid DNA patterns and poor outcomes of PTC[140,141]. Several types of oncogene alterations have been described in PTC, including the ret/PTC rearrangement, tyrosine-receptor kynase rearrangement and N-ras point mutation[142]. To date, knowledge regarding the participation of special oncogenes in PTC has not led to novel prognostic indicators applicable to present clinical practice[143].

Immunocytochemistry. CD44 has been shown to be expressed selectively in thyroid papillary carcinoma. Of the 16 papillary carcinomas studied by Chhieng, 88% stained intensely for CD44 in a membranous pattern. Of the 14 non-papillary thyroid carcinoma cases, only 1 (7%), a Hürthle cell adenoma, featured membranous CD44 staining.[94]

The monoclonal antibody HBME-1, generated against the microvillous surface of mesothelial cells, has been shown to have significant reactivity in histological sections of follicular-derived thyroid malignancies. Sack et al[49] examined the diagnostic utility of HBME-1 in thyroid FNACs. The cell-block and direct-smear preparations were positive in 5 of 7 papillary carcinomas (1 follicular variant. HBME-1 can be applied effectively to thyroid FNAC specimens and can be a valuable adjunct in the cytological diagnosis of thyroid malignancies.[49]

CD57 (HNK-1) is an oligosaccharide antigen that is expressed by cells of several lineages. It is present on multipotential neuroepithelial cells during embryogenesis, and tumours of epithelial, neuroectodermal and nerve sheath origin also express CD57. Its role in the diagnosis of thyroid tumours is controversial. The follicular variant of papillary thyroid carcinoma is reported to show significantly higher CD57 expression than colloid nodules or follicular adenomas.[131]

The ribonucleoprotein telomerase has been documented in 67% of the papillary carcinomas with no positivity in benign nodules. The telomerase assay appears useful in the distinction of benign from malignant thyroid lesions that have FNAC suspicious for but not diagnostic of papillary carcinoma.[50]

Differential diagnosis of papillary carcinoma includes papillary proliferation in multinodular goitre and Hashimoto's thyroiditis where other features of papillary carcinoma are absent. Adenomatoid nodules with focal papillary hyperplasia where the presence of focal papillary aggregates, the presence of a psammoma body within a background of copious colloid and scattered follicular cells may lead to diagnostic confusion.[59] Papillary carcinoma may be cystic, causing diagnostic problems. In the follicular variant of papillary carcinoma nuclear vacuoles may suggest the appropriate diagnosis. If the appearance is predominantly of single tumour cells, the appearances can mimic a medullary carcinoma. A thymoma with a dominant epithelial component has to be considered in the differential diagnosis.[132] No single cytological feature should be used independently in the cytological diagnosis of thyroid lesions. Tumour cellularity and papillary tissue fragments should not be equated with neoplasia per se; all cytomorphological features should be evaluated.[133]

Follicular carcinoma

Follicular carcinoma is an infrequently occurring thyroid gland tumour and represents 15% of all thyroid gland carcinomas. It presents as a solitary swelling in the gland and is never seen as an occult tumour. The mean age of presentation is 50 years.

Histologically, it is a minimally invasive carcinoma, which is macroscopically encapsulated and microscopically has a follicular, trabecular and cribriform and/or solid growth pattern. The cytological features of papillary carcinoma are not seen. The morphological appearances may vary between monomorphic and pleomorphic. The tumour has to be differentiated from benign follicular proliferations such as follicular adenoma and adenomatous hyperplastic nodule. Criteria for diagnosis of malignancy are capsular and/or vascular invasion. Nuclear atypia, mitoses and necrosis are not features of malignancy in follicular tumours.

The prognosis of follicular carcinoma with minimal invasion is good (10-year survival 85%). In contrast to papillary carcinoma, follicular carcinoma metastasises haematogenously with a preference for lung and bone. Metastases are often better differentiated than the primary tumour, and may be detected and treated by radioactive iodine.

Hürthle cell-variant follicular carcinoma has a less favourable prognosis. The diagnosis of malignancy in Hürthle cell tumours has the same general diagnostic criteria as for ordinary follicular carcinoma (capsular and/or vascular invasion). Clear cell variant is designated by some as a separate entity and by others as a variant of Hürthle cell type. The insular variant is a poorly circumscribed small cell microfollicular carcinoma, which has an unfavourable prognosis.

Cytological features. A well-differentiated follicular carcinoma has the same appearance as a microfollicular adenoma: cellular, follicular groups, follicles that are irregular in form with nuclear overlap, occasionally single cells and little or no colloid (Fig. 3.28). If colloid is present, it is present in particles. In these cases the diagnosis of 'follicular proliferation' is appropriate. In follicular carcinoma, haemorrhage,

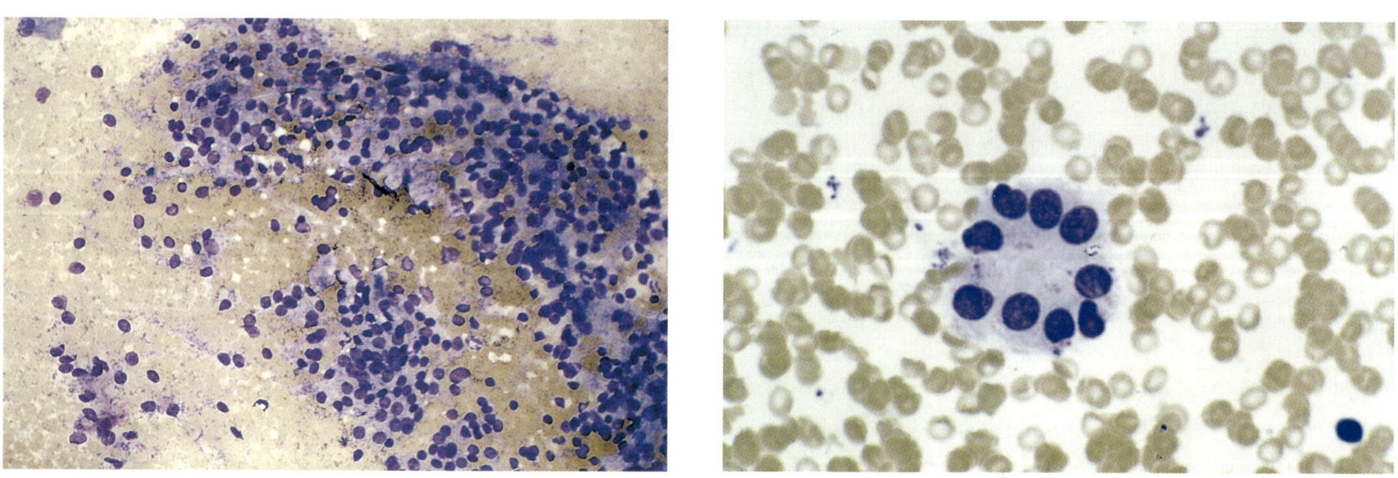

A B

Figure 3.28 Follicular carcinoma. **A,B.** Well-differentiated follicular carcinoma has the same appearance as a microfollicular adenoma: cellular, follicular groups, follicles that are irregular in form with nuclear overlap, occasionally single cells and little or no colloid (MGG ×200, ×600 oil).

necrosis and calcifications may be seen. If the cells have the appearance of clear cells than it is more likely that the tumour is a carcinoma than an adenoma. Clear cell carcinoma is fat-negative in contrast with metastases of renal cell carcinoma, with which it may be confused. In moderately or poorly differentiated follicular carcinoma with obvious nuclear atypia and nucleoli, the cytological diagnosis of malignancy is easy to make (Fig. 3.29). Oncocytic (Hürthle cell) adenoma cannot be differentiated from oncocytic carcinoma. These cells may show anisocytosis, anisonucleosis and large nucleoli whether they originate from Hashimoto's thyroiditis, oncocytic adenoma or carcinoma (Fig. 3.23). Pure oncocytic proliferations are indication for surgery.

The *insular variant* of follicular carcinoma shows high cellularity, with large sheets of tumour cells showing a microfollicular pattern or smaller sheets showing a solid or trabecular pattern, intermingled with predominantly single cells on a bloodstained background with very scanty colloid. Nuclear overlapping is constant. When present, the cytoplasm is poorly outlined. Nuclear hyperchromasia is always present, with coarsely or finely granular chromatin. The variation in nuclear shape and size is moderate, with small nucleoli and occasional mitoses. A papillary arrangement, with the presence of intranuclear cytoplasmic inclusions (vacuoles) and nuclear grooves, is also visible.[134–136]

Medullary carcinoma

Medullary carcinoma represents 4–5% of all thyroid carcinomas and arises from C-cells. The mean age at presentation is 50 years. In 10–20% of cases this type of carcinoma is familial when it can present at a younger age. The tumour is often multicentric and associated with tumours in other endocrine organs, as part of the multiple endocrine neoplasia (MEN) syndrome.

Histologically, the commonest type of medullary carcinoma has a monomorphic, small epithelial (plasmacytoid/carcinoid like) or spindle cell type and a solid or trabecular growth pattern with hyaline stroma containing amyloid present between the epithelial islands. There are variations in growth pattern (papillary, glandular), in cell type (giant cell, small cell) and histochemical variants (mucin producing, melanin containing without amyloid). All these variants are classified as medullary carcinoma on the basis of positive staining for calcitonin. The 10-year survival rate for

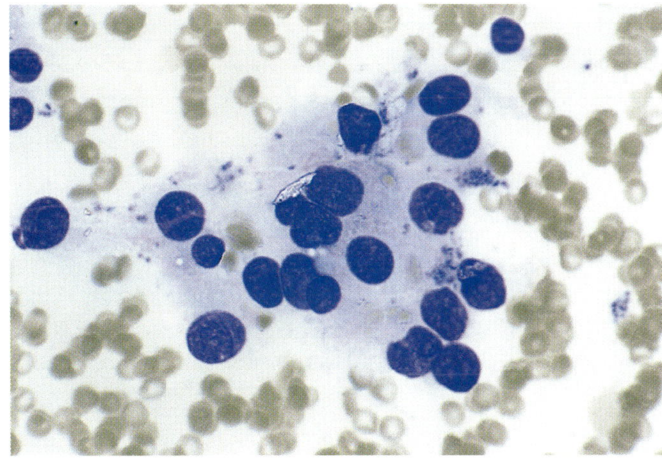

A

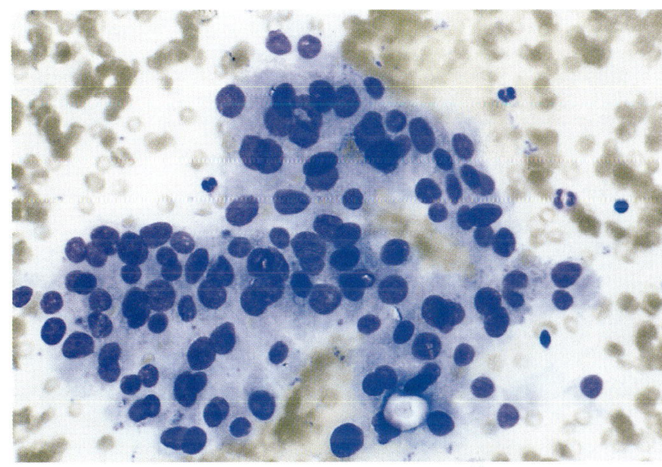

B

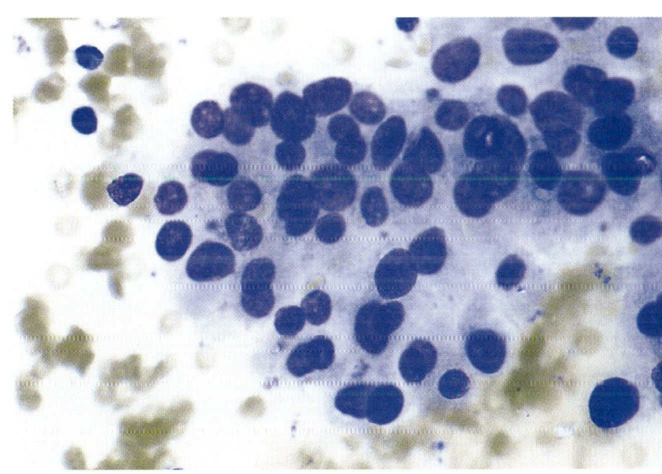

C

Figure 3.29 Follicular carcinoma. **A,B,C**. In moderately or poorly differentiated follicular carcinoma with obvious nuclear atypia and nucleoli, the cytological diagnosis of malignancy is easy to make (MGG ×600, ×400, ×600 oil).

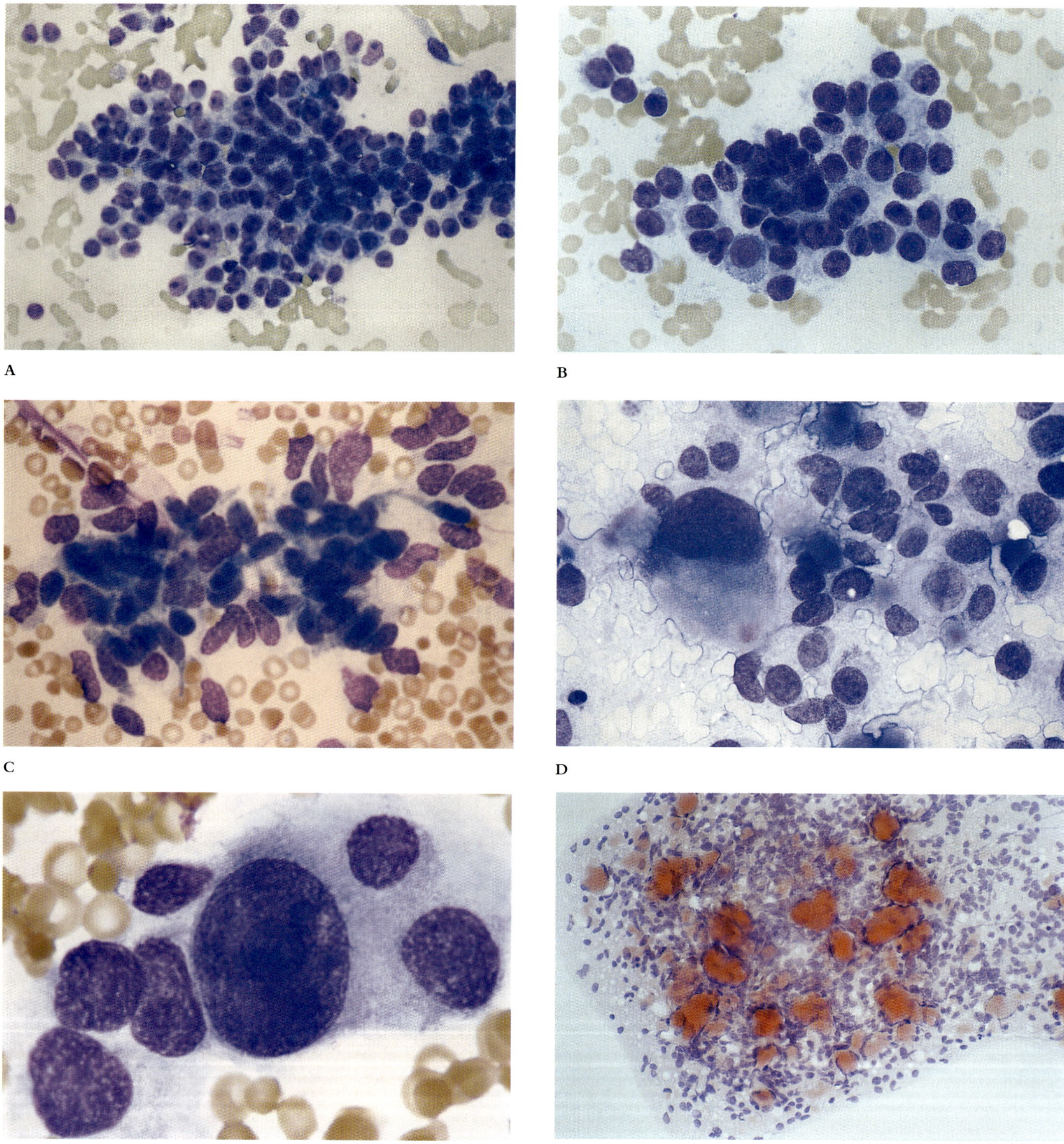

Figure 3.30 Medullary carcinoma. **A.** Cellular aspirates usually contain single cells but may have cell aggregates (MGG ×400). **B.** The cells may be small and round, **C.** elongated or **D,E.** pleomorphic, depending on the type of medullary carcinoma (MGG ×600 oil). The cytoplasm may have fine red granulation which may also be seen in follicular carcinoma. Occasional cells are binucleate or multinucleate with pleomorphic nuclei. **F.** Intracellular and extracellular amyloid may be seen. In MGG-stained preparations it is blue/violet and is congo red positive (congo red ×200).

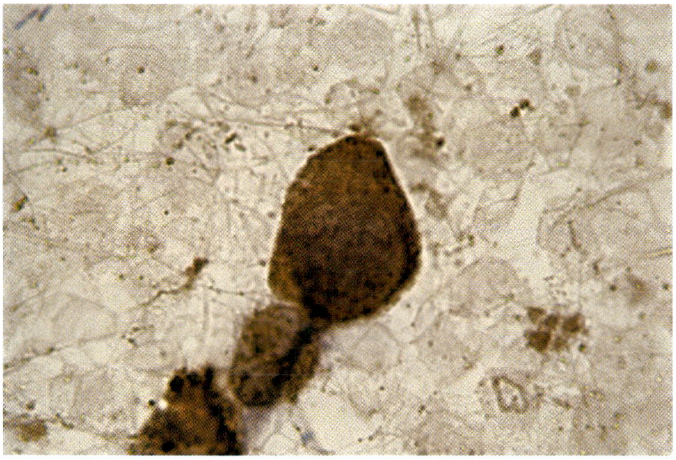

G

Figure 3.30 (*continued*). G. Tumour cells are positive for calcitonin (anticalcitonin, IP ×1000 oil).

medullary carcinoma is 50%. Among patients without initial distant metastatic involvement and with complete resection of the tumour, 20-year survival free of distant metastatic lesions is 81%. Overall 10- and 20-year survival rates are 63% and 44% respectively.[137]

A preoperative diagnosis of medullary carcinoma of the thyroid allows for the investigation of associated Multiple Endocrine Neoplasia and planning of definitive surgery without the need for frozen section. Criteria for cytodiagnosis are well known but variable patterns of presentation may cause diagnostic difficulty. Although correct diagnosis is made by cytology in the majority of instances, other tumours may show cytological findings similar to medullary carcinoma. Electron microscopy (EM) of FNAC material was found to be the most definitive method of proving or excluding medullary carcinoma of the thyroid. Immunocytochemistry may be misleading for rarely performed tests.[138,139]

Cytological features. Cellular aspirates usually contain single cells but may have cell aggregates. The cells may be small and round, elongated or pleomorphic, depending on the type of medullary carcinoma (Fig. 3.30). Nuclei are oval and eccentric. There are prominent nucleoli. Triangular shaped cells are characteristic. The cytoplasm may have fine red granulation, which may also be seen in follicular carcinoma and metastases of breast carcinoma. Occasional cells are binucleate or multinucleate with pleomorphic nuclei. Nuclear vacuoles may be seen. Intracellular and extracellular amyloid may be seen. In MGG-stained preparations it is blue/violet and is congo red positive.[140–144]

Medullary carcinoma can be easily recognised as malignant on FNAC. Immunocytochemically, tumour cells react with keratin, calcitonin and chromogranin. Thyroglobulin is usually negative. Grimelius staining is positive.

C-cell hyperplasia can mimic medullary carcinoma biochemically. The possible role of FNAC to distinguish between the two is in patients with elevated serum calcitonin and absence of a discrete thyroid nodule. The finding of clusters of calcitonin-positive cells intermixed with normal follicular cells by fine needle aspiration may provide a means of making a presurgical diagnosis of C-cell hyperplasia.[145]

Anaplastic carcinoma

Anaplastic carcinoma of the thyroid is one of the most aggressive tumour types in humans. Histologically it is composed of pleomorphic large cells, often partly spindle celled (pseudosarcomatous) and/or giant cells (often with numerous osteoclast-type giant cells). It presents in an older age group (usually over 60 years) as a rapidly progressive, indurated, asymmetric swelling, which may arise in a longstanding goitre or be associated with a variety of more well-differentiated thyroid carcinomas.[126,146,147] It may cause dyspnoea due to tracheal compression. Nearly all patients die shortly after the diagnosis is made due to local tumour extension.

Cytological features. FNAC smears from anaplastic carcinoma are usually cellular with abundant cell dissociation (Fig. 3.31). In the largest series of anaplastic carcinomas, Us-Krasovec et al[148] described 3 different cell patterns: (1) pleomorphic cell; (2) round cell; and (3) spindle cell.[148,149] Cytomorphological features of anaplastic carcinoma are highly specific and easy to recognise.

Due to the simple technique and high diagnostic accuracy, FNAC is the method of choice in patients with anaplastic carcinoma. There are often large nucleoli, abundant mitoses, necrosis and occasionally numerous neutrophils. Leukophagocytosis may be seen in tumour cells, osteoclast-type giant cells and rarely sqamous type differentiation. In difficult cases of anaplastic carcinoma, differential diagnoses

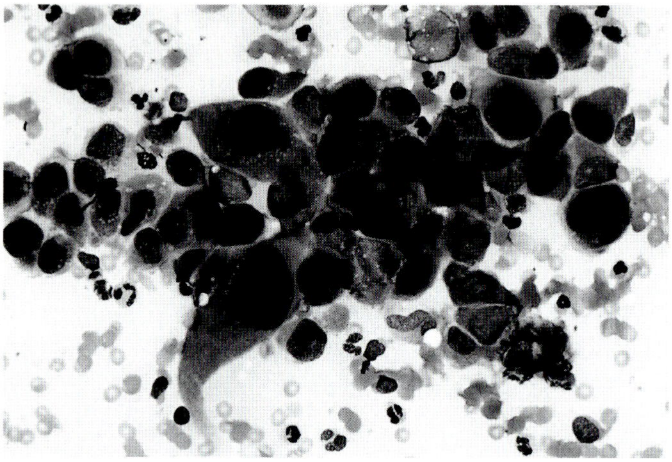

A

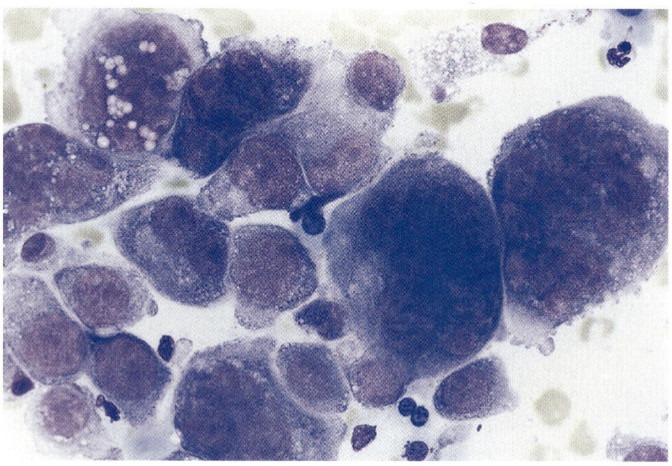

B

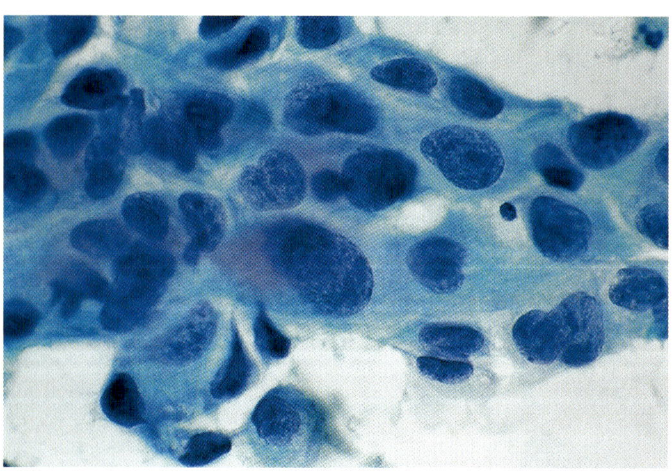

C

Figure 3.31 Anaplastic carcinoma. **A.** Smears from anaplastic carcinoma are usually cellular with abundant cell dissociation (MGG ×600 oil). **B.** There are often large nucleoli, abundant mitoses, necrosis and occasionally numerous neutrophils (MGG ×1000 oil). **C.** Rarely, squamous type differentiation may be seen (PAP ×1000 oil).

may be sarcoma or lymphoma. Immunocytochemistry is essential to distinguish this type of tumour. Anaplastic carcinoma may be cytokeratin negative and vimentin positive.

Differential diagnosis of anaplastic carcinoma also includes active fibroblasts and histiocytes in granulomatous inflammation, regressive changes in follicular epithelial cells, particularly after I-131 treatment (Fig. 3.12), medullary carcinoma, metastases of a poorly differentiated carcinoma, e.g. squamous cell carcinoma and purulent thyroiditis.

The main reasons for inadequate or non-representative FNAC sampling are: (1) tumour regressive changes (necrosis, haemorrhage, leukocytic infiltration); (2) extensive tumour fibrosis; and (3) distinct differentiated and anaplastic patterns in the same tumour.[148]

Thyroid lymphoma

Thyroid lymphomas are rare and almost always arise in the background of chronic lymphocytic thyroiditis (Hashimoto's thyroiditis) (Fig. 3.32).[150–153] They occur predominantly in elderly females. Most patients have a short history of an enlarging thyroid or a neck mass causing tracheal compression (Fig. 3.32a).[154] The conventional approach to treatment is a combination of radiation therapy and multiagent chemotherapy. There is no significant role for extirpative surgery in the management of thyroid lymphoma.[155] The prognosis of localised tumours (stage IE, Ann Arbor classification) is excellent. Extrathyroidal involvement (stage IIE–IVE) reduces the 5-year survival rate to about 70%, provided that current therapy regimens are respected.[150] Thyroid lymphoma may represent a neoplasm of mucosa-associated lymphoid tissue (MALT).[156] Large cell lymphoma is an aggressive disease and usually is not a significant diagnostic challenge from the pathological point of view. Small cell lymphoma, however, can sometimes be difficult to distinguish from chronic lymphocytic thyroiditis. In the past, most thyroid lymphomas were considered to be of follicle centre cell origin. Today, after the introduction of the MALT and the extranodal lymphoid tissue (ELT) concepts, most of the lymphomas in the extranodal sites are thought to originate from the marginal zone of the lymphoid follicles. The distinction between the different types of lymphomas has significant impact on the patient's prognosis, treatment and follow-up.[157–159] It is imperative that clinicians (endocrinologists and surgeons)

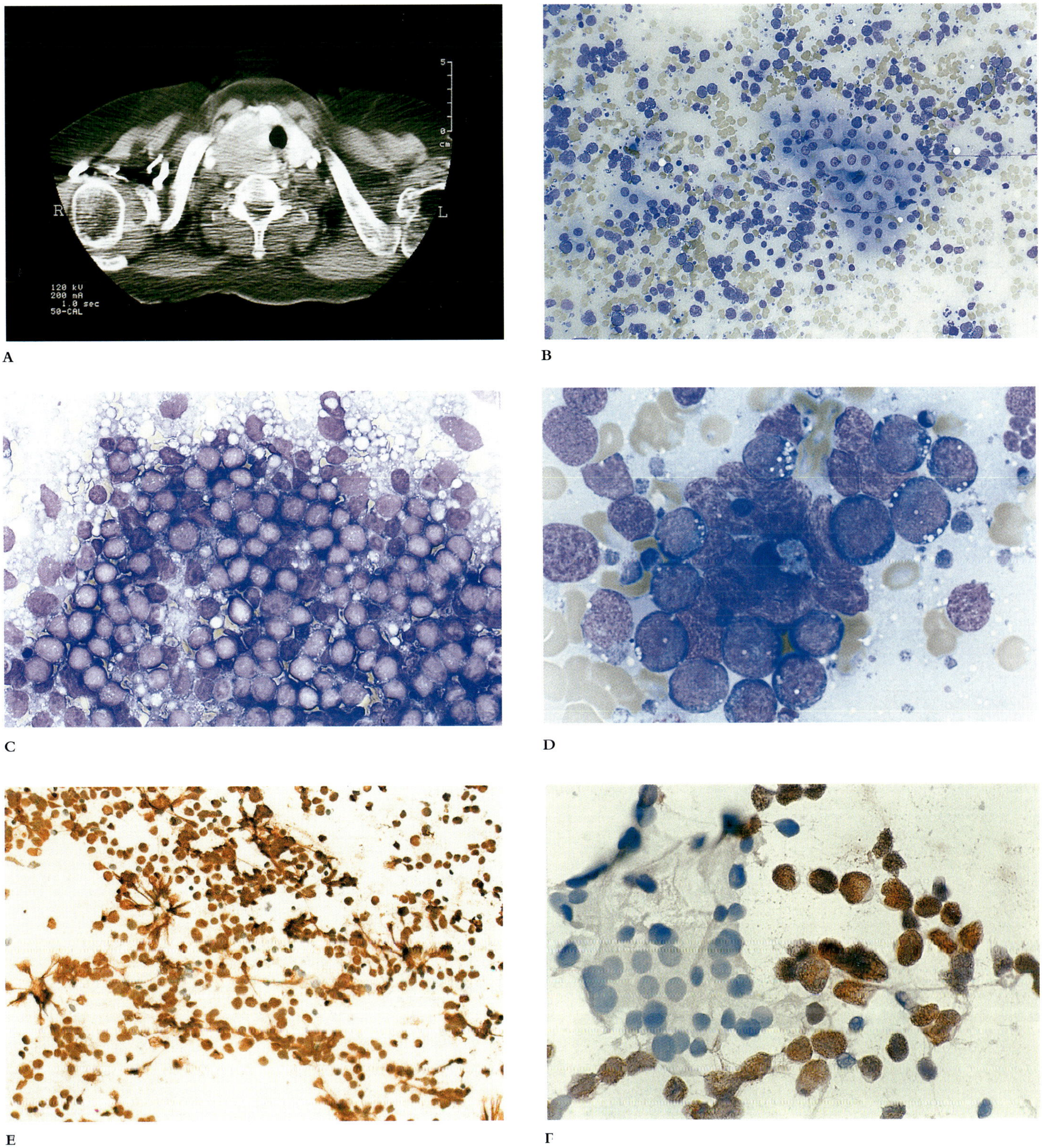

Figure 3.32 Thyroid lymphoma. **A.** CT scan of the neck in a 75-year-old patient with mass in the neck and deviation of trachea. **B.** Island of thyroid epithelium showing oncocytic change, surrounded by numerous lymphoid cells with predominance of blasts (MGG ×400). **C,D.** Lymphoid cells have a thin rim of basophilic cytoplasm and intracytoplasmic vacuolation (MGG ×600, ×1000, oil immersion). **E.** Proliferation marker (Ki-67) shows all lymphoid cells to be in cycle and epithelium negative (MIB 1, IP ×400, ×600, oil immersion).

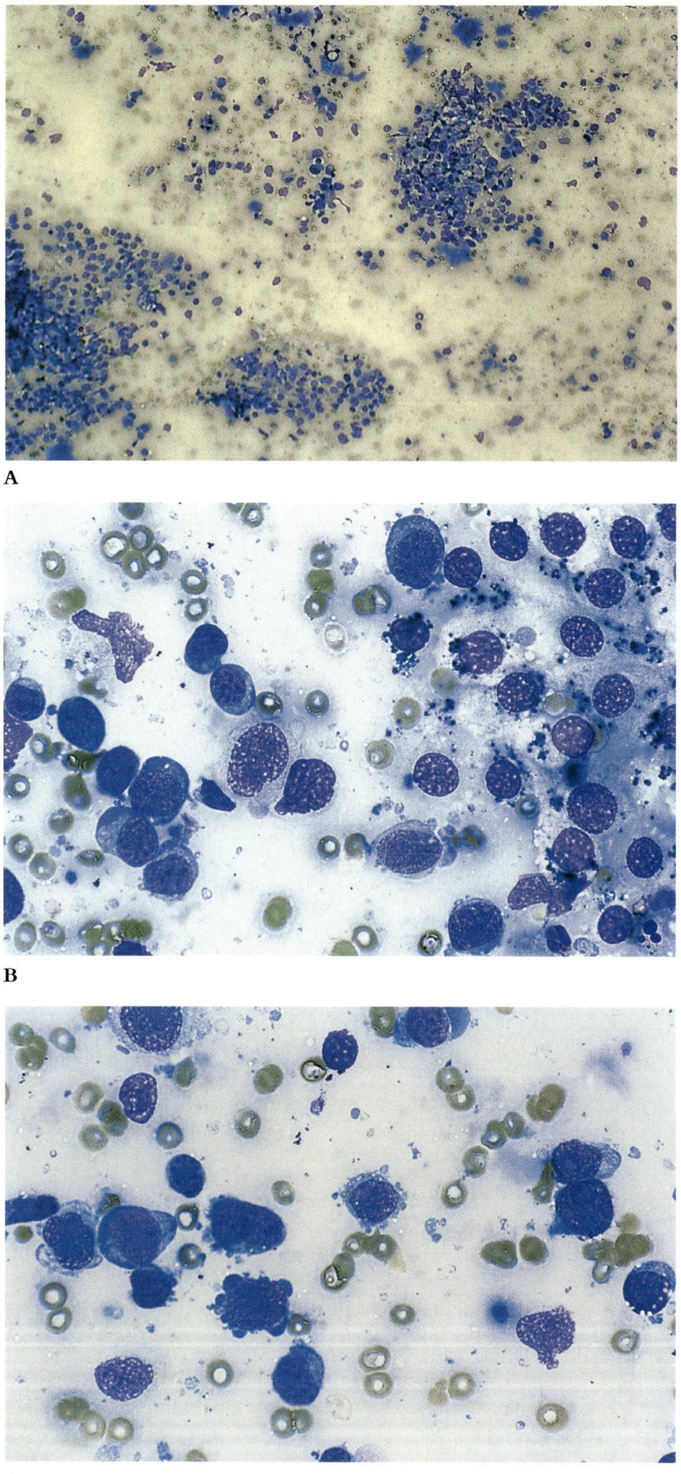

Figure 3.33 Post-transplant lymphadenopathy. Thyroid may be the site of this lymphoproliferative disorder (see chapter 4). **A.** Low power view shows islands of thyroid epithelium and lymphoid cells in the background (MGG ×200). **B.** Lymphoid cells range from mature lymphocytes to plasma cells but also include atypical immunoblast-type cells (MGG ×600, oil immersion). **C.** Detail of atypical lymphoid infiltrate. As discussed in chapter 4, the morphology is not adequate for establishing the presence or absence of lymphoma. Condition is potentially reversible after withdrawal of immunosuppression (MGG ×600).

and pathologists are aware of these types of lymphomas for the most appropriate diagnostic procedures to be selected, specific staging principles to be applied and appropriate disease-specific treatment to be implemented (see Chapter 4).[160–164]

In addition to morphological evaluation performed on direct smears, immunophenotyping, flow cytometry and molecular studies can be performed on the aspirated material. These additional studies make a clear distinction between lymphoma and Hashimoto's thyroiditis, which may present a similar cytological picture.[165,166]

Diagnostic pitfalls include anaplastic carcinoma of the small-cell type, chronic thyroiditis[167,168] and post-transplant lymphadenopathy disorder (PTLS) (see p. 143) (Fig. 3.33).

METASTATIC TUMOURS IN THYROID

Metastases may simulate primary malignant tumours of the thyroid, causing problems in the diagnosis and management of patients with a history of carcinoma. Chacho et al found that during a 7-year period 1.5% of thyroid FNAC contained metastatic carcinoma.[169] The primary sites of origin are most commonly breast, kidney, colon and stomach as well as lymphoma. The cytological features in the FNAC material are characteristic of the primary tumours. It is of critical importance that primary thyroid neoplasms occurring in patients known to have primary tumours elsewhere be distinguished from disseminated tumours involving the thyroid. Fine needle aspiration is of considerable value in this differential diagnosis. Needle aspirates of the thyroid are also of value in leading to the diagnosis of unsuspected non-thyroidal primary cancer.[170,171]

REFERENCES

1. Gharib H. Changing concepts in the diagnosis and management of thyroid nodules. *Endocrinol Metab Clin North Am* 1997; 26(4): 777–800.
2. Gharib H, Goellner JR. Fine-needle aspiration biopsy of the thyroid: an appraisal [see comments]. *Ann Intern Med* 1993; 118(4): 282–9.
3. Frable WJ. The treatment of thyroid cancer. The role of fine-needle aspiration cytology. *Arch Otolaryngol Head Neck Surg* 1986; 112(11): 1200–3.
4. Tambouret R, Szyfelbein WM, Pitman MB. Ultrasound-guided fine-needle aspiration biopsy of the thyroid. *Cancer* 1999; 87(5): 299–305.

5. Takashima S, Fukuda H, Kobayashi T. Thyroid nodules: clinical effect of ultrasound-guided fine-needle aspiration biopsy. *J Clin Ultrasound* 1994; 22(9): 535–42.

6. Shen PU, Kuhel WI, Yang GC, Hoda SA. Intraoperative touch-imprint cytological diagnosis of follicular variant of papillary thyroid carcinoma [letter]. *Diagn Cytopathol* 1997; 17(1): 80–3.

7. Tworek JA, Giordano TJ, Michael CW. Comparison of intraoperative cytology with frozen sections in the diagnosis of thyroid lesions. *Am J Clin Pathol* 1998; 110(4): 456–61.

8. Frankel KA. Correspondence re: Basolo F, Baloch ZW, Baldanzi A, Miccolo P, Livolsi VA. Usefulness of ultrafast Papanicolaou-stained scrape preparations in intraoperative management of thyroid lesions. [letter] *Mod Pathol* 1999; 12: 653–7. *Mod Pathol* 2000; 13(2): 210–1.

9. Cap J, Ryska A, Rehorkova P, Hovorkova E, Kerekes Z, Pohnetalova D. Sensitivity and specificity of the fine needle aspiration biopsy of the thyroid: clinical point of view. *Clin Endocrinol (Oxf)* 1999; 51(4): 509–15.

10. Altavilla G, Pascale M, Nenci I. Fine needle aspiration cytology of thyroid gland diseases. *Acta Cytol* 1990; 34(2): 251–6.

10a. Hundahl SA, Cady B, Cunningham MP, Mazzafem E, McKee RF et al. Initial results from a prospective cohort study of 5583 cases of thyroid treated in the United States during 1996. U.S. and German Thyroid Cancer Group. An American College of Surgeons Commission on Cancer Patient Evaluation Study. *Cancer* 2000; 89(1): 202–17.

11. Hawkins F, Bellido D, Bernal C et al. Fine needle aspiration biopsy in the diagnosis of thyroid cancer and thyroid disease. *Cancer* 1987; 59(6): 1206–9.

12. Hussain ST, Beeby I, Missan A, Buxton-Thomas MS. Use of fine needle aspiration cytology in the management of the solitary cold thyroid nodule. *Nucl Med Commun* 1993; 14(4): 335–8.

13. Merchant WJ, Thomas SM, Coppen MJ, Prentice MG. The role of thyroid fine needle aspiration (FNA) cytology in a district general hospital setting. *Cytopathology* 1995; 6(6): 409–18.

14. Franc B, Allory Y, Hejblum G. [Cytopuncture in tumors of the thyroid]. *Rev Prat* 1996; 46(19): 2315–20.

15. Dwarakanathan AA, Ryan WG, Staren ED, Martirano M, Economou SG. Fine-needle aspiration biopsy of the thyroid. Diagnostic accuracy when performing a moderate number of such procedures. *Arch Intern Med* 1989; 149(9): 2007–9.

16. Anderson JB, Webb AJ. Fine-needle aspiration biopsy and the diagnosis of thyroid cancer. *Br J Surg* 1987; 74(4): 292–6.

17. Bultrago Ramirez F, Saenz de Santamaria Morales J, Moreno Casado J. [Cytological diagnosis of thyroid nodules by fine needle aspiration. A study of 385 cases from primary care]. *Aten Primaria* 1989; 6(10): 714–8.

18. Guimaraes EM, Morais DM, Da Silva SJ, Cremonini NC. The impact of fine needle aspiration biopsy: diagnostic accuracy study. *Rev Assoc Med Bras* 1996; 42(1): 2–6.

19. Moisson-Meer A, Franc B, Duprey J et al. Reliability of needle biopsy of solitary thyroid nodules in view of surgical indications. *Rev Med Interne* 1996; 17(9): 732–7.

20. Klemi PJ, Joensuu H, Nylamo E. Fine needle aspiration biopsy in the diagnosis of thyroid nodules. *Acta Cytol* 1991; 35(4): 434–8.

21. Perez JA, Pisano R, Kinast C, Valencia V, Araneda M, Mera ME. Needle aspiration cytology in euthyroid uninodular goiter. *Rev Med Chil* 1991; 119(2): 158–63.

22. Akerman M, Tennvall J, Biorklund A, Martensson H, Moller T. Sensitivity and specificity of fine needle aspiration cytology in the diagnosis of tumors of the thyroid gland. *Acta Cytol* 1985; 29(5): 850–5.

23. Layfield LJ, Reichman A, Bottles K, Giuliano A. Clinical determinants for the management of thyroid nodules by fine-needle aspiration cytology. *Arch Otolaryngol Head Neck Surg* 1992; 118(7): 717–21.

24. Baloch ZW, Sack MJ, Yu GH, Livolsi VA, Gupta PK. Fine-needle aspiration of thyroid: an institutional experience. *Thyroid* 1998; 8(7): 565–9.

25. Cusick EL, MacIntosh CA, Krukowski ZH, Williams VM, Ewen SW, Matheson NA. Management of isolated thyroid swellings: a prospective six year study of fine needle aspiration cytology in diagnosis. *BMJ* 1990; 301(6747): 318–21.

26. Godinho-Matos L, Kocjan G, Kurtz A. Contribution of fine needle aspiration cytology to diagnosis and management of thyroid disease. *J Clin Pathol* 1992; 45(5): 391–5.

27. Castro MR, Gharib H. Thyroid nodules and cancer. When to wait and watch, when to refer. *Postgrad Med* 2000; 107(1): 113–6, 119–20, 123–4.

28. Tyler DS, Winchester DJ, Caraway NP, Hickey RC, Evans DB. Indeterminate fine-needle aspiration biopsy of the thyroid: identification of subgroups at high risk for invasive carcinoma. *Surgery* 1994; 116(6): 1054–60.

29. Gagneten CB, Roccatagliata G, Lowenstein A, Soto F, Soto R. The role of fine needle aspiration biopsy cytology in the evaluation of the clinically solitary thyroid nodule. *Acta Cytol* 1987; 31(5): 595–8.

30. Behnia M, Gharib H. Primary care diagnosis of thyroid disease. *Hosp Pract (Off Ed)* 1996; 31(6): 121–6, 131–4.

31. Khurana KK, Labrador E, Izquierdo R, Mesonero CE, Pisharodi LR. The role of fine-needle aspiration biopsy in the management of thyroid nodules in children, adolescents, and young adults: a multi-institutional study. *Thyroid* 1999; 9(4): 383–6.

32. Gharib H, Goellner JR, Johnson DA. Fine-needle aspiration cytology of the thyroid. A 12-year experience with 11,000 biopsies. *Clin Lab Med* 1993; 13(3): 699–709.

33. Harach HR. Usefulness of fine needle aspiration of the thyroid in an endemic goiter region. *Acta Cytol* 1989; 33(1): 31–5.

34. Gharib H. Fine-needle aspiration biopsy of thyroid nodules: advantages, limitations, and effect. *Mayo Clin Proc* 1994; 69(1): 44–9.

35. Schlinkert RT, van Heerden JA, Goellner JR et al. Factors that predict malignant thyroid lesions when fine-needle aspiration is 'suspicious for follicular neoplasm'. *Mayo Clin Proc* 1997; 72(10): 913–6.

36. Chadwick DR, Harrison BJ. The role of fine-needle aspiration cytology and frozen section histology in management of differentiated thyroid cancer: the UK experience. *Langenbecks Arch Surg* 1998; 383(2): 164–6.

37. Bugis SP, Young JE, Archibald SD, Chen VS. Diagnostic accuracy of fine-needle aspiration biopsy versus frozen section in solitary thyroid nodules. *Am J Surg* 1986; 152(4): 411–6.

38. Schmid KW, Ladurner D, Zechmann W, Feichtinger H. Clinicopathologic management of tumors of the thyroid gland in an endemic goiter area. Combined use of preoperative fine needle aspiration biopsy and intraoperative frozen section. *Acta Cytol* 1989; 33(1): 27–30.

39. Mulcahy MM, Cohen JI, Anderson PE, Ditamasso J, Schmidt W. Relative accuracy of fine-needle aspiration and frozen section in the diagnosis of well-differentiated thyroid cancer. *Laryngoscope* 1998; 108(4 pt 1): 494–6.

40. Kopald KH, Layfield LJ, Mohrmann R, Foshag LJ, Giuliano AE. Clarifying the role of fine-needle aspiration cytologic evaluation and frozen section examination in the operative management of thyroid cancer. *Arch Surg* 1989; 124(10): 1201–4, discussion 1204–5.

41. McHenry CR, Rosen IB, Walfish PG, Bedard Y. Influence of fine-needle aspiration biopsy and frozen section examination on the management of thyroid cancer. *Am J Surg* 1993; 166(4): 353–6.

42. Hamming JF, Vriens MR, Goslings BM, Songun I, Fleuren GJ, van de Velde CJ. Role of fine-needle aspiration biopsy and frozen section examination in determining the extent of thyroidectomy. *World J Surg* 1998; 22(6): 575–9, discussion 579–80.

43. Aguilar-Diosdado M, Contreras A, Gavilan I et al. Thyroid nodules. Role of fine needle aspiration and intraoperative frozen section examination. *Acta Cytol* 1997; 41(3): 677–82.

44. Boyd LA, Earnhardt RC, Dunn JT, Frierson HF, Hanks JB. Preoperative evaluation and predictive value of fine-needle aspiration and frozen section of thyroid nodules. *J Am Coll Surg* 1998; 187(5): 494–502.

45. Morosini PP, Mancini V, Filipponi S et al. [Comparison between the diagnostic accuracy in diagnosis of thyroid nodules with fine needle biopsy and intraoperative histological evaluation of frozen tissue]. *Minerva Endocrinol* 1997; 22(1): 1–5.

46. Chen H, Zeiger MA, Clark DP, Westra WH, Udelsman R. Papillary carcinoma of the thyroid: can operative management be based solely on fine-needle aspiration? *J Am Coll Surg* 1997; 184(6): 605–10.

47. Davoudi MM, Yeh KA, Wei JP. Utility of fine-needle aspiration cytology and frozen-section examination in the operative management of thyroid nodules. *Am Surg* 1997; 63(12): 1084–9, discussion 1089–90.

48. Ross JS, del Rosario AD, Sanderson B, Bui HX. Selective expression of CD44 cell-adhesion molecule in thyroid papillary carcinoma fine-needle aspirates. *Diagn Cytopathol* 1996; 14(4): 287–91.

49. Sack MJ, Astengo-Osuna C, Lin BT, Battifora H, LiVolsi VA. HBME-1 immunostaining in thyroid fine-needle aspirations: a useful marker in the diagnosis of carcinoma. *Mod Pathol* 1997; 10(7): 668–74.

50. Saji M, Westra WH, Chen H et al. Telomerase activity in the differential diagnosis of papillary carcinoma of the thyroid. *Surgery* 1997; 122(6): 1137–40.

51. Hales MS, Hsu FS. Needle tract implantation of papillary carcinoma of the thyroid following aspiration biopsy. *Acta Cytol* 1990; 34(6): 801–4.

52. Lopez JI, Pereda E, Rodil MA, Fernandez-Larrinoa A. Histological changes mimicking papillary carcinoma following fine needle aspiration of the thyroid gland. *Arch Anat Cytol Pathol* 1996; 44(2–3): 98–100.

53. Layfield LJ, Lones MA. Necrosis in thyroid nodules after fine needle aspiration biopsy. Report of two cases. *Acta Cytol* 1991; 35(4): 427–30.

54. Hurley DL, Gharib H. Evaluation and management of multinodular goiter. *Otolaryngol Clin North Am* 1996; 29(4): 527–40.

55. Lucas A, Llatjos M, Salinas I, Reverter J, Pizarro E, Sanmarti A. Fine-needle aspiration cytology of benign nodular thyroid disease. Value of re-aspiration. *Eur J Endocrinol* 1995; 132(6): 677–80.

56. Franklyn JA, Daykin J, Young J, Oates GD, Sheppard MC. Fine needle aspiration cytology in diffuse or multinodular goitre compared with solitary thyroid nodules. *BMJ* 1993; 307(6898): 240.

57. Cooper DS, Tiamson E, Ladenson PW. Psammoma bodies in fine needle aspiration biopsies of benign thyroid nodules. *Thyroidology* 1988; (1): 55–9.

58. Riazmontazer N, Bedayat G. Psammoma bodies in fine needle aspirates from thyroids containing nontoxic hyperplastic nodular goiters. *Acta Cytol* 1991; 35(5): 563–6.

59. Fiorella RM, Isley W, Miller LK, Kragel PJ. Multinodular goiter of the thyroid mimicking malignancy: diagnostic pitfalls in fine-needle aspiration biopsy. *Diagn Cytopathol* 1993; 9(3): 351–5, discussion 355–7.

60. Jayaram G, Singh B, Marwaha RK. Grave's disease. Appearance in cytologic smears from fine needle aspirates of the thyroid gland. *Acta Cytol* 1989; 33(1): 36–40.

61. Deshpande V, Kapila K, Sai KS, Verma K. Follicular neoplasms of the thyroid. Decision tree approach using morphologic and morphometric parameters. *Acta Cytol* 1997; 41(2): 369–76.

62. Shabb NS, Tawil A, Gergeos F, Saleh M, Azar S. Multinucleated giant cells in fine-needle aspiration of thyroid nodules: their diagnostic significance. *Diagn Cytopathol* 1999; 21(5): 307–12.

63. Luca IC, Zamfir C. Fine-needle biopsy cytology in autoimmune thyroiditis [in process citation]. *Rev Med Chir Soc Med Nat Iasi* 1998; 102(3–4): 150–1.

64. Nguyen GK, Ginsberg J, Crockford PM, Villanueva RR. Hashimoto's thyroiditis: cytodiagnostic accuracy and pitfalls. *Diagn Cytopathol* 1997; 16(6): 531–6.

65. Kumarasinghe MP, De Silva S. Pitfalls in cytological diagnosis of autoimmune thyroiditis. *Pathology* 1999; 31(1): 1–7.

66. MacDonald L, Yazdi HM. Fine needle aspiration biopsy of Hashimoto's thyroiditis. Sources of diagnostic error. *Acta Cytol* 1999; 43(3): 400–6.

67. Oertel YC, Oertel JE. Diagnosis of malignant epithelial thyroid lesions: fine needle aspiration and histopathologic correlation. *Ann Diagn Pathol* 1998; 2(6): 377–400.

68. Blumenfeld W, Nair R, Mir R. Diagnostic significance of papillary structures and intranuclear inclusions in Hurthle-cell neoplasms of the thyroid.

69. Nguyen GK, Husain M, Akin MR. Cytodiagnosis of benign and malignant Hurthle cell lesions of the thyroid by fine-needle aspiration biopsy. *Diagn Cytopathol* 1999; 20(5): 261–5.

70. Busseniers AE, Oertel YC. 'Cellular adenomatoid nodules' of the thyroid: review of 219 fine-needle aspirates. *Diagn Cytopathol* 1993; 9(5): 581–9.

71. Tuttle RM, Lemar H, Burch HB. Clinical features associated with an increased risk of thyroid malignancy in patients with follicular neoplasia by fine-needle aspiration. *Thyroid* 1998; 8(5): 377–83.

72. Karak AK, Sahoo M, Bhatnagar D. Hyalinizing trabecular adenoma – a case report with FNAC histologic, MIB-1 proliferative index and immunohistochemical findings. *Indian J Pathol Microbiol* 1998; 41(4): 479–84.

73. Bondeson L, Bondeson AG. Clue helping to distinguish hyalinizing trabecular adenoma from carcinoma of the thyroid in fine-needle aspirates. *Diagn Cytopathol* 1994; 10(1): 25–9.

74. Boccato P, Mannara GM, La Rosa F, Rinaldo A, Ferlito A. Hyalinizing trabecular adenoma of the thyroid diagnosed by fine-needle aspiration biopsy [clinical conference]. *Ann Otol Rhinol Laryngol* 2000; 109(2): 235–8.

75. Strong CJ, Garcia BM. Fine needle aspiration cytologic characteristics of hyalinizing trabecular adenoma of the thyroid. *Acta Cytol* 1990; 34(3): 359–62.

76. Kaleem Z, Davila RM. Hyalinizing trabecular adenoma of the thyroid. A report of two cases with cytologic, histologic and immunohistochemical findings. *Acta Cytol* 1997; 41(3): 883–8.

77. Hirokawa M, Shimizu M, Manabe T, Kuroda M, Mizoguchi Y. Hyalinizing trabecular adenoma of the thyroid: its unusual cytoplasmic immunopositivity for MIB1. *Pathol Int* 1995; 45(5): 399–401.

78. Goellner JR, Carney JA. Cytologic features of fine-needle aspirates of hyalinizing trabecular adenoma of the thyroid. *Am J Clin Pathol* 1989; 91(2): 115–9.

79. Cerasoli S, Tabarri B, Farabegoli P et al. Hyalinizing trabecular adenoma of the thyroid. Report of two cases, with cytologic, immunohistochemical and ultrastructural studies. *Tumori* 1992; 78(4): 274–9.

80. Fornes P, Lesourd A, Dupuis G et al. [Hyalinizing trabecular adenoma of the thyroid gland. Histologic and immunohistochemical study. Report of 2 cases]. *Arch Anat Cytol Pathol* 1990; 38(5–6): 203 7.

81. Schmid KW, Mesewinkel F, Bocker W. Hyalinizing trabecular adenoma of the thyroid – morphology and differential diagnosis. *Acta Med Austriaca* 1996; 23(1–2): 65–8.

82. Akin MR, Nguyen GK. Fine-needle aspiration biopsy cytology of hyalinizing trabecular adenomas of the thyroid. *Diagn Cytopathol* 1999; 20(2): 90–4.

83. Vassko V, Garcia S, Henry JF, De Micco C. Expression of proliferating cell nuclear antigen in follicular thyroid tumors: correlation with clinicopathological findings. *Oncol Rep* 1999; 6(2): 359–64.

84. Huss LJ, Mendelsohn G. Medullary carcinoma of the thyroid gland: an encapsulated variant resembling the hyalinizing trabecular (paraganglioma-like) adenoma of thyroid. *Mod Pathol* 1990; 3(5): 581–5.

85. Cameselle-Teijeiro J, Febles-Perez C, Sobrinho-Simoes M. Cytologic features of fine needle aspirates of papillary and mucoepidermoid carcinoma of the thyroid with anaplastic transformation. A case report. *Acta Cytol* 1997; 41(4 suppl): 1356–60.

86. Layfield LJ, Mohrmann RL, Kopald KH, Giuliano AE. Use of aspiration cytology and frozen section examination for management of benign and malignant thyroid nodules. *Cancer* 1991; 68(1): 130–4.

87. Harach HR, Saravia Day E, Zusman SB. Occult papillary microcarcinoma of the thyroid – a potential pitfall of fine needle aspiration cytology? [see comments]. *J Clin Pathol* 1991; 44(3): 205–7.

88. Kini SR, Miller JM, Hamburger JI, Smith MJ. Cytopathology of papillary carcinoma of the thyroid by fine needle aspiration. *Acta Cytol* 1980; 24(6): 511–21.

89. Kaur A, Jayaram G. Thyroid tumors: cytomorphology of papillary carcinoma. *Diagn Cytopathol* 1991; 7(5): 462–8.

90. Ellison E, Lapuerta P, Martin SE. Psammoma bodies in fine-needle aspirates of the thyroid: predictive value for papillary carcinoma. *Cancer* 1998; 84(3): 169–75.

91. Francis IM, Das DK, Sheikh ZA, Sharma PN, Gupta SK. Role of nuclear grooves in the diagnosis of papillary thyroid carcinoma. A quantitative assessment on fine needle aspiration smears. *Acta Cytol* 1995; 39(3): 409–15.

92. Shurbaji MS, Gupta PK, Frost JK. Nuclear grooves: a useful criterion in the cytopathologic diagnosis of papillary thyroid carcinoma. *Diagn Cytopathol* 1988; 4(2): 91–4.

93. Rupp M, Ehya H. Nuclear grooves in the aspiration cytology of papillary carcinoma of the thyroid. *Acta Cytol* 1989; 33(1): 21–6.

94. Chhieng DC, Ross JS, McKenna BJ. CD44 immunostaining of thyroid fine-needle aspirates differentiates thyroid papillary carcinoma from other lesions with nuclear grooves and inclusions. *Cancer* 1997; 81(3): 157–62.

95. Akhtar M, Ali MA, Huq M, Bakry M. Fine-needle aspiration biopsy of papillary thyroid carcinoma: cytologic, histologic, and ultrastructural correlations. *Diagn Cytopathol* 1991; 7(4): 373–9.

96. Ruiz-Velasco R, Waisman J, Van Herle AJ. Cystic papillary carcinoma of the thyroid gland. Diagnosis by needle aspiration with transmission electron microscopy. *Acta Cytol* 1978; 22(1): 38–42.

97. Tabbara SO, Acoury N, Sidawy MK. Multinucleated giant cells in thyroid neoplasms. A cytologic, histologic and immunohistochemical study. *Acta Cytol* 1996; 40(6): 1184–8.

98. Martinez-Parra D, Campos Fernandez J, Hierro-Guilmain CC, Sola Perez J, Perez-Guillermo M. Follicular variant of papillary carcinoma of the thyroid: to what extent is fine-needle aspiration reliable? *Diagn Cytopathol* 1996; 15(1): 12–16.

99. Zacks JF, de las Morenas A, Beazley RM, O'Brien MJ. Fine-needle aspiration cytology diagnosis of colloid nodule versus follicular variant of papillary carcinoma of the thyroid. *Diagn Cytopathol* 1998; 18(2): 87–90.

100. Kumar PV, Talei AR, Malekhusseini SA, Monabati A, Vasei M. Follicular variant of papillary carcinoma of the thyroid. A cytologic study of 15 cases. *Acta Cytol* 1999; 43(2): 139–42.

101. Gallagher J, Oertel YC, Oertel JE. Follicular variant of papillary carcinoma of the thyroid: fine-needle aspirates with histologic correlation. *Diagn Cytopathol* 1997; 16(3): 207–13.

102. Hugh JC, Duggan MA, Chang-Poon V. The fine-needle aspiration appearance of the follicular variant of thyroid papillary carcinoma: a report of three cases. *Diagn Cytopathol* 1988; 4(3): 196–201.

103. Das DK, Jain S, Tripathi RP et al. Marginal vacuoles in thyroid aspirates. *Acta Cytol* 1998; 42(5): 1121–8.

104. Goodell WM, Saboorian MH, Ashfaq R. Fine-needle aspiration diagnosis of the follicular variant of papillary carcinoma. *Cancer* 1998; 84(6): 349–54.

105. Harach HR, Zusman SB. Cytologic findings in the follicular variant of papillary carcinoma of the thyroid. *Acta Cytol* 1992; 36(2): 142–6.

106. Baloch ZW, Gupta PK, Yu GH, Sack MJ, LiVolsi VA. Follicular variant of papillary carcinoma. Cytologic and histologic correlation. *Am J Clin Pathol* 1999; 111(2): 216–22.

107. Das DK, Khanna CM, Tripathi RP et al. Solitary nodular goiter. Review of cytomorphologic features in 441 cases. *Acta Cytol* 1999; 43(4): 563–74.

108. Hirokawa M, Shimizu M, Terayama K, Kanahara T, Sonoo H, Manabe T. Macrofollicular variant of papillary thyroid carcinoma. Report of a case with fine needle aspiration biopsy findings. *Acta Cytol* 1998; 42(6): 1441–3.

109. Mesonero CE, Jugle JE, Wilbur DC, Nayar R. Fine-needle aspiration of the macrofollicular and microfollicular subtypes of the follicular variant of papillary carcinoma of the thyroid. *Cancer* 1998; 84(4): 235–44.

110. Cameselle-Teijeiro J, Febles-Perez C, Cameselle-Teijeiro JF, Alfonsin-Barreiro N, Moldes-Boullosa J, Barreiro F. Cytologic clues for distinguishing the tall cell variant of thyroid papillary carcinoma. A case report. *Acta Cytol* 1997; 41(4 suppl): 1310–6.

111. Hui PK, Chan JK, Cheung PS, Gwi E. Columnar cell carcinoma of the thyroid. Fine needle aspiration findings in a case. *Acta Cytol* 1990; 34(3): 355–8.

112. Gamboa-Dominguez A, Candanedo-Gonzalez F, Uribe-Uribe NO, Angeles-Angeles A. Tall cell variant of papillary thyroid carcinoma. A cytohistologic correlation. *Acta Cytol* 1997; 41(3): 672–6.

113. Perez F, Llobet M, Garijo G, Barcelo C, Castro P, Bernado L. Fine-needle aspiration cytology of columnar-cell carcinoma of the thyroid: report of two cases with cytohistologic correlation. *Diagn Cytopathol* 1998; 18(5): 352–6.

114. Harach HR, Zusman SB. Cytopathology of the tall cell variant of thyroid papillary carcinoma. *Acta Cytol* 1992; 36(6): 895–9.

115. Kaw YT. Fine needle aspiration cytology of the tall cell variant of papillary carcinoma of the thyroid [letter]. *Acta Cytol* 1994; 38(2): 282.

116. Pilotti S, Collini P, Sampietro G, Manzari A, Marubini E, Rilke F. Thyroid papillary carcinoma of columnar cell type: a clinicopathologic study of 16 cases [letter, comment]. *Cancer* 1998; 83(11): 2421–3.

117. Putti TC, Bhuiya TA, Wasserman PG. Fine needle aspiration cytology of mixed tall and columnar cell papillary carcinoma of the thyroid. A case report. *Acta Cytol* 1998; 42(2): 387–90.

118. Dina R, Capitanio A, Damiani S. A morphometric analysis of cytological features of tall cell variant and classical papillary carcinoma of the thyroid [in process citation]. *Cytopathology* 2000; 11(2): 124–8.

119. Jayaram G. Cytology of columnar-cell variant of papillary thyroid carcinoma [in process citation]. *Diagn Cytopathol* 2000; 22(4): 227–9.

120. Doria MI, Jr., Attal H, Wang HH, Jensen JA, DeMay RM. Fine needle aspiration cytology of the oxyphil variant of papillary carcinoma of the thyroid. A report of three cases. *Acta Cytol* 1996; 40(5): 1007–11.

121. Vasei M, Kumar PV, Malekhoseini SA, Kadivar M. Papillary Hurthle cell carcinoma (Warthin-like tumor) of the thyroid. Report of a case with fine needle aspiration findings. *Acta Cytol* 1998; 42(6): 1437–40.

122. Chen KT. Fine-needle aspiration cytology of papillary Hurthle-cell tumors of thyroid: a report of three cases. *Diagn Cytopathol* 1991; 7(1): 53–6.

123. Caruso G, Tabarri B, Lucchi I, Tison V. Fine needle aspiration cytology in a case of diffuse sclerosing carcinoma of the thyroid. *Acta Cytol* 1990; 34(3): 352–4.

124. Kumarasinghe MP. Cytomorphologic features of diffuse sclerosing variant of papillary carcinoma of the thyroid. A report of two cases in children. *Acta Cytol* 1998; 42(4): 983–6.

125. Chan JK, Carcangiu ML, Rosai J. Papillary carcinoma of thyroid with exuberant nodular fasciitis-like stroma. Report of three cases. *Am J Clin Pathol* 1991; 95(3): 309–14.

126. Vinette DS, MacDonald LL, Yazdi HM. Papillary carcinoma of the thyroid with anaplastic transformation: diagnostic pitfalls in fine-needle aspiration biopsy. *Diagn Cytopathol* 1991; 7(1): 75–8.

127. Us-Krasovec M, Golouh R. Papillary thyroid carcinoma with exuberant nodular fasciitis-like stroma in a fine needle aspirate. A case report. *Acta Cytol* 1999; 43(6): 1101–4.

128. Yang YJ, LiVolsi VA, Khurana KK. Papillary thyroid carcinoma with nodular fasciitis-like stroma. Pitfalls in fine-needle aspiration cytology. *Arch Pathol Lab Med* 1999; 123(9): 838–41.

129. Woyke S, al-Jassar AK, al-Jarallah MA, Temmim L. Papillary carcinoma of the thyroid with numerous spindle-shaped tumor cells in fine needle aspiration smears. A case report. *Acta Cytol* 1994; 38(2): 226–30.

130. Leung CS, Hartwick RW, Bedard YC. Correlation of cytologic and histologic features in variants of papillary carcinoma of the thyroid. *Acta Cytol* 1993; 37(5): 645–50.

131. Khan A, Baker SP, Patwardhan NA, Pullman JM. CD57 (Leu-7) expression is helpful in diagnosis of the follicular variant of papillary thyroid carcinoma. *Virchows Arch* 1998; 432(5): 427–32.

132. Oertel YC. Thymoma mimicking thyroid papillary carcinoma: another pitfall in fine-needle aspiration. *Diagn Cytopathol* 1997; 17(1): 61–3.

133. Faser CR, Marley EF, Oertel YC. Papillary tissue fragments as a diagnostic pitfall in fine-needle aspirations of thyroid nodules. *Diagn Cytopathol* 1997; 16(5): 454–9.

134. Sironi M, Collini P, Cantaboni A. Fine needle aspiration cytology of insular thyroid carcinoma. A report of four cases. *Acta Cytol* 1992; 36(3): 435–9.

135. Guiter GE, Auger M, Ali SZ, Allen EA, Zakowski MF. Cytopathology of insular carcinoma of the thyroid. *Cancer* 1999; 87(4): 196–202.

136. Kuhel WI, Kutler DI, Santos-Buch CA. Poorly differentiated insular thyroid carcinoma. A case report with identification of intact insulae with fine needle aspiration biopsy. *Acta Cytol* 1998; 42(4): 991–7.

137. Gharib H, McConahey WM, Tiegs RD et al. Medullary thyroid carcinoma: clinicopathologic features and long-term follow-up of 65 patients treated during 1946 through 1970. *Mayo Clin Proc* 1992; 67(10): 934–40.

138. Forrest CH, Frost FA, de Boer WB, Spagnolo DV, Whitaker D, Sterrett BF. Medullary carcinoma of the thyroid: accuracy of diagnosis of fine-needle aspiration cytology. *Cancer* 1998; 84(5): 295–302.

139. Kini SR, Miller JM, Hamburger JI, Smith MJ. Cytopathologic features of medullary carcinoma of the thyroid. *Arch Pathol Lab Med* 1984; 108(2): 156–9.

140. Bauman A, Strawbridge HT, Bauman WA. The clinical value of fine needle aspiration biopsy in a patient with medullary thyroid carcinoma and pseudofollicular carcinoma. *N Y State J Med* 1989; 89(9): 527–9.

141. Zeppa P, Vetrani A, Marino M et al. Fine needle aspiration cytology of medullary thyroid carcinoma: a review of 18 cases. *Cytopathology* 1990; 1(1): 35–44.

142. Collins BT, Cramer HM, Tabatowski K, Hearn S, Raminhos A, Lampe H. Fine needle aspiration of medullary carcinoma of the thyroid. Cytomorphology, immunocytochemistry and electron microscopy. *Acta Cytol* 1995; 39(5): 920–30.

143. Gomez-Fernandez C, Kraemer HJ, Ganjei P. Metastatic medullary thyroid carcinoma in liver diagnosis by aspiration cytology. *Diagn Cytopathol* 1994; 11(3): 277–80.

144. Kaur A, Jayaram G. Thyroid tumors: cytomorphology of medullary, clinically anaplastic, and miscellaneous thyroid neoplasms [see comments]. *Diagn Cytopathol* 1990; 6(6): 383–9.

145. Aulicino MR, Szporn AH, Dembitzer R et al. Cytologic findings in the differential diagnosis of C-cell hyperplasia and medullary carcinoma by fine needle aspiration. A case report. *Acta Cytol* 1998; 42(4): 963–7.

146. Brooke PK, Hameed M, Zakowski MF. Fine-needle aspiration of anaplastic thyroid carcinoma with varied cytologic and histologic patterns: a case report. *Diagn Cytopathol* 1994; 11(1): 60–3.

147. Bauman ME, Tao LC. Cytopathology of papillary carcinoma of the thyroid with anaplastic transformation. A case report. *Acta Cytol* 1995; 39(3): 525–9.

148. Us-Krasovec M, Golouh R, Auersperg M, Besic N, Ruparcic-Oblak L. Anaplastic thyroid carcinoma in fine needle aspirates. *Acta Cytol* 1996; 40(5): 953–8.

149. Schneider V, Frable WJ. Spindle and giant cell carcinoma of the thyroid: cytologic diagnosis by fine needle aspiration. *Acta Cytol* 1980; 24(3): 184–9.

150. Fehr-Merhof A, Flury R, Ruttimann S. [From Hashimoto thyroiditis to B-cell lymphoma of the thyroid gland]. *Schweiz Med Wochenschr* 1999; 129(23): 883–9.

151. Scholefield JH, Quayle AR, Harris SC, Talbot CH. Primary lymphoma of the thyroid, the association with Hashimoto's thyroiditis. *Eur J Surg Oncol* 1992; 18(2): 89–92.

152. Zeman V. [Hashimoto's lymphocytic thyroiditis and simultaneous malignant tumors of the thyroid gland]. *Vnitr Lek* 1979; 25(4): 360–5.

153. Fenton JE, Stack J, Kelly P, O'Dwyer TP. Lymphoma and Hashimoto's thyroiditis. *J Laryngol Otol* 1995; 109(8): 781–3.

154. Paraf F, Brousse N. [Primary lymphoma of the thyroid: terminology, diagnostic criteria and relationship to Hashimoto's thyroiditis (letter)]. *Presse Med* 1992; 21(21): 997.

155. Matsuzuka F, Miyauchi A, Katayama S et al. Clinical aspects of primary thyroid lymphoma: diagnosis and treatment based on our experience of 119 cases. *Thyroid* 1993; 3(2): 93–9.

156. Anscombe AM, Wright DH. Primary malignant lymphoma of the thyroid – a tumour of mucosa-associated lymphoid tissue: review of seventy-six cases. *Histopathology* 1985; 9(1): 81–97.

157. Das DK, Gupta SK, Francis IM, Ahmed MS. Fine-needle aspiration cytology diagnosis of non-Hodgkin lymphoma of thyroid: a report of four cases. *Diagn Cytopathol* 1993; 9(6): 639–45.

158. Matsuda M, Sone H, Koyama H, Ishiguro S. Fine-needle aspiration cytology of malignant lymphoma of the thyroid. *Diagn Cytopathol* 1987; 3(3): 244–9.

159. Jayaram G, Rani S, Raina V, Singh CH, Chandra M, Marwaha RK. B cell lymphoma of the thyroid in Hashimoto's thyroiditis monitored by fine-needle aspiration cytology. *Diagn Cytopathol* 1990; 6(2): 130–3.

160. Kossev P, Livolsi V. Lymphoid lesions of the thyroid. review in light of the revised European-American lymphoma classification and upcoming World Health Organization classification. *Thyroid* 1999; 9(12): 1273–80.

161. Garcia Erce JA, Alvarez Alegret R, Damborenea Tajada J, Garcia Barrado AI, Garcia Zueco JC. [The limitations of fine-needle aspiration puncture in the diagnosis of primary thyroid lymphoma (letter, comment)]. *Rev Clin Esp* 1999; 199(10): 693.

162. Zdziarska B, Zuk E, Listewnik M. [A case of centroblastic lymphoma of the thyroid gland]. *Pol Merkuriusz Lek* 1998; 4(19): 29–31.

163. Kuma K, Matsuzuka F. [Diagnosis and therapy of malignant thyroid lymphoma]. *Nippon Naika Gakkai Zasshi* 1997; 86(7): 1190–5.

164. Herranz MT, Corrales A, Molina MA, Redondo E, Almagro M, Marti J. Thyroid lymphoma in a 51-year-old woman. *An Med Interna* 1993; 10(3): 132–4.

165. Detweiler RE, Katz RL, Alapat C, el-Naggar A, Ordonez N. Malignant lymphoma of the thyroid: a report of two cases diagnosed by fine-needle aspiration. *Diagn Cytopathol* 1991; 7(2): 163–71.

166. Takashima S, Tomiyama N, Morimoto S, Kozuka T, Ichihara K. Nonpalpable primary thyroid lymphoma diagnosed by ultrasound-guided fine needle biopsy. *J Clin Ultrasound* 1992; 20(2): 142–5.

167. Matsuda M, Sone H, Koyama H, Shiba E, Tahara H, Kimura K. [Needle aspiration cytology of malignant lymphoma of the thyroid]. *Gan No Rinsho* 1987; 33(1): 21–6.

168. Aozasa K, Takakuwa T. Differential diagnosis of Hashimoto's thyroiditis from thyroidal neoplastic diseases. *Nippon Rinsho* 1999; 57(8): 1894–8.

169. Chacho MS, Greenebaum E, Moussouris HF, Schreiber K, Koss LG. Value of aspiration cytology of the thyroid in metastatic disease. *Acta Cytol* 1987; 31(6): 705–12.

170. Lasser A, Rothman JG, Calamia VJ. Renal-cell carcinoma metastatic to the thyroid. Aspiration cytology and histologic findings. *Acta Cytol* 1985; 29(5): 856–8.

171. Smith SA, Gharib H, Goellner JR. Fine-needle aspiration. Usefulness for diagnosis and management of metastatic carcinoma to the thyroid. *Arch Intern Med* 1987; 147(2): 311–2.

4

Lymph nodes

Introduction
Non-neoplastic lymphoproliferative conditions
Hodgkin's lymphoma
Non-Hodgkin's lymphoma
Metastatic carcinoma

INTRODUCTION

The role of FNAC in the initial diagnosis of primary lymphadenopathies is: first, to confirm that the lesion is a lymph node; second, to exclude metastatic disease or specific infection; and third, to distinguish between benign and malignant lymphoid proliferations. Used in the proper setting, FNAC will provide a definitive diagnosis in the majority of cases, especially relating to lymphoid versus non-lymphoid pathology, metastatic disease and infection.[1] While primary diagnosis of lymphoma by FNAC is still controversial, it is helpful in triaging the patients who may require excision biopsy (Fig. 4.1).[2] Patients with a definitive cytological diagnosis may be spared unnecessary surgery and reviewed through follow-up.[3]

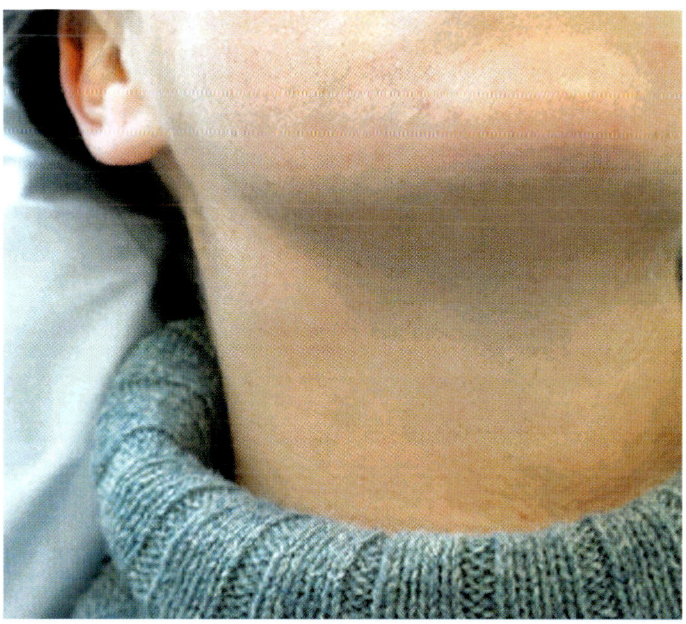

Figure 4.1 FNAC of cervical swelling aims to distinguish between the lymphoid and non-lymphoid pathology. This 29-year-old patient presented with history of anterior triangle swelling of several weeks duration. Clinically, it was thought to be a branchial cleft cyst. FNAC revealed lymphoid cells consistent with lymph node hyperplasia. There was no evidence of infection, lymphoma or metastases.

Distribution of lymph node pathology

In a survey of 1064 FNAC specimens during a 10-year period in our practice,[4] we have observed that patients most frequently presented with a lump of unknown origin, persistent lymphadenopathy, as a follow-up of a known clinical

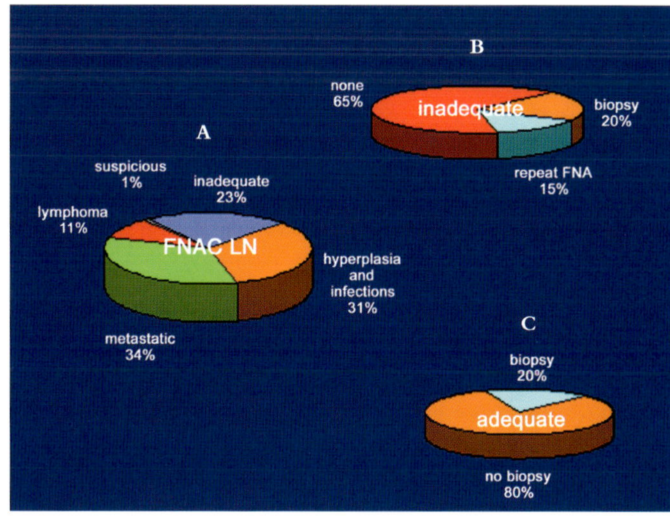

Figure 4.2 A. Relative proportions of FNAC diagnoses in a survey of 1043 FNAC of lymph nodes in the past 10 years. Metastatic carcinoma and hyperplasias/infections represent the majority of lymph node FNAC diagnoses. **B.** Management of inadequate FNAC. (top right) Total 234 (23%). Repeat FNAC 15%, biopsy 20%, follow-up 65%. **C.** Total number of LN biopsies avoided in 80% of patients with adequate FNAC.

condition or staging of a known malignant tumour. Of the specimens adequate for assessment (77%), the most commonly diagnosed categories were metastatic carcinoma (33%) followed by reactive/inflammatory (31%) and lymphoma (11%).[4] Similarly, in a survey of the role of FNAC in Nigeria, Thomas et al[5] found that the most common diagnosis was reactive change/non-specific inflammation (33.4%), tuberculosis and metastatic lesions (25.7% and 22.4% respectively) and lymphoma (16.9%).[5] Following the FNAC, biopsies were performed on the 18% of patients with adequate FNAC material. Biopsies were performed in 10% of reactive/inflammatory conditions and in 47% of lymphomas, both categories guided by the appropriate clinical setting and the patient's history .

Diagnostic accuracy

With an overall accuracy rate of 96–99% and a typing accuracy rate of 96.5%, FNAC yields a high rate of conclusive cytological diagnoses in the assessment of metastatic malignancies,[4,6–8] a high rate of conclusive diagnoses in the assessment of high-grade non-Hodgkin's lymphomas (79–90%) and Hodgkin's disease (with the exception of the lymphocytic predominance variant of the latter), but has significant limitations in the assessment of low-grade non-Hodgkin's lymphomas.[4,9,10]

Diagnostic pitfalls

Diagnostic pitfalls in FNAC of the lymph nodes can broadly be listed in 7 categories: differentiating low-grade B- and T-cell lymphomas from reactive hyperplasia;[11] distinguishing between the small lymphocytic lymphomas (lymphocytic lymphoma, mantle zone lymphoma, marginal zone lymphoma, lymphocyte-predominant Hodgkin's disease, progressive transformation of lymph nodes); overlooking lymphoma when metastases are suspected; Hodgkin's disease (lymphocyte depleted) versus anaplastic large cell (Ki-1, CD30 positive) lymphoma; Ki-1 anaplastic large cell lymphoma versus other non-lymphoid tumours; lymphoma versus other malignancies, and problems with immunophenotyping.[12] The most commonly encountered diagnostic difficulty is in distinguishing low-grade lymphoma from reactive hyperplasia. This is particularly evident with follicular lymphomas. In the case of low-grade non-Hodgkin's lymphomas, morphological and immunocytochemical (T- and B-cell differentiation markers) methods need to be supplemented by dual-parameter flow cytometry, evaluation of proliferative activity by Ki-67 and molecular techniques in order to achieve conclusive diagnoses.[11]

Ancillary techniques

Immunocytochemistry

Immunocytochemical studies performed on FNAC material in conjunction with the cytological diagnosis lead to an increase in diagnostic accuracy as well as providing means for subclassification of neoplastic lymphoid cells. This technique gives results comparable to those obtained by histopathological and immunohistochemical analysis on surgically removed lymph nodes.[13] Apart from phenotypic markers, proliferation markers appear to predict biological behaviour and responses to therapy in non-Hodgkin's lymphoma. The antibody against Ki-67, a marker for cycling cells, measured by either visual scoring or image analysis, correlates positively with increasing grade of lymphoma.[14] The excellent correlation between histological and cytological preparations indicates that FNAC material is suitable for the immunocytochemical assessment of the growth fraction of non-Hodgkin's lymphoma.[9,15] Immunophenotyping facilitates patient management in the setting of the recurrence or suspected recurrence of a known lymphoproliferative disorder.[16]

Flow cytometry

Immunophenotyping can be accomplished via immunocytochemistry or flow cytometry (FCM).[17,18] In the experience of Simsir et al,[17] 85% of the cases were immunophenotyped by both techniques. The advantage of immunocytochemistry is the preservation of cytomorphology, particularly in cases with very few well-preserved cells. The advantages of flow cytometry are in the detection of a small population of monoclonal cells in a background of reactive cells (particularly useful in effusion samples in which the predominant cell population is often reactive T-lymphocytes), in the increased diagnostic precision through evaluation of objective parameters and in the use of multiple markers with dual labelling. Flow cytometry enables clonality analysis and immunophenotyping and is therefore a helpful addition in the diagnosis and classification of reactive lymphoid hyperplasia and malignant lymphoma.[19,20] Clonality analysis is achieved measuring the

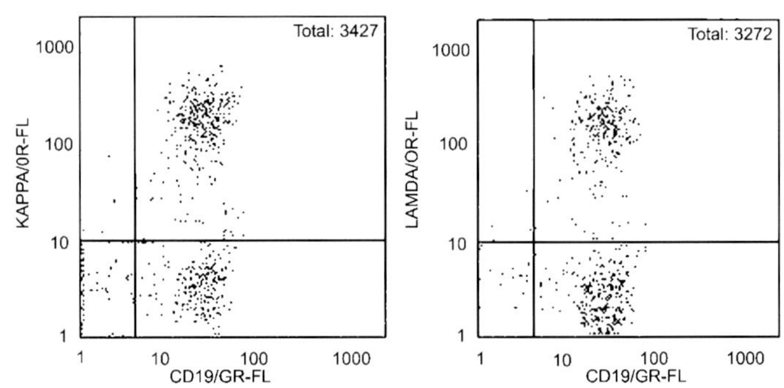

Figure 4.3 Flow cytometry. Reactive lymph node hyperplasia. 22% CD19+/kappa+, 16%
CD19+/lambda +, LCR-1,4:1. (From Jeffers MD et al: J Clin Pathol 1998; 51:189–196). (With permission from BMJ Publishing.)

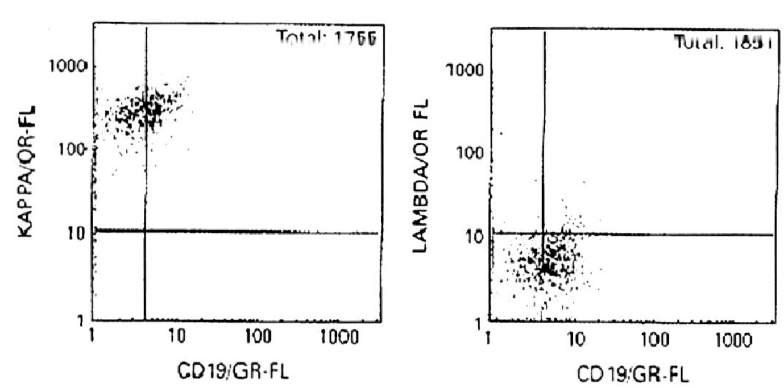

Figure 4.4 Flow cytometry. Non-Hodgkin's lymphoma. 37% CD19=/kappa+, 1.7% CD/lambda + (LCR 22.1). (From Jeffers MD et al: J Clin Pathol 1998; 51:189–196).(With permission from BMJ Publishing.)

immunoglobulin light chain ratio (LCR). Reactive lymphoid hyperplasia is polyclonal by FCM (LCR <2/1). Most of B-cell non-Hodgkin's lymphomas are monoclonal (LCR > 3/1)[21] (Figs 4.3 and 4.4). Analysis of CD5, CD10 and CD23 expression by flow cytometry enables subclassification of mantle cell lymphoma, small lymphocytic lymphoma and some lymphomas of follicle centre cell origin (Figs 4.5–4.7).[21–23] When comparing the cytospin analysis and flow cytometry, both appear equally capable of immunotyping aspirated lymphoid samples reliably.[19,23–26]

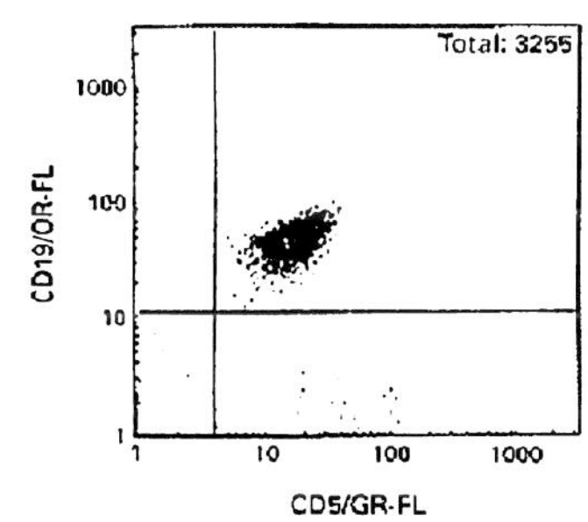

Figure 4.5 Flow cytometry. Mantle zone lymphoma. 96% CD19+/CD5+ (LCR 18.1). (From Jeffers MD et al: J Clin Pathol 1998; 51:189–196). (With permission from BMJ Publishing.)

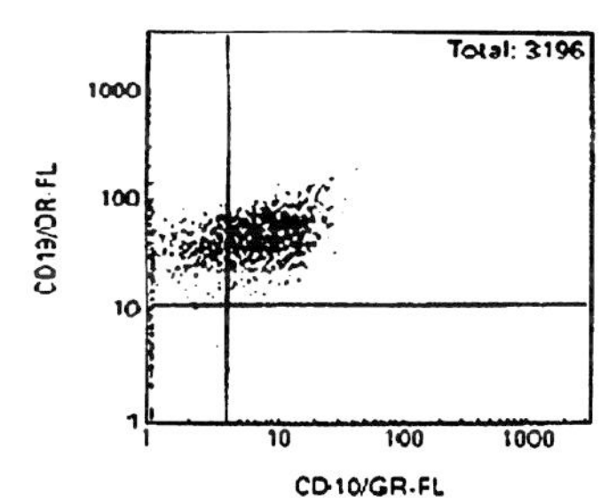

Figure 4.6 Flow cytometry. Follicular lymphoma. 51% CD19=/CD10+ (LCR 18:1). (From Jeffers MD et al: J Clin Pathol 1998; 51:189–196). (With permission from BMJ Publishing.)

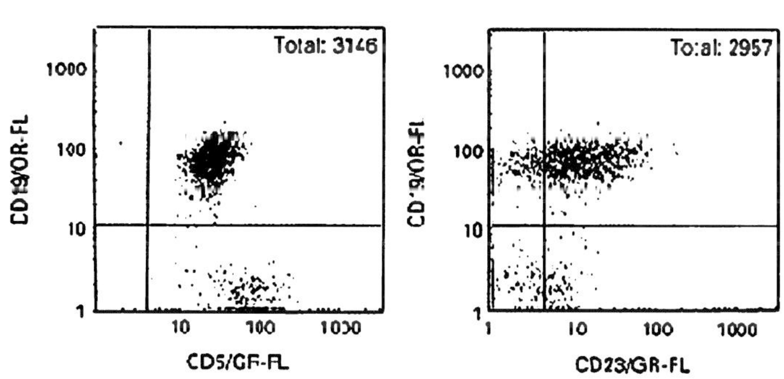

Figure 4.7 Flow cytometry. Small lymphocytic lymphoma. 82% CD19+/CD5+, 64% CD19=/CD23+. (From Jeffers MD et al: J Clin Pathol 1998; 51:189–196). (With permission from BMJ Publishing.)

The successful primary classification of most intra-abdominal non-Hodgkin's lymphomas can be achieved with a combination of cytology and flow cytometry, and this can be the initial approach in patients with deep-seated lesions.[27]

Molecular techniques

The application of *polymerase chain reaction* (PCR) to cytological material represents a promising, relatively non-invasive approach to clinical molecular genetic analysis.[28] It can be used to identify monoclonal rearrangements of the immunoglobulin heavy chain gene, T-cell receptor and translocations involving the bcl-1 and bcl-2 genes.[29] The detection rate of the t(14;18), the most common translocation in B-cell lymphomas, which results in rearrangement of the immunoglobulin heavy chain and BCL2 genes, has been examined in fresh and archival cytological smears (Fig. 4.8).[30–32] The results of the technique on FNAC material are highly comparable to those from excision biopsies.[33] The infrequent identification of monoclonal rearrangements and translocations in reactive processes requires cautious application of molecular data.[32,33] Katz et al[34] suggest that genotyping for lineage assignment and/or clonality be performed to include cases of atypical lymphoid proliferations, T-cell malignant neoplasms, lymphoid malignant neoplasms with equivocal markers and differentiation between lymphoid and non-lymphoid neoplasms. Genotyping by antigen-receptor gene rearrangement appears to be redundant in cases with mature B-cell phenotypes that demonstrate monoclonality by immunophenotyping.[34]

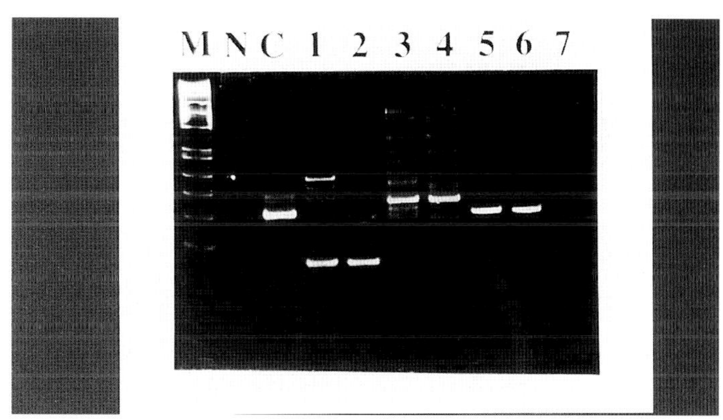

Figure 4.8 Detection of B-cell clonality: Ethidium bromide stained 10% gel of FR3 PCR products performed in duplicate to confirm clonality. Lanes: M = molecular weight marker ϕX/Hinfl [sizes in base pairs (bp)] N = negative control, C = positive control t(14;18), Lanes 1–6 B-cell lymphomas. All B-cell lymphomas cases were represented as discrete monoclonal bands.

More recently, human herpesvirus-8 (HHV-8) has been identified by PCR amplification of DNA from FNAC samples isolated from various forms of Kaposi's sarcoma. All of the cases diagnosed as Kaposi's sarcoma and 1 of the lymphoid hyperplasia cases were PCR positive for HHV-8 DNA, while all other cases of spindle cell lesions were negative. The molecular demonstration of HHV-8 DNA may be a useful adjunct in the diagnosis of Kaposi's sarcoma by fine needle aspiration.[35]

In situ hybridisation: Southern blot analysis is a useful technique for establishing tumour cell lineage, clonality, and the presence of oncogene rearrangements in fine-needle aspiration specimens of non-Hodgkin's lymphoma.[36] The assessment of immunoglobulin light chain expression is a useful adjunct to morphology of reactive and malignant lymphoid proliferations.[37]

The relative contribution of immunocytochemistry, in situ hybridisation for immunoglobulin light chain mRNA and polymerase chain reaction for immunoglobulin heavy chain gene rearrangement towards the final clinicopathological diagnosis is estimated to be: immunocytochemistry, 86%; in situ hybridisation, 77%; PCR, 62%. With the help of ancillary techniques, FNAC accurately distinguished reactive lymphoid hyperplasia from malignant lymphoma in 97% of cases.[38] The sensitivity of PCR and FNAC in diagnosis of neoplastic B-cell proliferations was 92% and 78% respectively.[39]

NON-NEOPLASTIC LYMPHOPROLIFERATIVE CONDITIONS

Follicular hyperplasia

Lymph nodes of the head and neck are often the site of lymph node enlargement. This may be as a response to known local antigenic stimuli (e.g. tonsilitis) or part of generalised lymphadenopathy due to systemic disease (e.g. rheumatoid arthritis) (Fig. 4.9). In follicular hyperplasia, lymph node follicles increase both in size and in number. Enlarged germinal centres may contain mitoses and tingible body macrophages as a result of high cell turnover.

Cytological features. FNAC material from an enlarged lymph node reflects germinal centres ('secondary follicles') which are often present in large numbers and are seen as residual follicle centre fragments (RFCFs) (Fig. 4.10a, b).

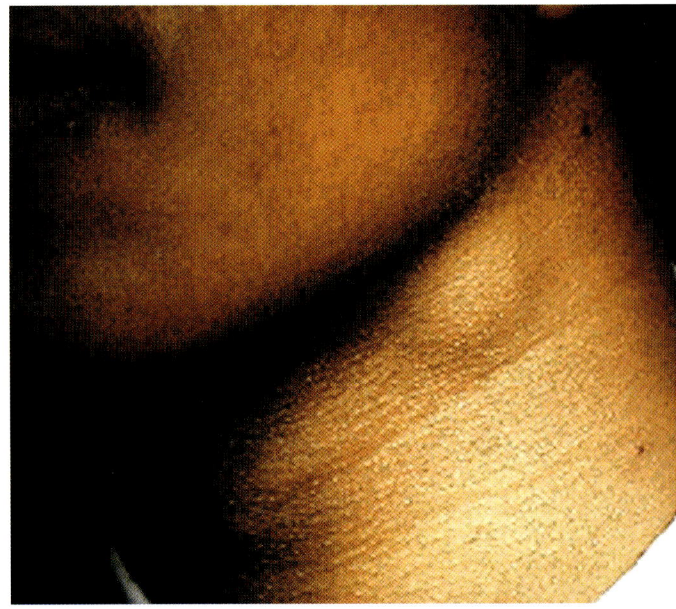

Figure 4.9 Lymph node hyperplasia. 23-year-old patient presented with a 1-month history of swelling in the left side of the neck. Clinically, it was mobile and soft. Patient was referred to the FNAC clinic for investigation.

These aggregates are centred around dendritic reticulum cells (follicular dendritic cells) and are composed mainly of centroblasts and centrocytes (Fig. 4.11). Centroblasts are large, round cells with a thin rim of evenly spaced basophilic cytoplasm (MGG) and a nucleus containing several visible nucleoli. Centrocytes are smaller than centroblasts and contain irregularly shaped nuclei with coarse chromatin. Follicular dendritic cells have oval nuclei, prominent nucleoli and ill defined interlacing cytoplasm which appears to encompass RFCFs. This is particularly well visible on medium-power view at the initial screen. These areas stand out as pale blue zones (MGG) in whose network the concentration of follicle centre cells is seen. Their presence can be confirmed with immunocytochemistry (CD21) (Fig. 4.12). The non-lymphoid cells in the lymph node, sinus macrophages and tingible body macrophages are also seen. Hyperplastic germinal centres often contain plasma cells and immunoblasts, sometimes in large numbers (Figs 4.13 and 4.14). In cases of protracted follicular hyperplasia, enlarged germinal centres appear to disintegrate. The expanded node is occupied mainly by small lymphocytes and some larger lymphocytes. This process is known as *progressive transformation of germinal centres*.

Distinguishing between reactive lymph node hyperplasia and low-grade nonHodgkin's lymphoma is the most

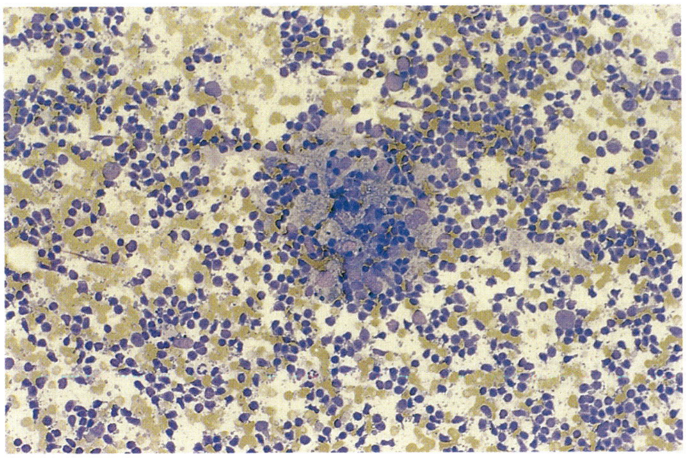

A

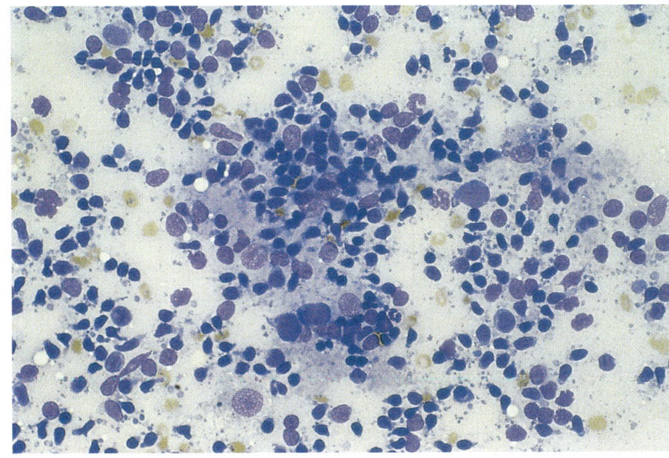

B

Figure 4.10 Lymph node hyperplasia. Same patient as in Figure 4.9. **A.** Low magnification of the FNAC material from an enlarged lymph node reflects the large germinal centres ('secondary follicles') which are often present in large numbers and are seen as residual follicle centre fragments (RFCFs). These aggregates are centred around dendritic reticulum cells (follicular dendritic cells). **B.** Higher power reveals residual follicle centre fragment.

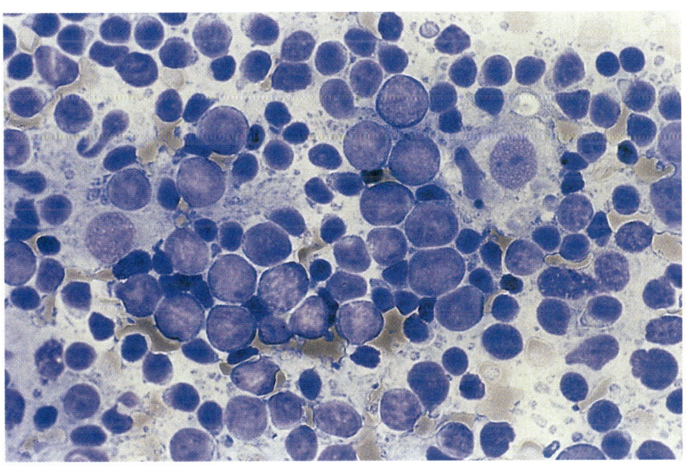

A

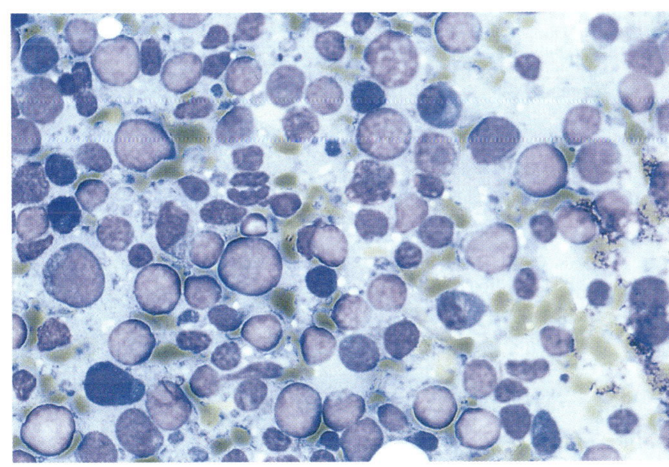

B

Figure 4.11 Lymph node hyperplasia. **A** Residual follicle centre fragment aggregates are centred around dendritic reticulum cells (follicular dendritic cells) and are composed mainly of centroblasts and centrocytes. **B** Centroblasts are large round cells with thin rim of evenly spaced basophilic cytoplasm and nucleus containing several visible nucleoli. Centrocytes are smaller than centroblasts and contain irregularly shaped nuclei with coarse chromatin and nucleoli and large, ill-defined interlacing cytoplasm, which appears to encompass the RFCFs.

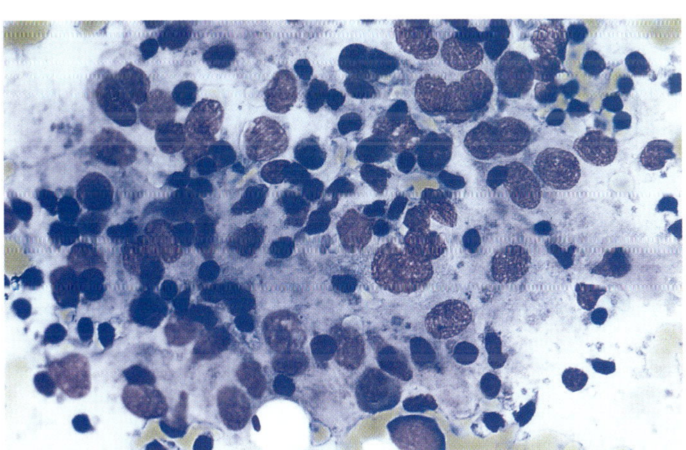

A

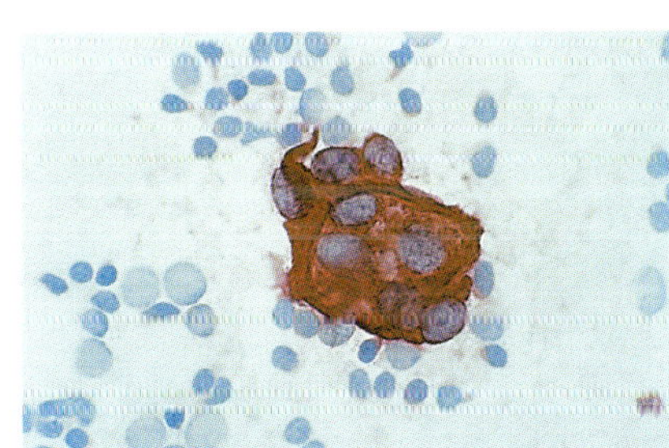

B

Figure 4.12 Lymph node hyperplasia. **A** Follicular dendritic cells have oval nuclei, prominent nucleoli and ill-defined interlacing cytoplasm which appears to encompass RFCFs. These areas stand out as pale blue zones (MGG) in whose network the concentration of follicle centre cells is seen. **B** Their presence can be confirmed with immunocytochemistry (CD21, APAAP).

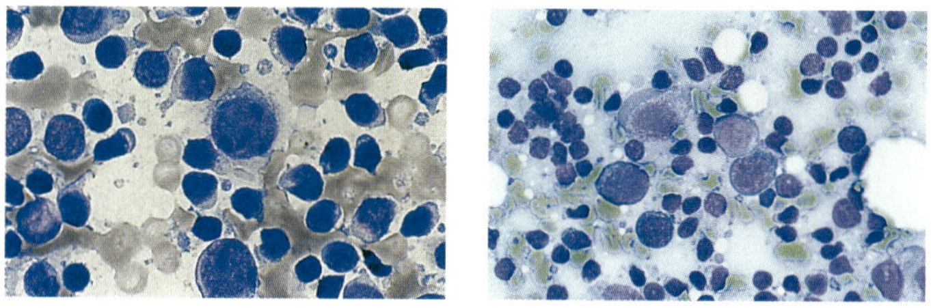

A B

Figure 4.13 Lymph node hyperplasia. **A** Hyperplastic germinal centres often contain plasma cells and immunoblasts. These may be misinterpreted. **B** The morphological suspicion of Hodgkin's cells may be falsely thought to be supported by immunocytochemistry.

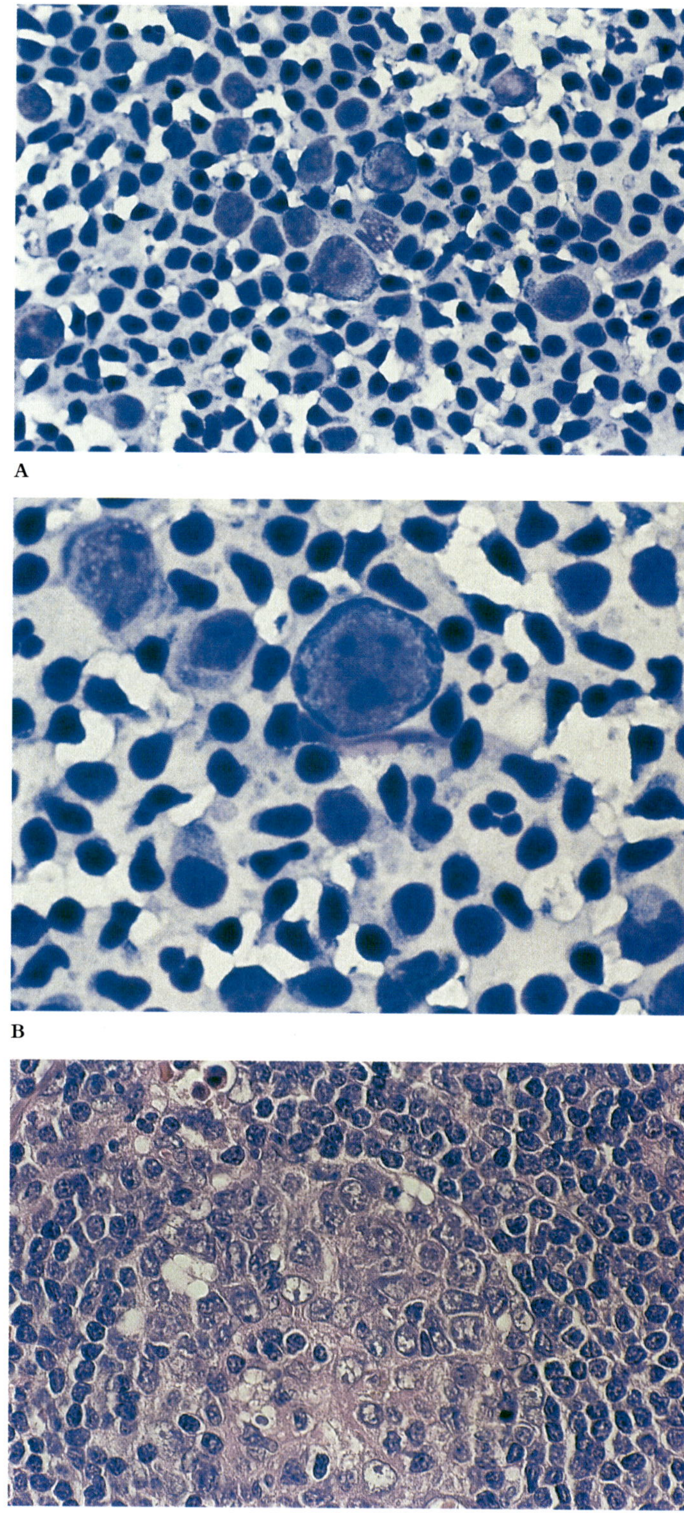

A B C

Figure 4.14 Lymph node hyperplasia. **A, B.** Rapid Giemsa stain performed in the outpatients' clinic, due to its rather crude tinctorial properties, may cause undue concern in interpretation of FNAC in hyperplastic lymph nodes with prominence of centroblasts and immunoblasts. **C.** Histological section of the lymph node shows follicular hyperplasia only. There is no evidence of lymphoma.

difficult area in lymph node FNAC. Diagnosis of low-grade lymphoma on cytological preparations is based on the finding of a monotonous cell population of lymphoid cells as contrasted with the typically polymorphous population seen in reactive proliferations.[40,41] Potential errors may occur when reactive conditions appear to contain atypical cells or when lymphomas contain an admixture of benign cells. For this reason, excision biopsy is advised in case of an inappropriately persisting lymphadenopathy for which no cause can be found. On the other hand, cytological diagnosis of lymph node hyperplasia, in an appropriate clinical setting, supports conservative management in many cases and reduces the need for biopsy.[38]

Sinus histiocytosis with massive lymphadenopathy (Rosai Dorfman)

Sinus histiocytosis with massive lymphadenopathy (SHML) is an uncommon entity of unknown aetiology affecting lymph nodes and extranodal sites. Originally it was described as occurring in young males. Since then over 423 histologically documented cases of SHML have been documented, including many extranodal sites. Sinuses of affected lymph nodes (usually cervical) are filled with very large distinctive macrophages, frequently containing engulfed lymphocytes in their cytoplasm. The condition is self-limiting but lymphadenopathy may persist for a long time. It is more common in black people.

Cytological features of SHML include increased numbers of large, non-cohesive histiocytes associated with a polymorphous, cellular background composed of mixed small mature lymphocytes and plasma cells. The large histiocytes (120–150 μm) have oval nuclei with smooth nuclear contour, one or two small but distinct nucleoli, abundant foamy cytoplasm and well-defined cytoplasmic margins. Many histiocytes contain lymphocytes, red cells or plasma cells in their cytoplasm.[42] Lymphophagocytosis (emperipolesis) is a prominent feature.[43–47] Emperipolesis is emphasised by a halo around the lymphocyte and fine vacuoles in the cytoplasm. Identification of an empty halo around engulfed lymphocyte is better seen on alcohol-fixed smears and histologically than on air-dried smears.[48,49] Immunophenotypic study of the histiocytes, performed on the FNAC smears and on paraffin-embedded sections shows reactivity for S-100 protein and alpha-1-antichymotrypsin and negativity for lysozyme.[50] Multinucleated histiocytes resembling Touton giant cells may be present. Neutrophils, eosinophils and aggregates of epithelioid cells are absent. A reactive lymphadenopathy may be diagnosed in the majority of cases on FNAC alone although occasionally histiocytes show atypia and may be mistaken for Hodgkin's cells.[51]

Differential diagnosis includes Langerhans' cell histiocytosis, granulomatous disease, large cell lymphoma, malignant histiocytosis, haemophagocytic syndrome, histoplasmosis and dermatopathic lymphadenopathy. Langerhans' cell histiocytosis, apart from having typical Langerhans' cells with nuclear folds, contains prominent eosinophilic infiltrate. Granulomatous lymphadenitis due to a variety of infectious agents usually presents as aggregates of cohesive histiocytes/epithelioid cells. These have ill-defined cytoplasm and elongated nuclei. Anaplastic large cell lymphoma and malignant histiocytosis have a more monotonous population of large atypical lymphoid cells. Haemophagocytosis may be seen in malignant histiocytosis and in haemophagocytic syndrome but emperipolesis is typical of sinus histiocytosis with massive lymphadenopathy and is not seen in other conditions. Histoplasmosis is characterised by finding the fungi in the cytoplasm. Dermatopathic lymphadenopathy is histologically characterised by preserved cortical follicles with hyperplastic germinal centres and progressive expansion of interdigitating reticulum cells associated with eosinophils and macrophages containing lipid and melanin pigment.

Cytological features of *dermatopathic lymphadenopathy* are consistent with lymph node hyperplasia. Finding of melanin pigment and appropriate clinical setting may help in reaching the diagnosis (Fig. 4.15). Difficulties arise when a node draining the area of skin involvement with mycosis fungoides is aspirated. Molecular techniques, in particular detection of the T-cell receptor gene rearrangement, may be helpful in distinguishing a low-grade T-cell lymphoma from dermatopathic lymphadenopathy (Fig. 4.55d).

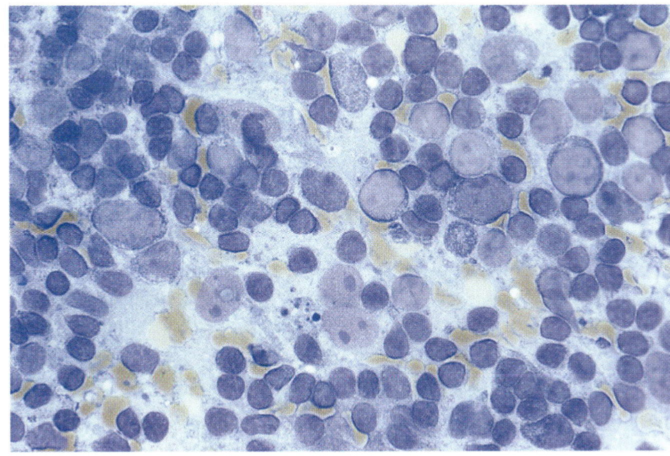

Figure 4.15 Dermatopathic lymphadenopathy. Cytological features of dermatopathic lymphadenopathy are consistent with lymph node hyperplasia. Finding of melanin pigment in the tingible body macrophages and the appropriate clinical setting may help in reaching the diagnosis (MGG ×600).

Given the rarity of sinus histiocytosis (Rosai Dorfman) and the clinical suspicion of lymphoma, biopsy of the node is advised. The morphological finding of emperipolesis and immunocytochemical staining for S-100 should, however, be sufficient to allow a confident diagnosis in the follow-up of patients with recurrent disease or extranodal progression.

Granulomatous lymphadenitis

Mycobacterial infection

Tuberculosis is the most frequent diagnosis in the FNAC of nodes in a developing country and is the most commonly diagnosed infective condition, particularly in those under the age of 20 years.[5] The posterior triangle of the neck is the most prevalent site.[47] In developing countries, where there are limited funds and facilities, FNAC has an important role in the investigation of peripheral lymphadenopathy as an alternative to surgical excision biopsy. However, tuberculous lymphadenopathy is a not infrequent finding in the UK, particularly among the inner city immigrant population and in the immunosuppressed (Figs 4.16–4.20). The sensitivity and specificity of lymph node FNAC in the diagnosis of tuberculosis is 78% and 99% respectively.[47,52] FNAC of peripheral lymph nodes of patients with tuberculosis is an effective diagnostic test.

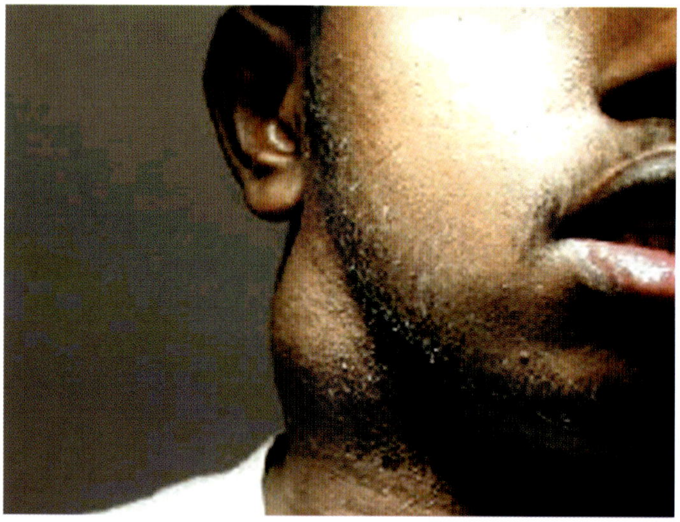

Figure 4.16 Tuberculous lymphadenopathy. Swelling of the nodes in the posterior triangle. The patient has night sweats and weight loss. The node is soft and fluctuant. FNAC is performed with pathologist and assistant wearing masks and protective clothing. Slides are not left in the air to dry but are contained in a transport box or handled in a grade 3 safety cabinet.

Cytological features include aggregates of epithelioid cells, multinuclear giant cells of Langhans' type and necrosis which can be seen in various ratios ranging from completely necrotic to more granulomatous (Figs 4.17 and 4.19). Acid-fast bacilli may be detected with Ziehl-Neelsen stain. FNAC material is routinely sent to microbiology for culture on Lowenstein culture medium. In the immunosuppressed, the infection with MAI (*Mycobacterium avium intracellulare*) may be detected through presence of numerous macrophages that contain acid-fast bacilli in large numbers (Fig. 4.20).

When comparing features of mycobacterial infection in HIV-positive and HIV-negative patients, Lapuerta et al[53] found that identification of granulomatous inflammation occurs at a similar rate in FNAC specimens from patients with HIV infection (16%) and without HIV infection (21%). Necrosis was the sole reported finding in a significant subset of cases (16%), occurring in patients with and without HIV infection. Authors conclude that the granulo-

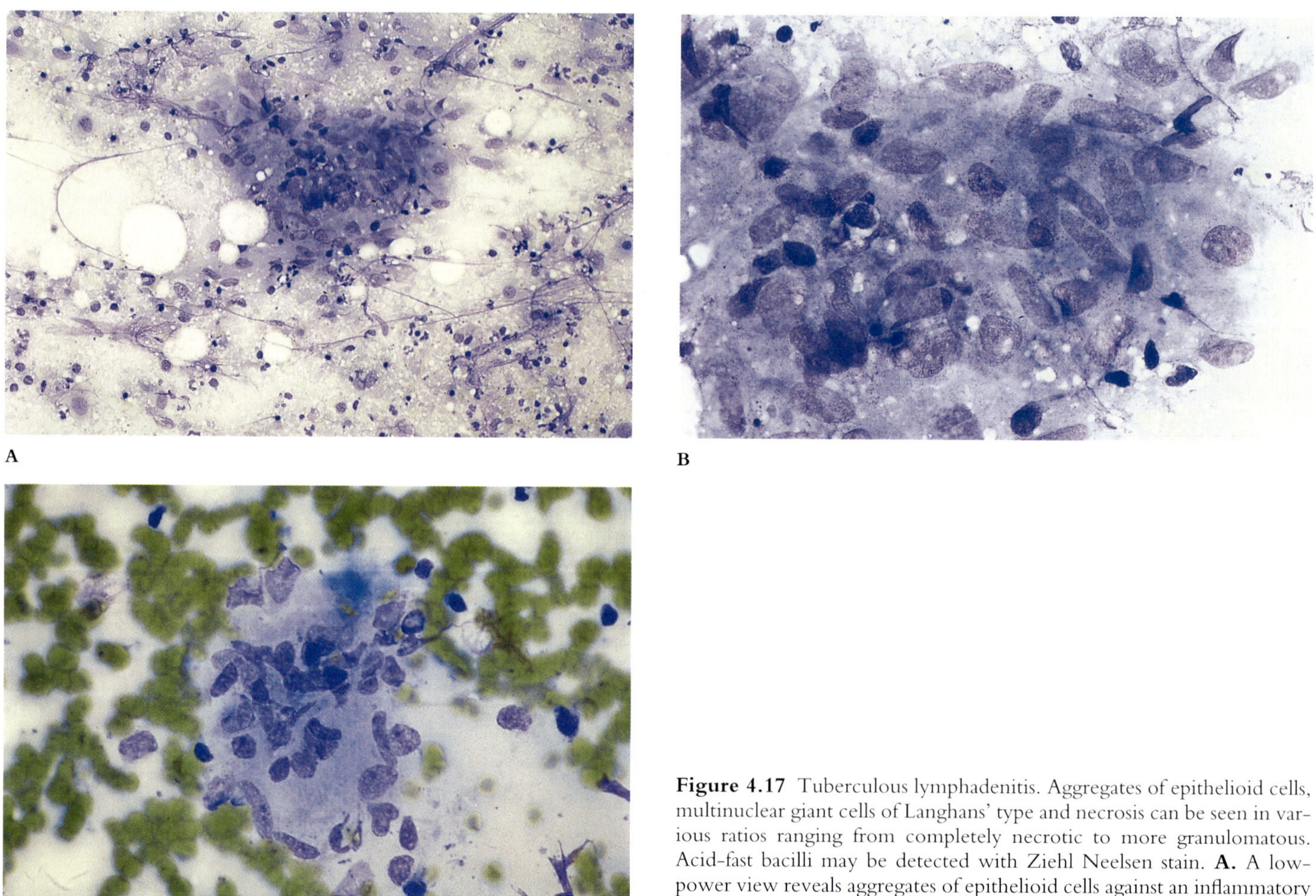

A

B

C

Figure 4.17 Tuberculous lymphadenitis. Aggregates of epithelioid cells, multinuclear giant cells of Langhans' type and necrosis can be seen in various ratios ranging from completely necrotic to more granulomatous. Acid-fast bacilli may be detected with Ziehl Neelsen stain. **A.** A low-power view reveals aggregates of epithelioid cells against an inflammatory lymphoid background (MGG ×200). **B, C.** High-power view shows epitheloid cells and Langhans' giant cells (MGG ×600 oil).

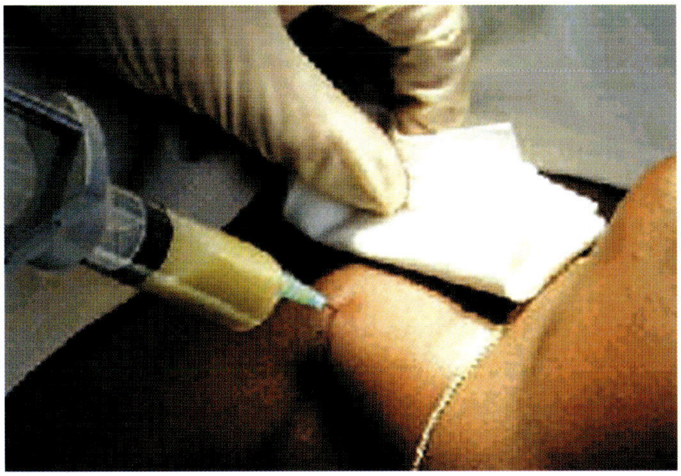

Figure 4.18 FNAC drainage of the necrotic tuberculous lymph node. Material is always sent for microbiology culture on LJ, medium.

matous inflammation and other FNAC findings in peripheral lymph nodes of patients with tuberculosis are similar in those with and those without HIV infection.[53]

Apart from tuberculosis, granulomatous lymphadenitis may be encountered in sarcoidosis (where it usually does not include necrosis), cat scratch disease, brucellosis, toxoplasmosis, some fungal infections, leishmaniasis, lepromatous and tuberculoid leprosy, primary syphilis, lymphogranuloma venereum, chronic tularaemia and rheumatoid arthritis (Fig. 4.21). Sarcoid-like granulomas may be seen in beryl-liosis and in reaction to other mineral substances including silicones (Fig. 4.22). Hodgkin's and rarely non-Hodgkin's lymphomas may provoke granulomatous reaction.

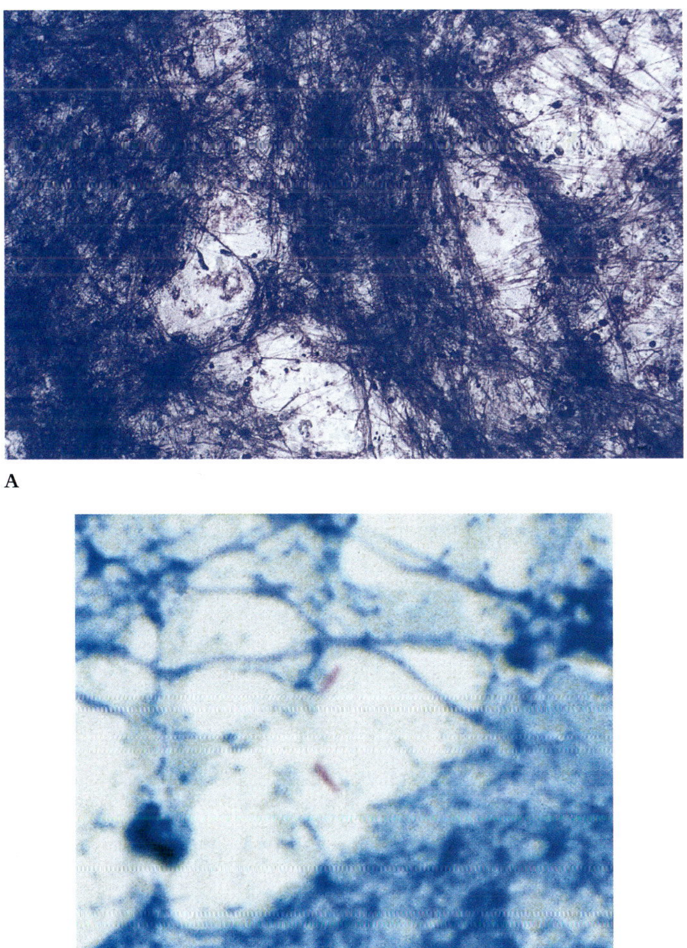

A

B

Figure 4.19 Tuberculous lymphadenitis. **A** Caseous necrosis produces necrotic background with no viable cells. Epithelioid cells and giant cells may not be seen in the centre of the necrotic node (×400, MGG). **B** ZN stain shows acid fast bacilli (×600, oil, ZN).

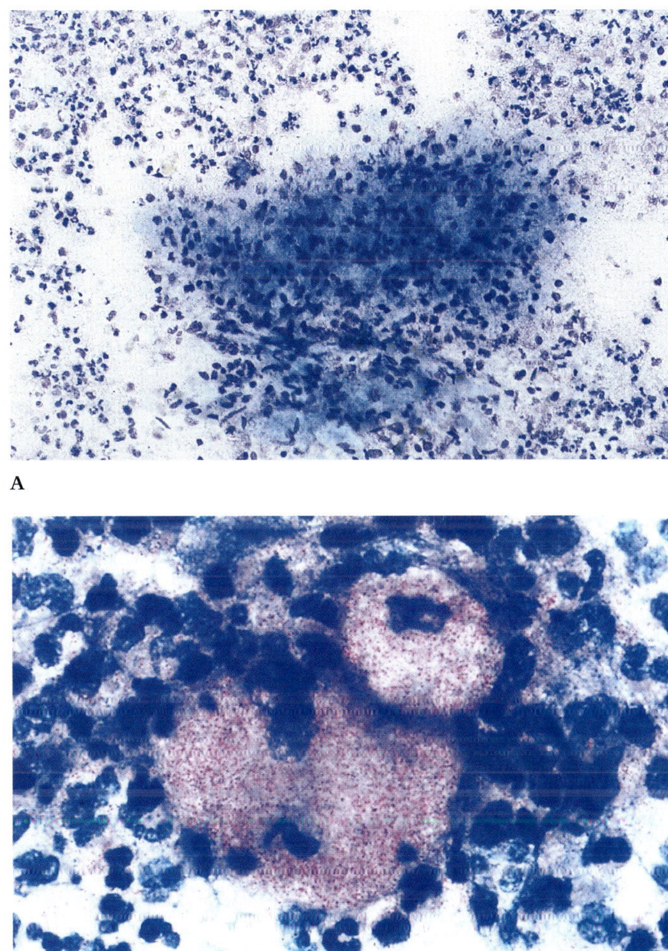

A

B

Figure 4.20 Mycobacterial infection. In HIV-positive patients, mycobacterial infection may be caused by other mycobacteria e.g. *M. Kansasii* or *M. avium intracellulare* (MAI). **A.** Low-power view of lymph node FNAC showing aggregate of pale staining macrophages (MGG ×200). **B.** High-power view of Ziehl-Neelsen stained slide shows numerous intracytoplamic acid fast-bacilli (ZN, ×1000).

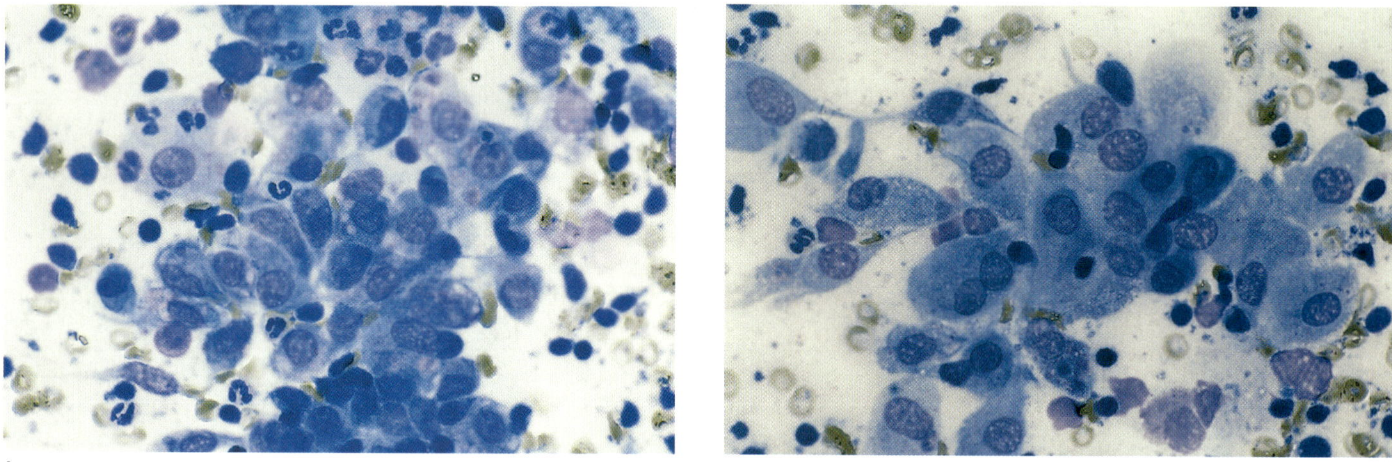

A B

Figure 4.21 Granulomatous lymphadenitis. Rheumatoid arthritis can sometimes provoke generalised or regional lymphadenopathy. Rheumatologists are usually aware of this phenomenon but patients may be seen by a different doctor who may not appreciate the relevance of this history and therefore not pass it on to the cytopathologist. Alternatively, an excessively large lymph node, even if the history is known, may require investigation. **A.** High-power view of an aggregate of histiocytes in a rheumatoid lymph node hyperplasia (MGG ×600 oil). **B.** Same patient, detail of histiocytic/epithelioid cells suggesting granuloma. No necrosis is seen.

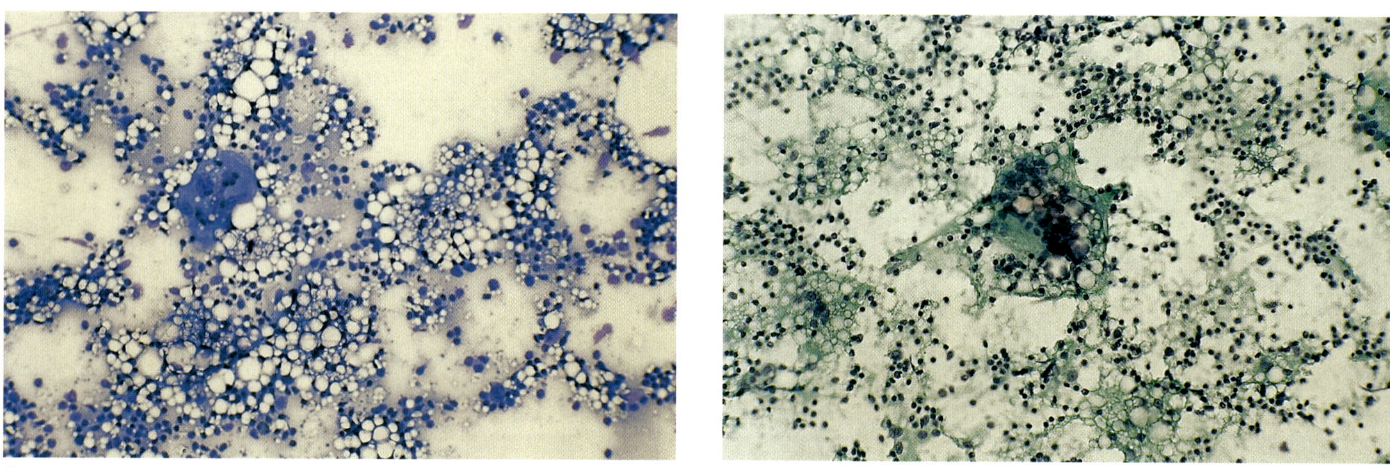

A B

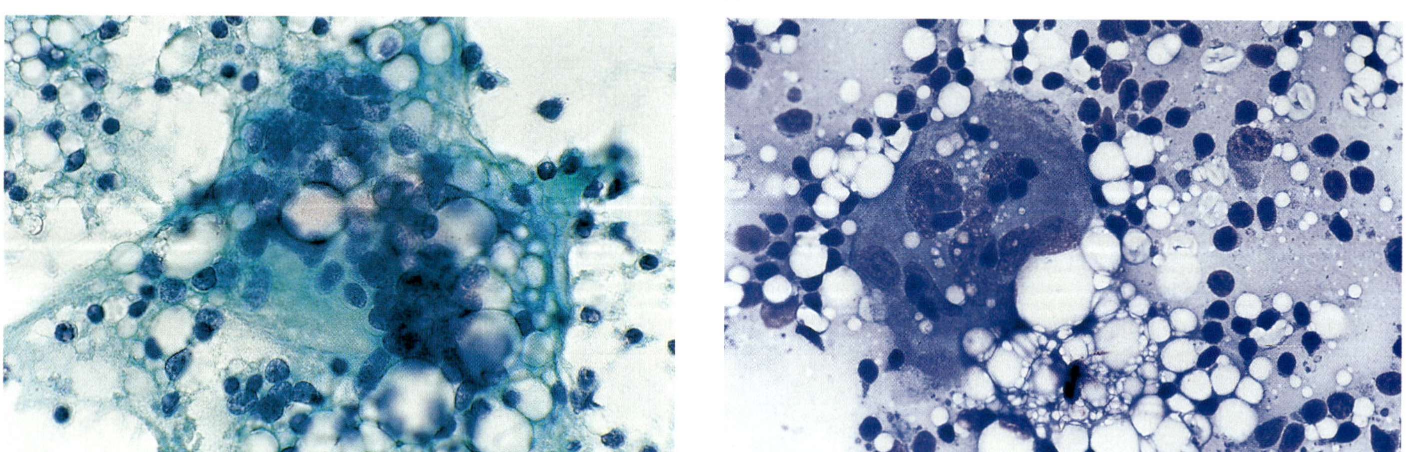

C D

Figure 4.22 Granulomatous lymphadenitis is provoked by silicone. This patient had a history of a silicone breast implant. She now presented with several small nodules in the supraclavicular fossa. **A, B.** Low-power view of lymphoid cells with a large multinucleate giant cell. Droplets of silicone are dispersed (PAP, MGG ×200). **C, D.** High-power view of the multinucleate giant cells with vacuolated material. It does not refract light (PAP, MGG ×600 oil immersion).

Cat scratch disease

Cat scratch disease is usually a benign, self-limited lymphadenitis, characterised by suppurative granulomas, caused by a small gram-negative bacillus. It affects children and adults, usually during the autumn and winter months and is usually associated with a cat scratch or bite 2–4 weeks prior to lymphadenopathy, although it can be acquired through the skin without a visible lesion. It may be associated with fever and a wide spectrum of generalised symptoms. Lymphadenopathy is most commonly parotid, cervical or axillary. In children, it may be dramatic and clinically mimic malignancy (Fig. 4.23). Neoplasia was initially suspected clinically in 38% of cases in one study.[54] Histologically, numerous abscesses or small areas of necrosis surrounded by

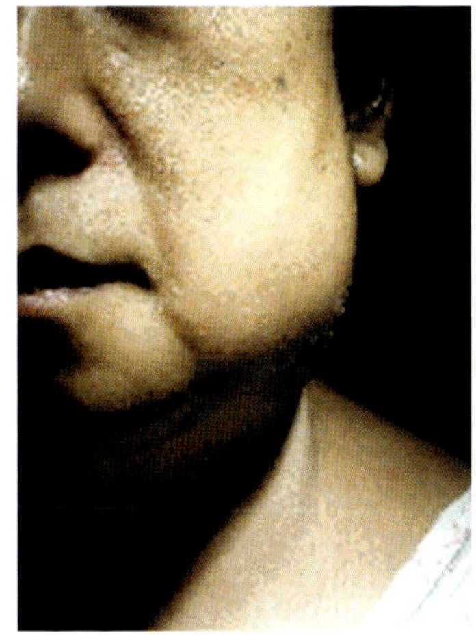

Figure 4.23 Cat scratch disease. This patient presented with a 4-week history of hard diffuse swelling at the angle of mandible which was clinically thought to be malignancy.

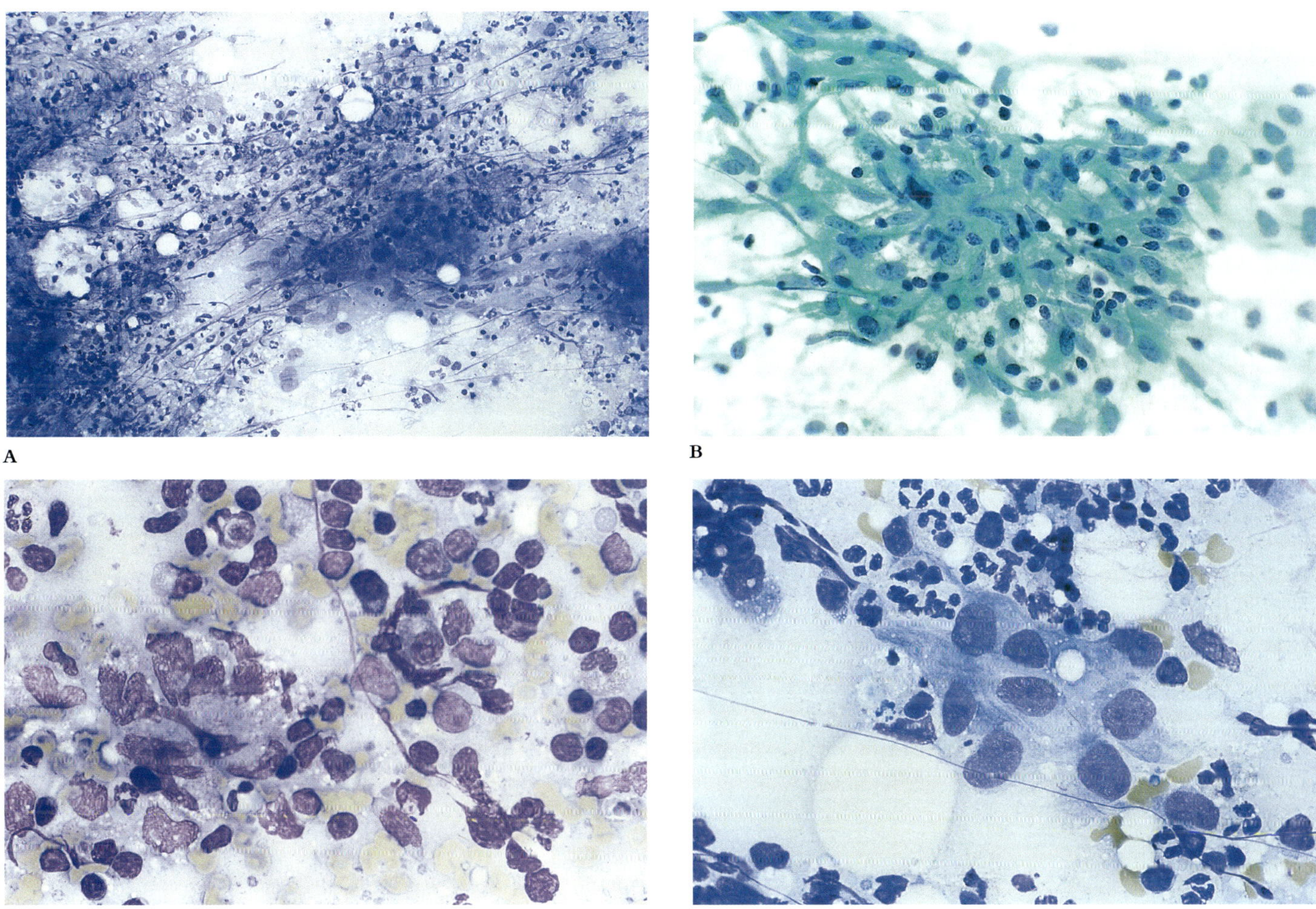

A B C

Figure 4.24 Cat scratch disease. **A.** Lower power view shows a heterogenous mix of cell types, confluent epithelioid cells admixed with neutrophils against a background of polymorphic inflammatory cells (MGG ×200). **B.** Alcohol fixed preparations show aggregates of epithelioid cells (PAP ×400). **C.** High power view shows lymphocytes, immunoblasts, plasma cells, neutrophils, histiocytes and rare eosinophils. Rare multinucleate giant cells may also be seen (×600 oil immersion). **D.** A varying number of medium-sized to large lymphoid cells with an appearance suggestive of monocytoid B-lymphocytes are associated with the epithelioid cells (×600 oil immersion).

histiocytic reaction, occasionaly granulomata are found. Diagnosis is confirmed by a positive intradermal skin test.

Cytological features include a heterogenous mix of cell types, confluent epithelioid cells admixed with neutrophils against a background of polymorphic inflammatory cells to include lymphocytes, immunoblasts, plasma cells, neutrophils, histiocytes and rare eosinophils (Fig. 4.24). Rare multinucleate giant cells may also be seen. A varying number of medium-sized to large lymphoid cells with an appearance suggestive of monocytoid B-lymphocytes are associated with the epithelioid cells.[55,56] Warthin-Starry silver stain-positive bacteria are detected in 69% of cases and are not limited to those preparations with suppurative granulomas.[54,55] The most distinctive cytological feature is that of a granuloma, present in 77% of cases; suppuration is present in 66%, epithelioid histiocytes in 46% and suppurative granulomata in 38%.[54] Neither granulomata nor suppurative inflammation are seen in all cases. The diagnosis is generally one of exclusion since cultures, smears and tissue staining may be negative.

The cytological differential diagnosis includes all lymphadenopathies with suppurative granulomas. These include lymphogranuloma venereum, yersinia lymphadenitis, tularaemia, brucellosis, listeriosis and meliodosis.[56]

Fungal diseases (mycoses)

These are rarely encountered in the UK except in travellers and in the immunosuppressed. The most frequently encountered infections are histoplasmosis and cryptococcosis. Histoplasmosis, although primarily affecting the lungs, may also affect lymph nodes causing necrotising granulomatous lesions which may calcify. Histoplasma capsulatum is readily demonstrated on MGG and PAS stained preparations as intracellular organisms (Fig. 4.25). Cryptoccocosis, although a disease of hot climates is seen in immunosuppressed individuals and may involve lymph nodes. Cryptococcus evokes little cellular response and is readily recognised on silver staining as oval budding spores (Fig. 4.26).

Toxoplasmosis

Toxoplasmosis is a disease caused by protozoan *Toxoplasma gondii*. In humans, the disease occurs as both congenital and

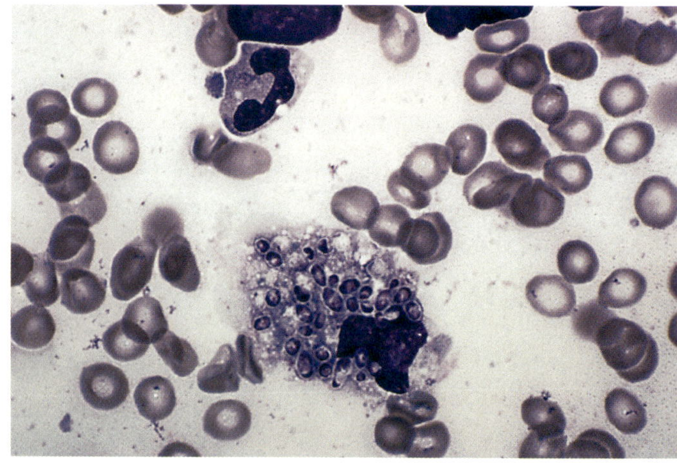

A

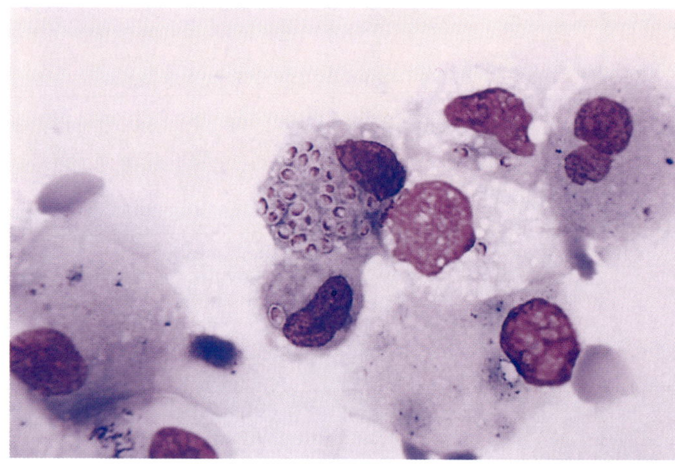

B

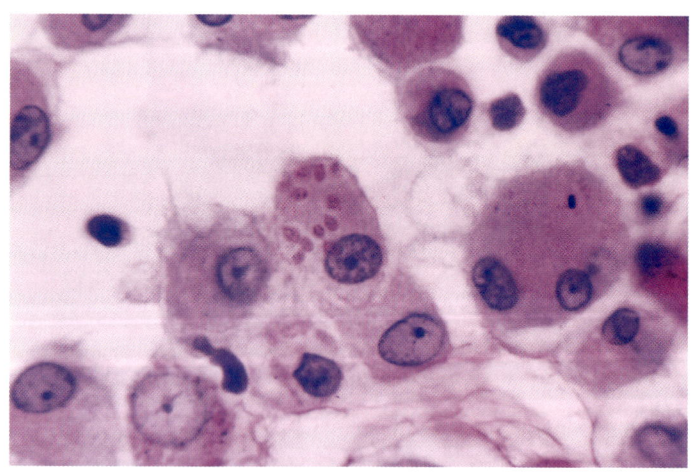

C

Figure 4.25 *Histoplasma capsulatum*. Organisms are readily seen in the cytoplasm of macrophages. **A.** MGG. **B.** Diff **C.** Quik (PAS, ×1000 oil immersion).

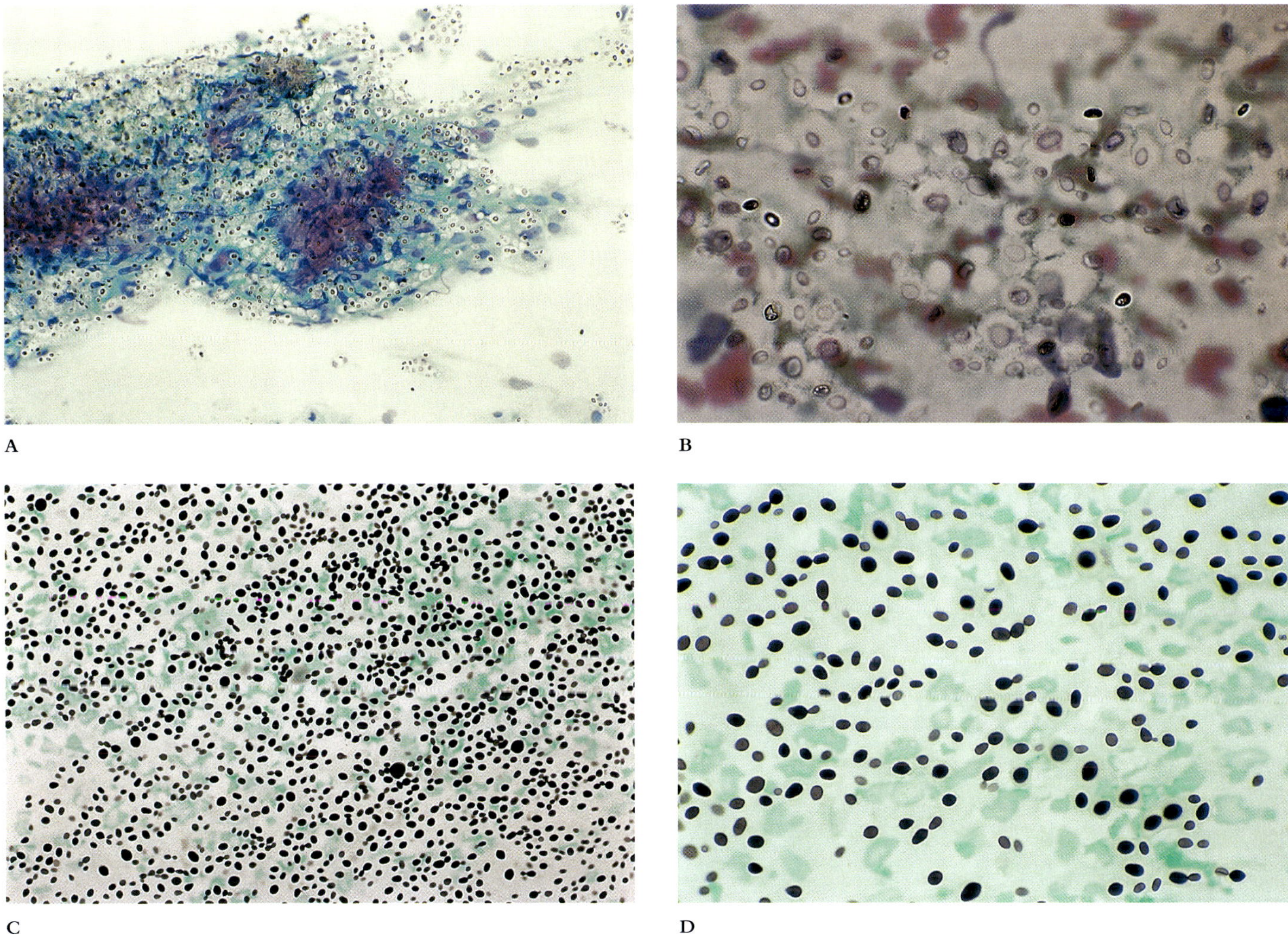

Figure 4.26 Cryptococcal infection. FNAC of lymph node in a HIV-positive patient. **A.** Low-power view shows scattered pale oval dots, easily confused with air bubbles under the covering glass (PAP ×200). **B.** High-power view reveals detail of the refractile, pale bodies (PAP ×1000 oil immersion). **C, D.** Methenamine silver (Grocott) shows numerous oval fungal spores with characteristic budding (MS ×200, ×1000 oil immersion).

acquired. The congenital form can cause fetal death, hydrocephaly, microcephaly, encephalitis or chorioretinitis. The acquired form usually presents as a mild, usually asymptomatic lymphadenopathy which occurs sporadically. Toxoplasmic lymphadenopathy is a fairly common (15%) cause of unexplained lymphadenopathy and surgical biopsy is often performed because of a suspicion of lymphoma. Since the disease is generally self-limiting, no treatment is necessary and fine needle aspiration can spare the patient unnecessary hospitalisation and surgery.[57] Disease presents as cervical lymphadenopathy either acutely or of some months duration, usually in children and young adults.[58] The main reservoir of infection is the domestic cat. The disease can be diagnosed by serological tests but the diagnosis is complicated by the high prevalence of antibodies in the normal population.

Cytological features include polymorphous population of lymphocytes which vary in size from small mature lymphocytes which predominate, to larger, transformed lymphocytes, plasma cells and immunoblasts (Fig. 4.27). Prominent follicular dendritic cells and germinal centre histiocytes filled with phagocytised karyorrhectic debris are also present. The characteristic finding is that of epithelioid cells seen in small, loose aggregates. Although not pathognomonic of toxoplasmosis, the finding of small aggregates of epithelioid cells against a background of lymph node hyperplasia, with an absence of giant cells and necrosis, is

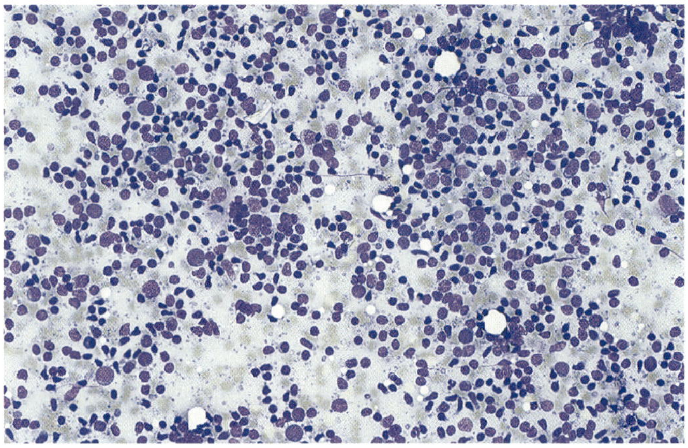
A

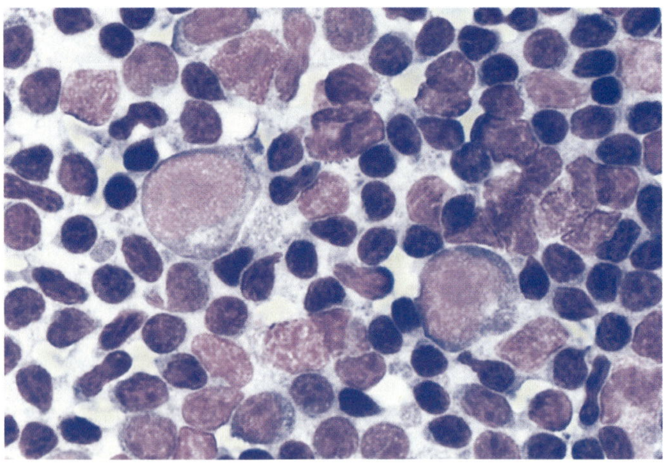
B

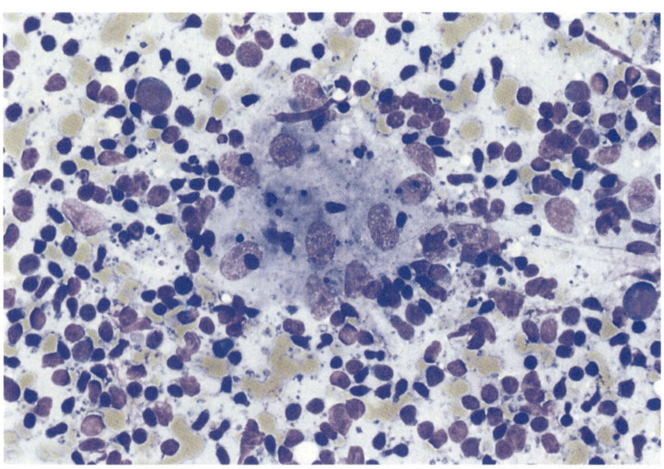
C

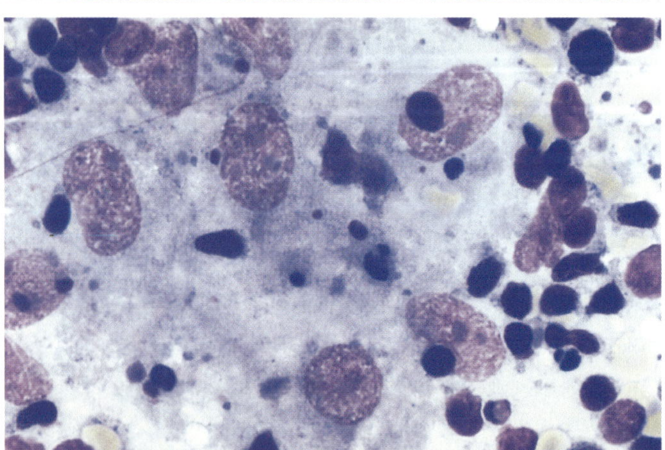
D

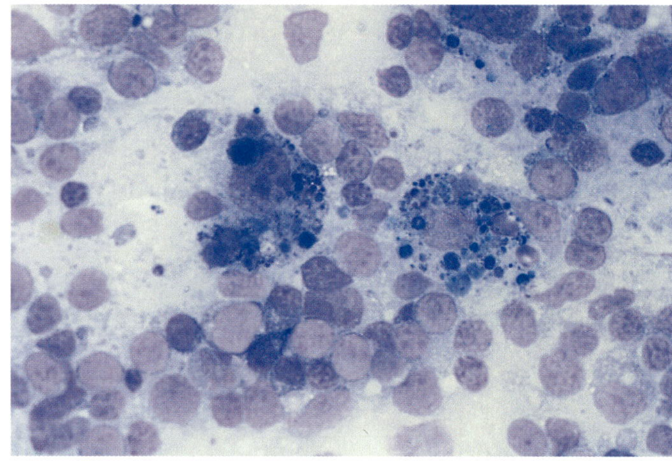
E

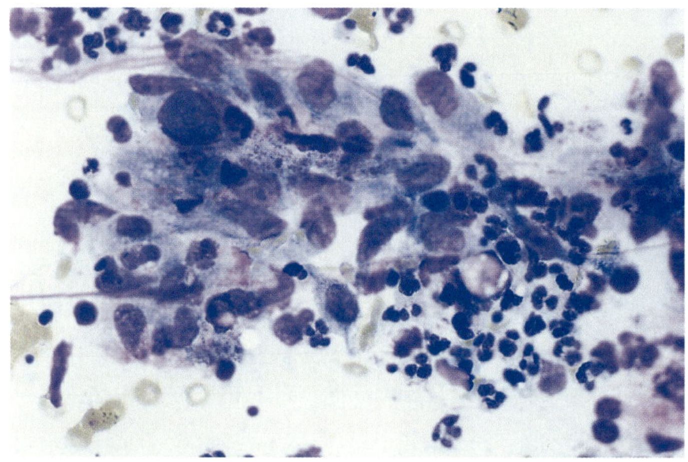
F

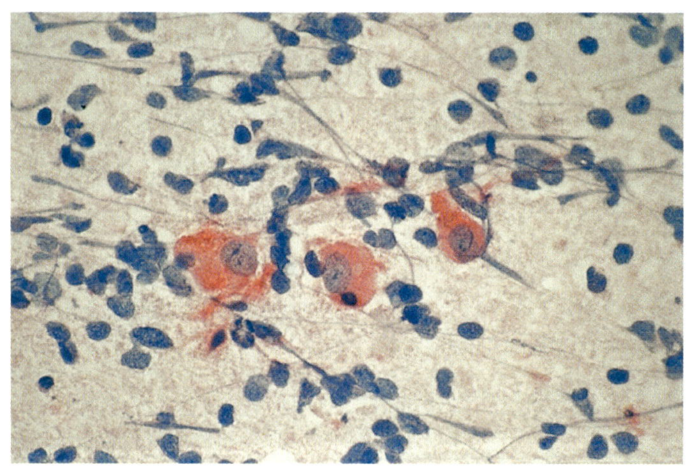
G

Figure 4.27 Toxoplasmosis. FNAC of a 9-year-old child presenting with large submandibular lymph node without any generalised symptoms. **A.** Low-power view showing polymorphous population of lymphocytes (MGG ×200). **B.** Lymphocytes vary in size from small mature lymphocytes, which predominate, to larger, transformed lymphocytes, plasma cells and immunoblasts (MGG ×600 oil immersion). **C,D,E.** Prominent follicular dendritic cells filled with phagocytised karyorrhectic debris (MGG ×600, ×1000 oil immersion). **F.** Epithelioid cells are seen in small, loose aggregates. This finding prompts the suggestion of toxoplasmosis. Occasionally, microorganisms can be identified in the cytological preparations. Rarely, numerous tachyzoites may be seen dispersed free in exudate, and also within cells, forming pseudocysts (MGG ×600). **G.** Immunocytochemistry for *Toxoplasma gondii* antigen is positive (APAAP ×600 oil immersion).

highly suggestive of toxoplasmosis. Occasionally microorganisms can be identified in the cytological preparations. Zaharopoulos[59] described toxoplasma cysts in Papanicolaou-stained smears and dispersed tachyzoites and a pseudocyst in MGG preparations.[59] As a fairly rare occurrence, numerous tachyzoites may be seen dispersed free in exudate, and also within cells, forming pseudocysts. Immunocytochemistry for *Toxoplasma gondii* antigen is positive. The tachyzoites seen in MGG preparations, when subjected to fluorescence microscopy, emit autofluorescence, facilitating their identification. Besides the use of immunocytochemistry in the diagnosis of the disease, air-dried preparations stained by the MGG method are valuable for the demonstration of such parasites through careful searching, along with the possible use of fluorescence microscopy.

Leishmaniasis

Leishmaniasis is a parasitosis caused by protozoa of the genus *Leishmania* that multiply in the cells of the reticuloendothelial system. Transmission of the parasite occurs through the vector (phlebotomus). The main reservoirs are humans and dogs. Leishmania has a worldwide distribution with 5 large known areas of location: Russia and China, South America, India and Pakistan, north and east Africa and countries of the Mediterranean. Clinically, the disease presents as cutaneous, mucocutaneous or visceral (kala-azar) infection. Patients present with lymphadenopathy. Histologically, lymph nodes show histiocytic microgranulomas confluent with epithelioid cells, multinucleated giant cells and occasionally areas of necrosis. Organism can be cultured on NNN medium, which takes approximately 2 weeks to grow, or by Leishmania skin test, which becomes positive 3 months after the onset of disease. Cytological material can be obtained either by scraping the skin lesions or by FNAC. However, FNAC is recommended as the method of choice of confirming the diagnosis.[60]

Cytological features. The pathognomonic cytological picture consists of lymphocytes, plasma cells and epithelioid granulomata intermingled with histiocytes. Multinucleated giant cells may be seen. Numerous *Leishmania* organisms are seen in the cytoplasm of histiocytes and extracellularly.[61] Under oil immersion, these Leishman-Donovan bodies measure 1.5–3 μm and are small, rounded cells with a fine membrane, a relatively large nucleus and a paranucleus (kinetoplast).[62] Some kinetoplasts are observed within the intracytoplasmic vesicles (phagolysosomes) and some extracellularly. Apart from lymph nodes, organisms can be found in the spleen and bone marrow.

Differential diagnosis includes all granulomatous lymphadenopathies (tuberculosis, atypical mycobacteria, toxoplasmosis, syphilis, leprosy, lymphogranuloma venereum, brucellosis and mycotic infections). In the case of skin disease, other skin diseases that contain parasitised macrophages are rhinoscleroma, lymphogranuloma venereum and histoplasmosis.

Chronic lymphadenitis of infective origin

Kikuchi's lymphadenitis

Kikuchi's lymphadenitis is a self-limiting condition typically affecting young women. Patients present with cervical lymphadenopathy affecting one or more lymph nodes, sometimes accompanied by malaise and pyrexia. Sometimes lymphadenopathy may be extensive, clinically mimicking lymphoma. Histologically, there are foci of necrosis in the lymph nodes with numerous nuclear fragments giving an impression of polymorphs, although polymorphs are conspicuously absent.

Cytological features. Characteristic FNAC findings are those of karyorrhectic and granular debris and distinctive phagocytic histiocytes. These phagocytic histiocytes have peripherally placed 'crescentic' nuclei and abundant cytoplasm containing phagocytosed karyorrhectic or eosinophilic granular debris, easily distinguishable from tingible body macrophages, which have centrally placed, round nuclei. Also found are plasmacytoid monocytes, medium-sized cells with eccentrically placed, round nuclei, condensed chromatin and a moderate amount of amphophilic cytoplasm. Non-phagocytic histiocytes with twisted nuclei and delicate chromatin and immunoblasts that sometimes show atypical features such as irregular foldings of the nuclei can also be seen (Fig. 4.28).[63] Neutrophils are sparse or absent. FNAC findings of lymph nodes involved by various reactive processes, tuberculosis and lymphoma for comparison show that although tingible body macrophages and debris are not uncommon, very few phagocytic histiocytes with crescentic nuclei or plasmacytoid monocytes are observed.

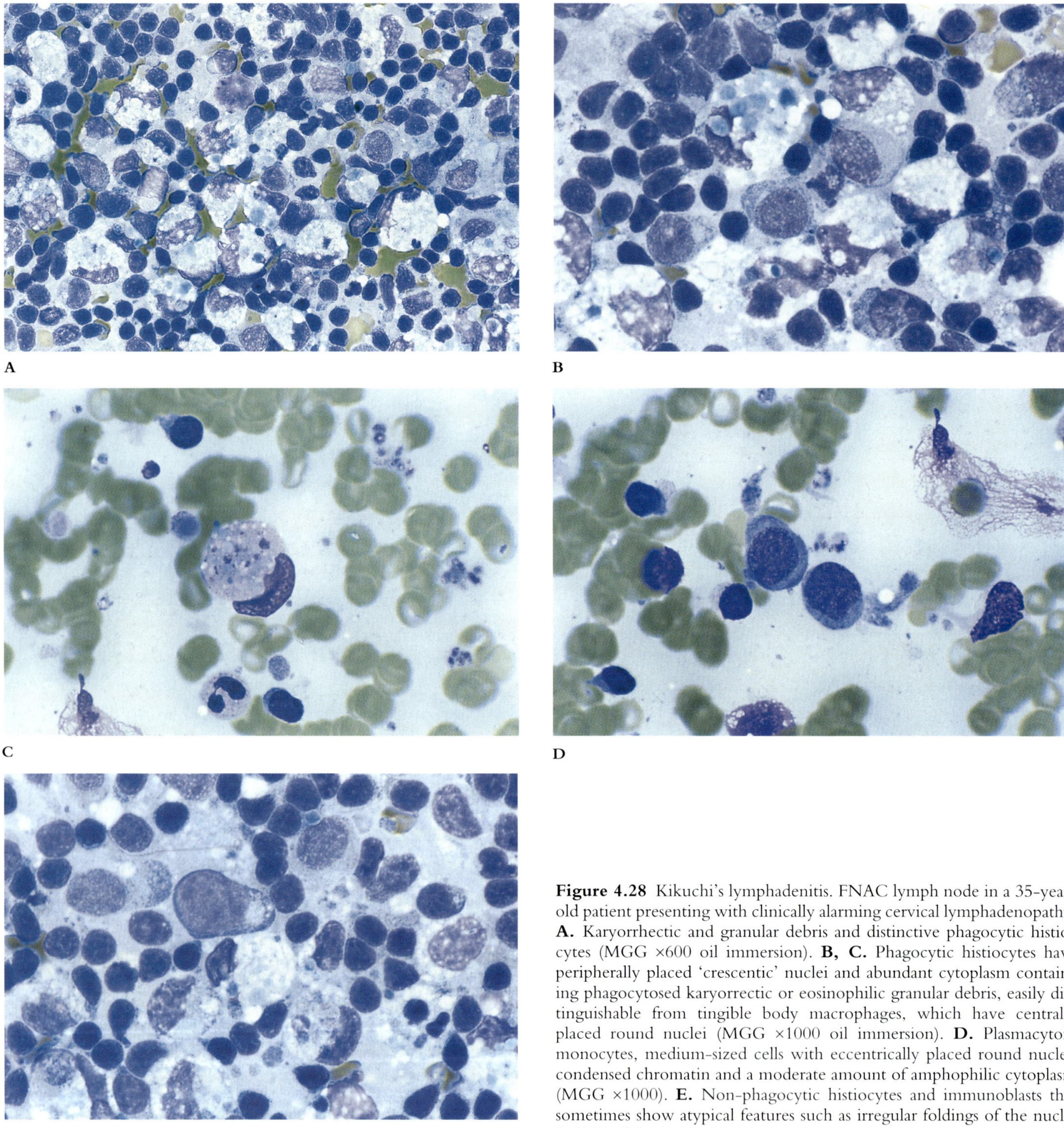

Figure 4.28 Kikuchi's lymphadenitis. FNAC lymph node in a 35-year-old patient presenting with clinically alarming cervical lymphadenopathy. **A.** Karyorrhectic and granular debris and distinctive phagocytic histiocytes (MGG ×600 oil immersion). **B, C.** Phagocytic histiocytes have peripherally placed 'crescentic' nuclei and abundant cytoplasm containing phagocytosed karyorrectic or eosinophilic granular debris, easily distinguishable from tingible body macrophages, which have centrally placed round nuclei (MGG ×1000 oil immersion). **D.** Plasmacytoid monocytes, medium-sized cells with eccentrically placed round nuclei, condensed chromatin and a moderate amount of amphophilic cytoplasm (MGG ×1000). **E.** Non-phagocytic histiocytes and immunoblasts that sometimes show atypical features such as irregular foldings of the nuclei (×1000 oil immersion).

The features described above permit diagnosis of Kikuchi's lymphadenitis by FNAC.[64] Because of morphological similarities between lupus lymphadenitis and Kikuchi's lymphadenitis, however, serological studies are warranted to exclude systemic lupus erythematosus.

Infectious mononucleosis

Infectious mononucleosis (glandular fever) is caused by Epstein-Barr virus (EBV), which is also associated with Burkitt's lymphoma and nasopharyngeal carcinoma. Disease may be subclinical or manifest itself as generalised lymphadenopathy and flu-like illness. Diagnosis is made by positive Paul Bunnel heterophil antibody test or monospot test. Histologically, there may be florid blast transformation of lymphocytes with blurring of normal architecture. Occasional large blasts may mimic Reed-Sternberg cells. Patients are referred for FNAC usually for clinically suspected malignant lymphoma, due to often sizeable, sometimes unilateral, cervical lymphadenopathy (Fig. 4.29).

Cytological features. Smears show greater numbers of large immunoblastic lymphocytes than are usually seen in the reactive lymph node. Features may be mistaken for a malignant lymphoma but include a considerable background of polymorphic immunoblasts. Since several reactive and neoplastic processes mimic this pattern, cases should be confirmed by confirmatory serological studies and/or resolution of lymphadenopathy (Fig. 4.30). Failing this, an excisional lymph node biopsy should follow.[65]

Acquired immunodeficiency syndrome (AIDS)

HIV-infected patients in the early stages of infection may present with a widespread painless lymphadenopathy accompanied with malaise and listlessness. This is known as persistent generalised lymphadenopathy (PGL) (Fig. 4.31).

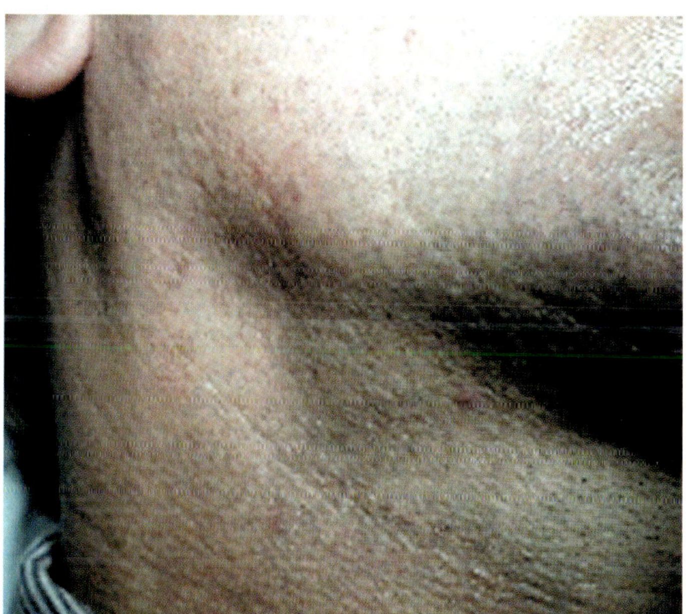

Figure 4.29 Infectious mononucleosis. The patient was referred for FNAC for clinically suspicious persistent, unilateral cervical lymphadenopathy.

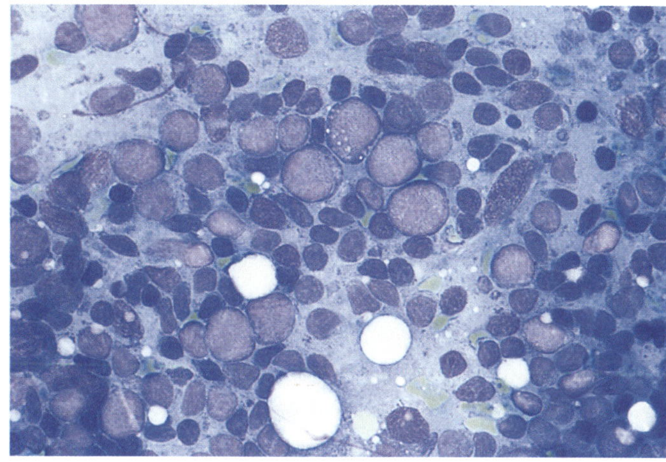

A

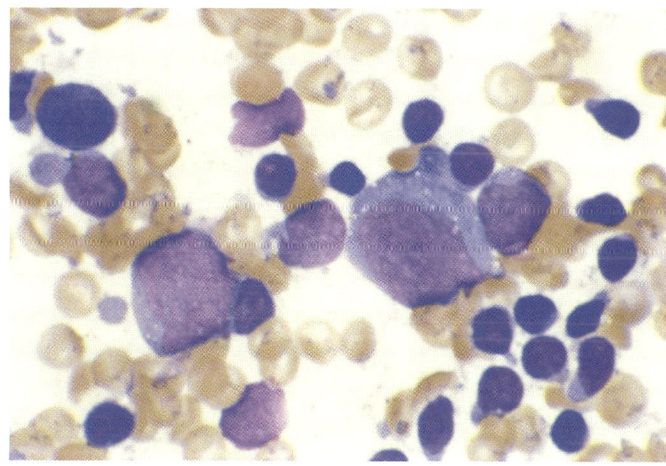

B

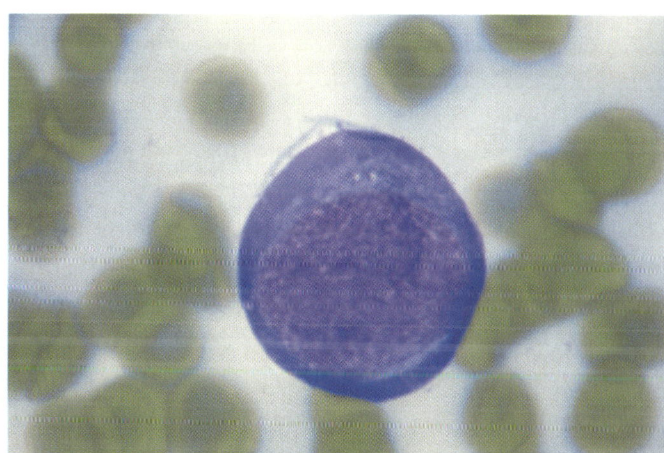

C

Figure 4.30 Infectious mononucleosis. **A.** Smears show greater numbers of immunoblasts than are usually seen in the reactive lymph node (×600 oil immersion). **B,C.** Features may be mistaken for a malignant lymphoma but include a considerable background of polymorphic immunoblasts (×1000 oil immersion). Since several reactive and neoplastic processes mimic this pattern, cases should be confirmed by either confirmatory serological studies and/or resolution of lymphadenopathy. Otherwise, they should be referred for excision.

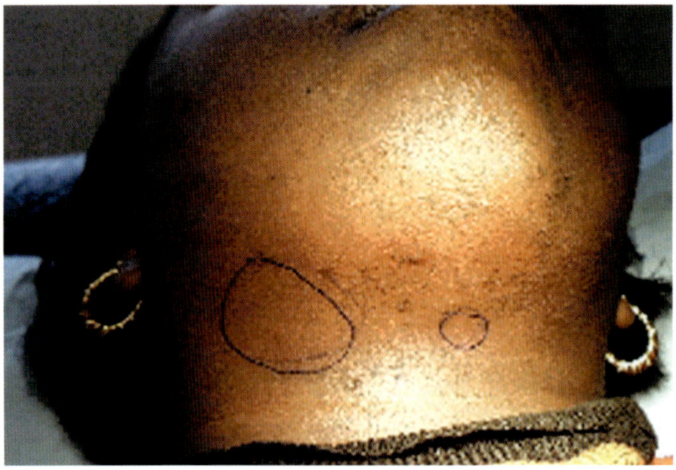

Figure 4.31 HIV-associated lymphadenopathy. The commonest site of FNAC in HIV-positive patients is the cervical lymph nodes. Patients may present at any stage of the disease with enlarged lymph nodes. Clinically, differential diagnosis is either PGL, specific infection, lymphoma or Kaposi's sarcoma. FNAC is useful in distinguishing between these entities and sparing the patient unnecessary biopsy.

Immunological function is still preserved although a progressive reversal of the TH:TS ratio may be observed. After a time, lymphadenopathy disappears and is superseded by the phase of immune deficiency where loss of weight, diarrhoea and cerebral impairment are common symptoms. Opportunistic infections are frequent in this phase. The lymph nodes in the terminal stage are small and difficult to find.

Histologically, lymph nodes in PGL show striking follicular hyperplasia with large and irregular germinal centres with poorly developed mantle zones and paracortex relatively depleted of lymphocytes. In the later stages, follicles shrink and disappear with scanty aggregates of B-lymphocytes in place of follicle centres (Fig. 4.32). Proliferation of endothelial venules in the paracortex is noted.

Palpable or radiologically identified masses in patients infected with HIV are amenable to FNAC to differentiate between the infections and neoplasms.[66] FNAC offers a rapid, simple and cost-effective approach to diagnosis. The commonest site of FNAC in HIV-positive patients is cervical lymph nodes (54%). Reactive lymphadenopathy (PGL) is the most commonly diagnosed condition, followed by infection, and malignancy.[67,68] Part of the FNAC specimen is sent for bacterial culture, fungal culture and acid-fast smear and culture. Some of the infections detected in FNAC include toxoplasmosis, histoplasmosis, tuberculosis, atypical mycobacterium, cryptococcosis and methicillin-resistant staphylococcal infection. Shapiro & Pincus[70] found that all patients with either unilateral lymphadenopathy or lymph nodes 3 cm or larger in size had positive aspirates. Tenderness and recent enlargement are important indicators.[69] A statistically significant difference between patients with lymph nodes smaller than 2 cm and those with nodes larger than 2 cm was found.[70] Cervical node biopsy is not indicated in HIV or AIDS patients with non-tender or non-enlarging nodes.[71]

Cytological features of lymphadenopathy associated with HIV infection vary depending on the stage of disease. In the initial stage, PGL may be reflected by a florid proliferation of follicle centre cells with many centroblasts, immunoblasts and tingible body macrophages reflecting the high cell turnover (Fig. 4.32). In the later stages, follicle depletion described in histology is reflected by relatively hypocellular aspirates with only the small lymphocytes and follicular dendritic cells remaining as a residue of follicles.

Drug reactions

Lymphadenopathy is a recognised feature of some drug hypersensitivity reactions, namely penicillin, sulphonamides, certain antimalarials and non-steroidal anti-inflammatory drugs. Generalised symptoms usually prompt the drug to be withdrawn and lymphadenopathy to subside before it has been further investigated. Some anticonvulsant drugs, in particular hydantoin and carbamazepine, may cause lymphadenopathy and gum hypertrophy as side-effects (Fig. 4.33).[72] Histologically and cytologically, the T-cells of the paracortex show blastic transformation similar to infectious mononucleosis. Atypical blasts may also be present. Histological features in the skin are those of a cutaneous pseudolymphoma, including CD30+ cells.[72] Development of malignant lymphoma in some of these nodes has been reported.[73]

Miscellaneous lymphadenopathies

Castleman's disease

Castleman's disease is a rare atypical lymphoproliferative disorder the morphology of which, soon after the original presentation of Castleman et al, has been subdivided into hyaline vascular and plasma cell histopathological patterns,

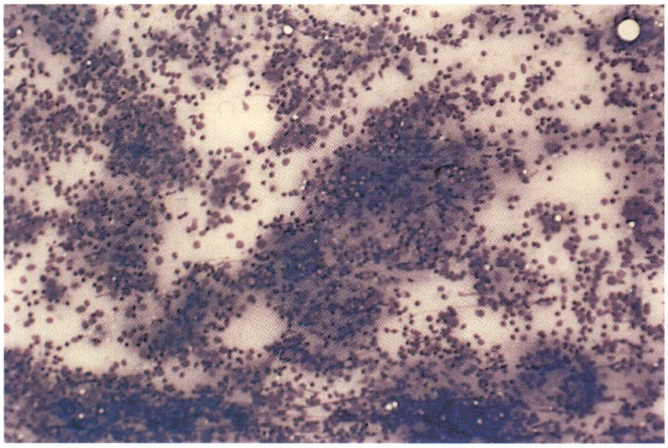

A

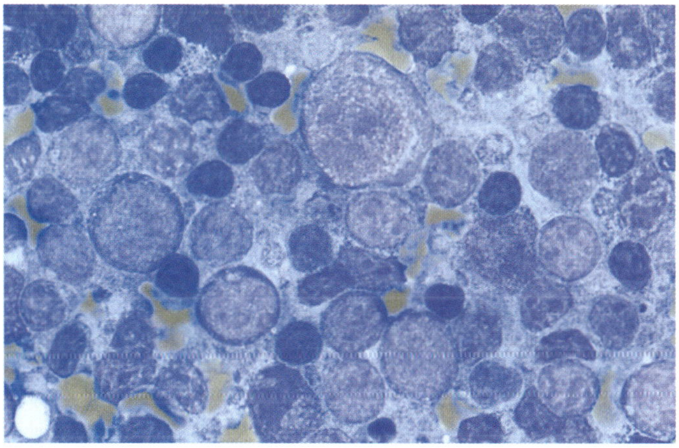

B

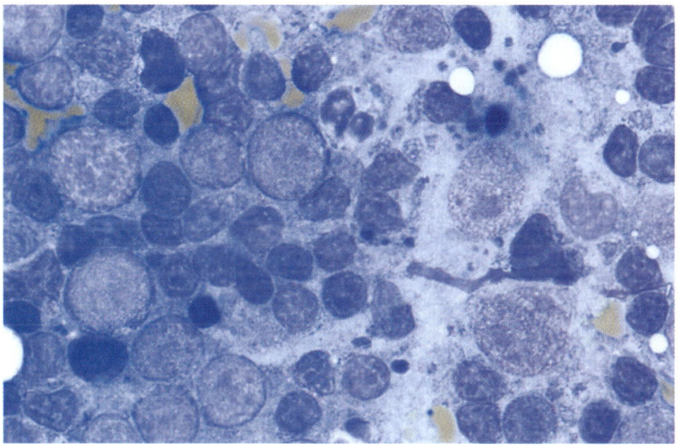

C

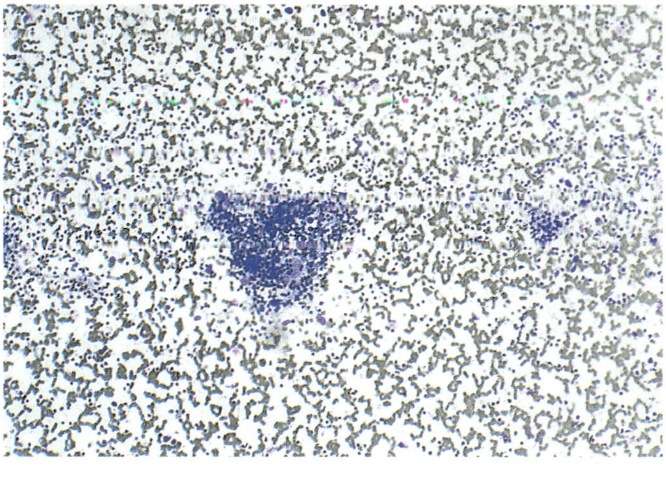

D

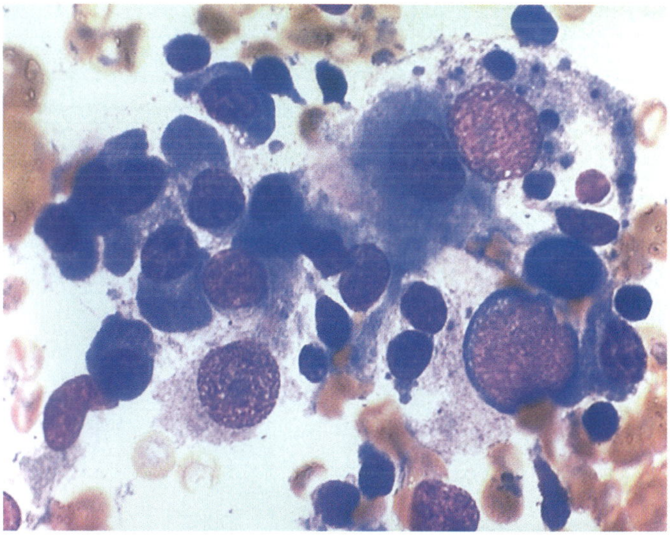

E

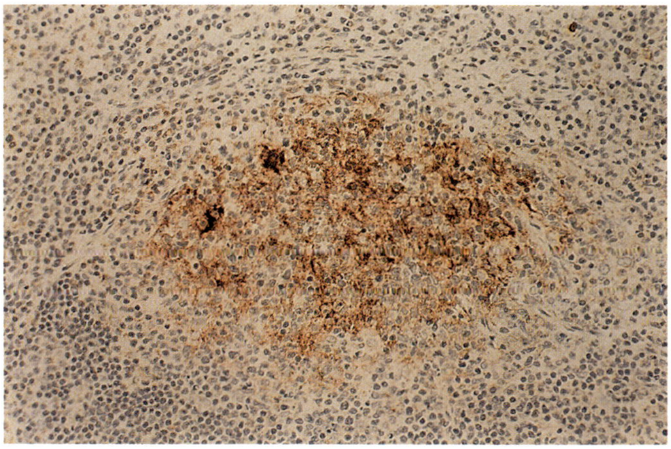

F

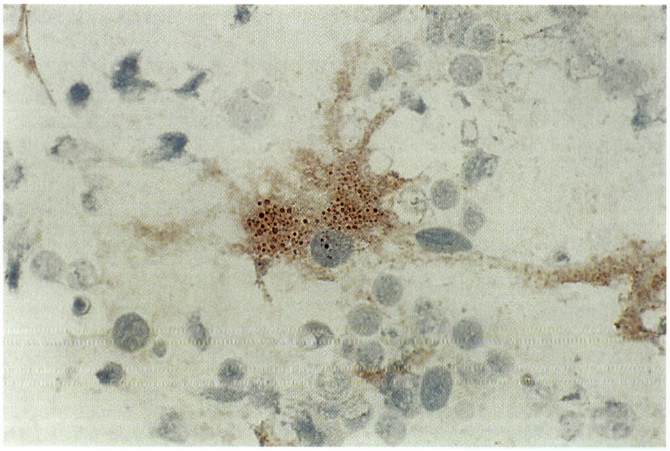

G

Figure 4.32 HIV-associated lymphadenopathy. **A,B,C.** In the initial stage, PGL may be represented in the FNAC material by a florid proliferation of follicle centre cells with many centroblasts, immunoblasts and tingible body macrophages reflecting the high cell turnover (MGG ×200, ×600 oil immersion). **D.** In later stages of disease, PGL may be seen as a sparsely cellular FNAC sample, composed of lymphoid cells mainly aggregated around the residual follicle centred fragments (MGG ×200). **E.** High power view of the same follicle centre as before, showing follicular dendritic cells, some lymphocytes and plasma cells (MGG ×600, oil immersion). **F.** Histological section of a lymph node shows P24 antiretroviral antibody is positive in dendritic reticulum cells (APAAP, ×400). **G.** Cytology shows P24 positivity in follicular dendritic cells (P24, IP, ×600, oil immersion).

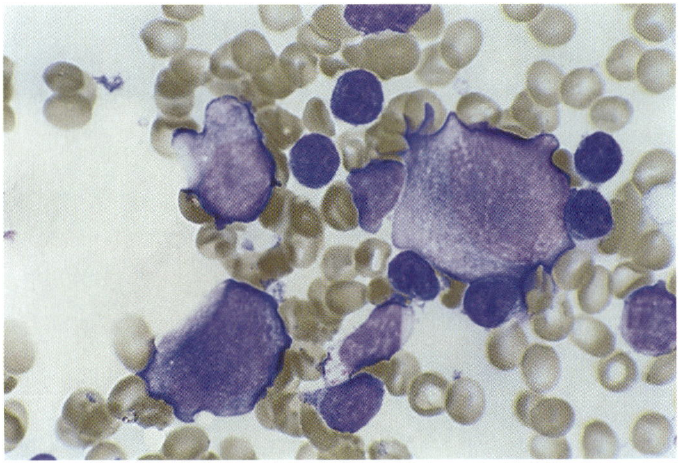

Figure 4.33 Phenytoin-induced lymphadenopathy. This patient was referred for unexplained cervical lymphadenopathy. Clinical history revealed that the patient was an epileptic on phenytoin treatment. Smears show blastic transformation similar to infectious mononucleosis. Atypical blasts are present (MGG ×100 oil immersion).

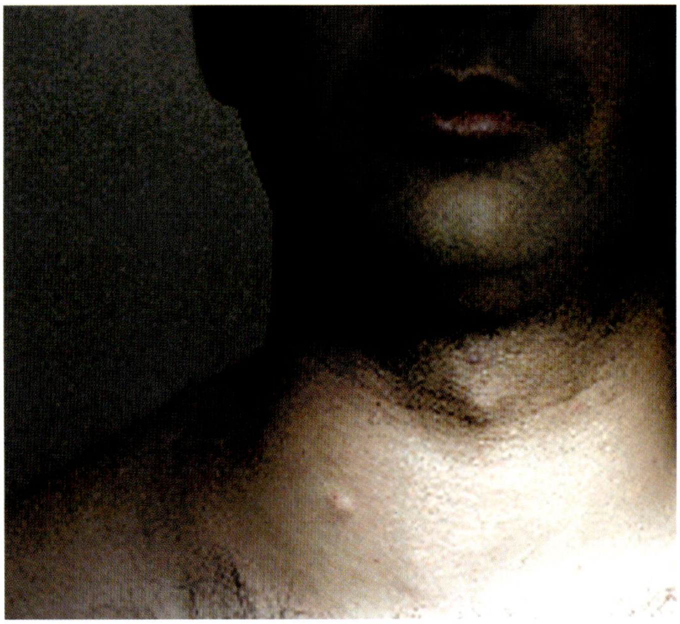

Figure 4.34 Castleman's disease. This 29-year-old patient presented with a painless diffuse swelling of the right side of the neck of some weeks duration. The FNAC findings are shown in Figure 4.35.

with intermediate variants. The former occurs much more frequently than the latter and is usually localised to the mediastinum or pulmonary hilum (Fig. 4.34). The latter involves lymph nodes separately or in aggregates and often displays multicentricity with systemic symptoms including autoimmune phenomena and an aggressive course. Infections are the most frequent cause of patient demise in these cases, followed by malignancies such as Kaposi's sarcoma, malignant lymphoma or carcinoma. Histologically, the hallmarks of Castleman's disease are: increase of follicular dendritic reticulum cells, often dysplastic, in the germinal centre and marginal zone; broad marginal zone expansion with prominence of immunophenotypically aberrant B-cells (Ki B3-negative, CD5-positive); possible predominance of paracortical plasma cells, often with clusters of clonal λ-light chain restricted plasma cells; and increase of paracortical plasmacytoid monocytes. The hyaline vascular type shows small hyalinised and hypervascular germinal centres with hypervascular interfollicular stroma and sinus effacement. The plasma cell pattern contains plasma cell aggregates in lymph node paracortex and partially spared sinuses. The two types are frequently concomitant. A key event in the pathogenesis of Castleman's disease has been suggested recently to be an abnormal production of a B-cell growth factor, such as IL-6, leading to lymphoproliferation and plasma cell differentiation and being involved in the oncogenesis of plasmacytoma. In this event, Kaposi's sarcoma associated virus (HHV-8), which has been found in many cases of Castleman's disease, especially in the multicentric form, could play a crucial role in both producing IL-6 and releasing angiogenic factors. A possible differentiation block may lead to the development of a malignant lymphoma, Kaposi's sarcoma or other malignant neoplasias and can be supposed to be consequences of the immunodeficiency typical of Castleman's disease.

Cytological features. Castleman's disease of the hyaline vascular subtype is an uncommon lesion; experience with fine needle aspiration of this tumour is limited to rare case reports.[74] In the clinical context of orophranygeal and mediastinal mass, hypercellular smears with mature small lymphoid population associated with larger atypical cells, which are consistent with follicular dendritic cells, can be suggestive of Castleman's disease (Fig. 4.35). Confirmation of a polytypic B-cell population by flow cytometry, supported by immunohistochemistry, is very helpful. Biopsy is advised.

Langerhans' cell histiocytosis (histiocytosis X)

Langerhans' cell histiocytosis is a non-neoplastic condition of unknown aetiology. It is regarded as a reactive disorder

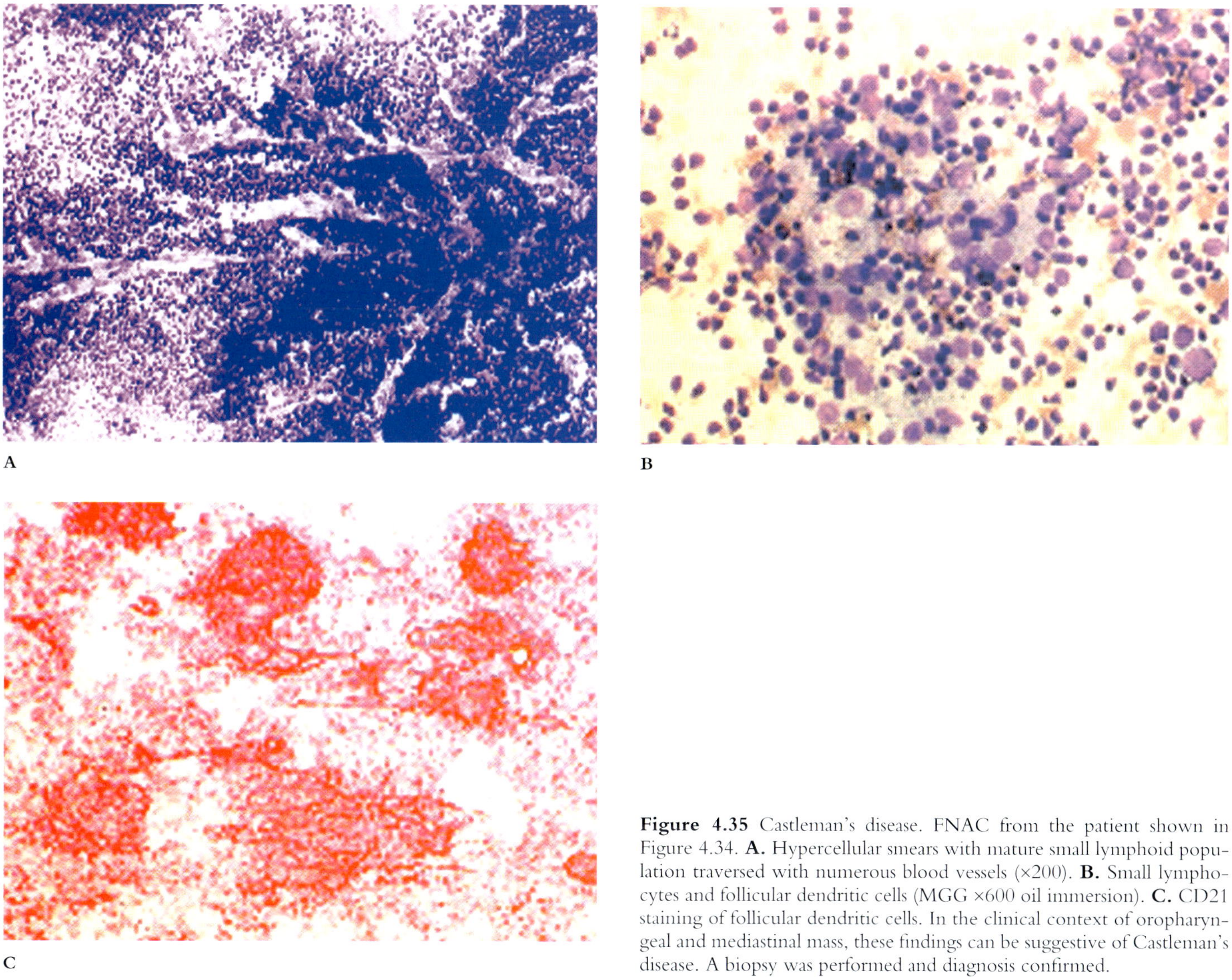

Figure 4.35 Castleman's disease. FNAC from the patient shown in Figure 4.34. **A.** Hypercellular smears with mature small lymphoid population traversed with numerous blood vessels (×200). **B.** Small lymphocytes and follicular dendritic cells (MGG ×600 oil immersion). **C.** CD21 staining of follicular dendritic cells. In the clinical context of oropharyngeal and mediastinal mass, these findings can be suggestive of Castleman's disease. A biopsy was performed and diagnosis confirmed.

reacting to an unknown inciting agent(s). Clinically, it includes a triad of related disorders, *Letterer-Siwe syndrome*, *Hand Schüller Christian* and *eosinophilic granuloma*, with variable organ involvement of infiltration and characteristic proliferation of Langerhans' cells, a special kind of histiocyte of dendritic type. Cytological material may be obtained from different sites including lymph nodes and bone marrow, as well as more unusual sites including thyroid[75–77] effusions[78] and solitary bone lesions (Fig. 4.36).[79–83] Lymph node involvement in Langerhans' cell histiocytosis can be seen as a component of the systemic form, or it may be the initial and sometimes exclusive manifestation of the disease.[84]

Cytological features of Langerhans' cell histiocytosis diagnosed by fine needle aspiration include numerous

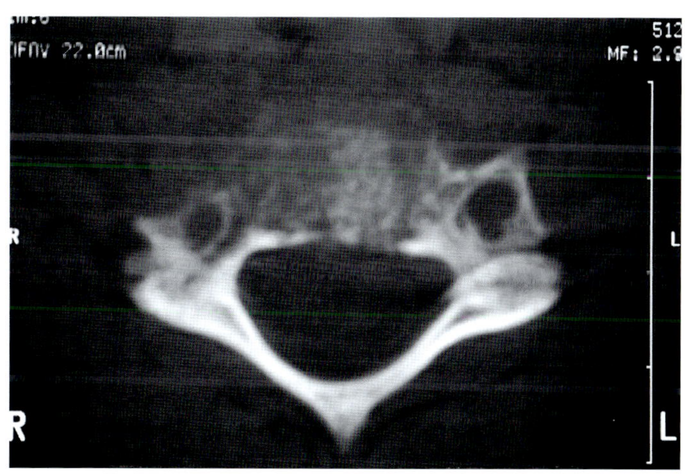

Figure 4.36 Langerhans' cell histiocytosis. Cervical vertebrum of a child showing translucent areas of bone involvement.

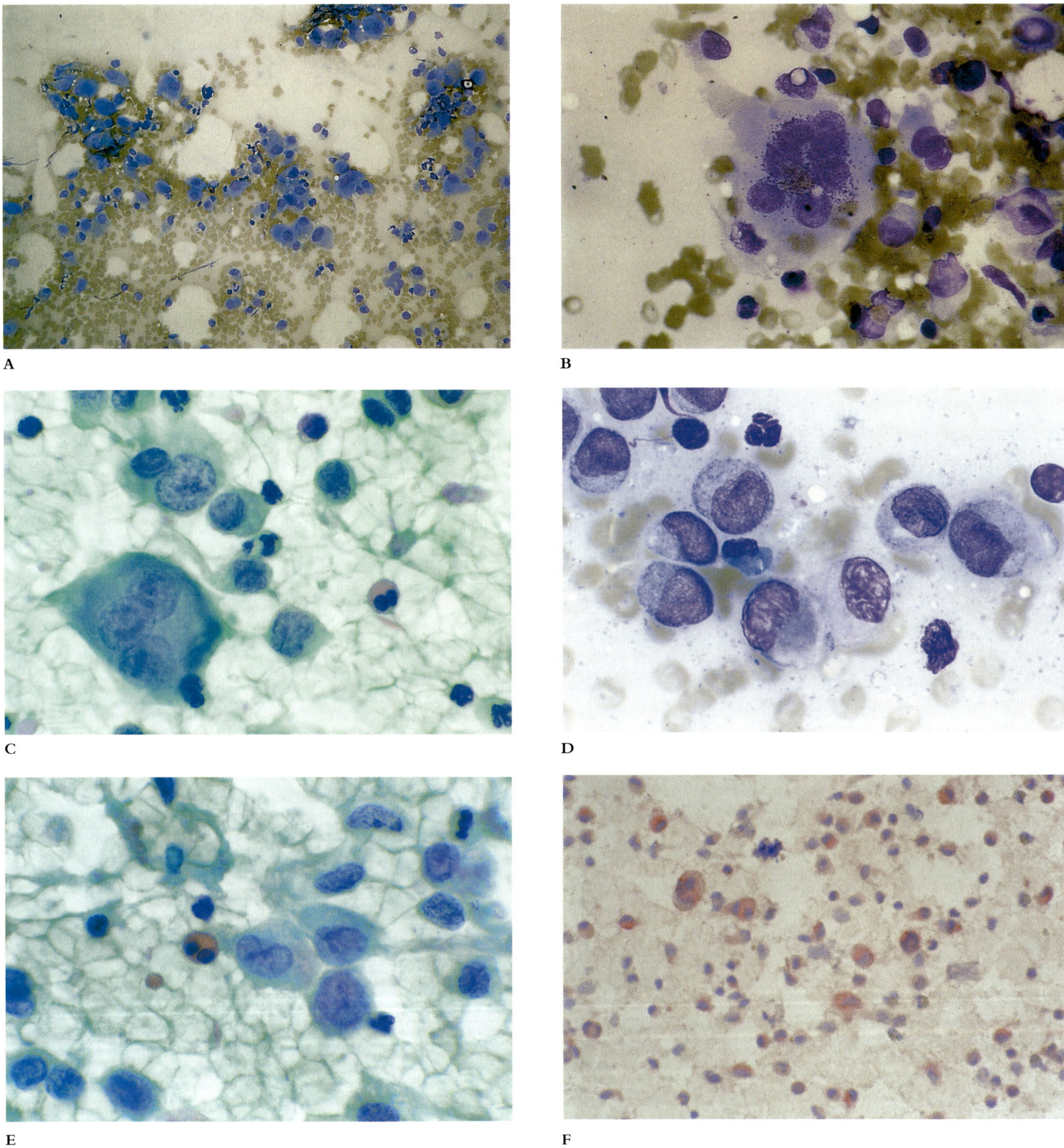

Figure 4.37 Langerhans' cell histiocytosis. **A,B,C.** FNAC shows numerous Langerhans' cells admixed with eosinophils, neutrophils, lymphocytes, macrophages and multinucleated giant cells (MGG ×200, MGG ×1000 oil, PAP ×1000 oil). **D,E.** Characteristic Langerhans' cells with abundant pale non-phagocytic cytoplasm and somewhat irregular folded or grooved nuclei. Immunocytochemistry shows positivity of these cells for S-100, CD1a (leu 6) and HLA-DR antibody (MGG, PAP ×1000 oil immersion). **F.** CD1 positive Langerhans' cells (APAAP ×400).

Langerhans' cells admixed with eosinophils, neutrophils, lymphocytes, macrophages and multinucleated giant cells. Characteristic Langerhans' cells have abundant, pale, non-phagocytic cytoplasm and somewhat irregular folded or grooved nuclei (Fig. 4.37).[85] Immunocytochemistry shows positivity of these cells for S-100 , CD1a (leu 6) and HLA-DR antibody.[86] They are generally negative for LCA, lysosyme, Leu-M1, LN1 and epithelial membrane antigen. Electron microscopy of the aspiration-derived specimen reveals Birbeck granules.[76,87] Patterns of cytological presentation may vary from Langerhans' cell predominant, eosinophil predominant and macrophage predominant.[88] Failure to recognise the diversity of presentations of disease may result in diagnostic errors. Differential diagnosis includes sinus histiocytosis with massive lymphadenopathy but the presence of characteristic cells and abundance of eosinophils is helpful in distinguishing the two conditions.

In the largest series of cases diagnosed on FNAC, Pohar Marinsek & Us-Krasovec[89] determined diagnostic accuracy in recognising Langerhans' cell histiocytosis in cytological smears. They diagnosed the condition in 27 out of 28 adequate FNAC samples with only 1 case suspected of malignancy.[89] The cytomorphological pattern of Langerhans' cell histiocytosis in FNAC smears is usually characteristic, and a correct diagnosis is possible, especially with the aid of electron microscopy and immunocytochemistry.

Post-transplant lymphadenopathy

Post-transplant lymphoproliferative disorder (PTLD) constitues a heterogenous spectrum of EBV-associated lymphoid proliferations that affect 2–4% of organ allograft recipients.[90,91] Histological features of PTLD vary from polymorphic to monomorphic, often requiring a combination of morphological and ancillary studies to gain diagnostic and prognostic information (Box 4.1). No reliable morphologic, immunophenotypic or genotypic criteria unequivocally distinguish between a monomorphic or monoclonal PTLD and malignant lymphoma. This distinction rests on the biological response of the individual. If withdrawal of immunosuppression fails to result in reduction in the size of the mass, the process is best considered malignant, requiring appropriate treatment.

PTLD has been described only rarely in cytological specimens.[90–92] However, cytological samples may provide the initial diagnosis of this potentially fatal disease and allow appropriate intervention.

Box 4.1 World Health Organization categories of post-transplant lymphoproliferative disorders (PTLD)[100]

1. Early lesions
Reactive plasmacytic hyperplasia
Infectious mononucleosis-like

2. PTLD: polymorphic
Polyclonal (rare)
Monoclonal

3. PTLD: monomorphic (classify according to lymphoma classification)
B-cell lymphomas
Diffuse large B-cell lymphoma (immunoblastic, centroblastic, anaplastic)
Burkitt/Burkitt-like lymphoma
Plasma cell myeloma

T-cell lymphomas
Peripheral T-cell lymphoma, not otherwise categorised
Other types (hepatosplenic, gamma-delta, T/NK)

4. Other types (rare)
Hodgkin's disease-like lesions (associated with methotrexate therapy)
Plasmacytoma-like lesions

Cytological features. The diagnosis of PTLD should be suggested when cytological specimens from organ allograft recipients show a polymorphous atypical lymphoid proliferation, frequently with plasmacytoid differentiation and necrosis (Fig. 4.38 and Chapter 3, Fig. 3.33). Morphological presentations of PTLD range from plasmacytoid lymphoproliferative disease to those of an immunoblastic or large-cell lymphoma.[92,93] Plasmacytoid lymphoproliferative disease is characterised by a mostly polymorphous population of lymphoid cells containing many large transformed lymphocytes, occasional immunoblast-like atypical lymphocytes, necrosis and, frequently, obvious plasmacytoid differentiation. Immunoblastic or large-cell lymphoma cytological presentation may be a monotonous population of large lymphoid cells consistent with malignant lymphoma, large-cell type.[91] The presence of EBV can be documented in the majority of cases by in situ hybridisation, PCR or Southern blot. Although this generally establishes a causal relationship of the tumour to EBV, it rarely provides useful diagnostic information.[94] In addition to morphology, flow cytometric immunophenotyping and, in selected cases, DNA polymerase chain

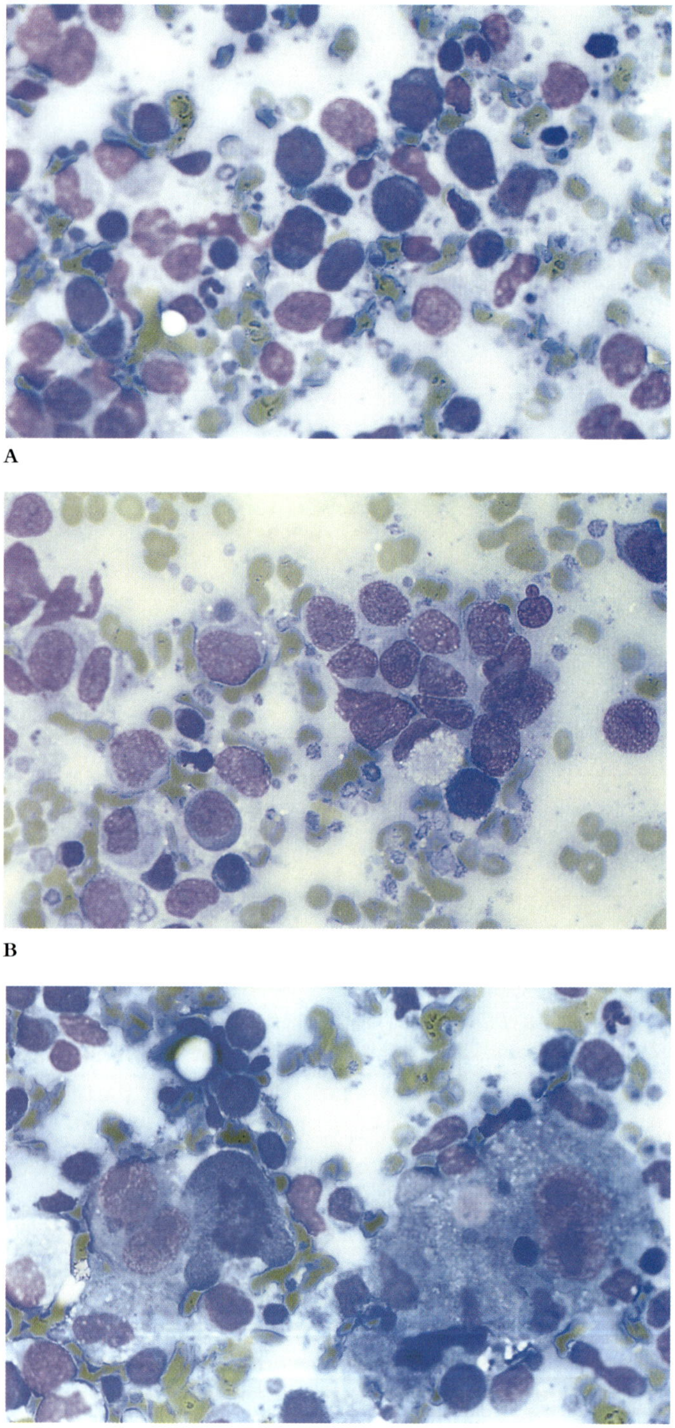

A

B

C

Figure 4.38 FNAC findings in Post transplant lymphadenopathy. **A.** Mostly polymorphous population of lymphoid cells containing many large transformed lymphocytes (MGG ×400). **B.** There are occasional immunoblast-like atypical lymphocytes, necrosis and obvious plasmacytoid differentiation (MGG ×600, oil immersion). **C.** Atypical immunoblasts with mistoses and prominent nucleoli (MGG ×1000, oil immersion).

reaction (PCR) can be performed on FNAC material to show monoclonal or polyclonal pattern.[94] DNA PCR analysis demonstrates a monoclonal rearrangement of the immunoglobulin heavy chain gene.

Differential diagnosis of a mass developing in a post-transplant immunosuppressed patient includes localised infections, malignant neoplasms and EBV-related neoplasms, in particular PTLD. The presence of PTLD in a body fluid specimen is a poor prognostic indicator.[90,95]

Kimura's disease

Kimura's disease is a chronic angioproliferative disorder of unknown aetiology, presenting usually as painless solitary or multiple benign subcutaneous swellings of the skin; it has a predilection for the periauricular and scalp regions, and is often associated with regional lymphadenopathy. Peripheral blood eosinophilia and raised serum IgE levels are features of the condition. It occurs endemically in the Far East and sporadically in the West. The overall prognosis is good. Treatment is either surgery or conservative with corticosteroids or radiation.[96] Complete surgical excision whenever feasible is the preferred treatment despite a high recurrence rate.

Histologically, the lesions are characterised by proliferating blood vessels with rich eosinophilic infiltrate. Hyperplastic lymph nodes show prominent germinal centres surrounded by concentrically arranged small lymphocytes. In the interfollicular areas there is a marked small vessel proliferation, presence of plasma cells, mast cells, lymphoid cells and eosinophils, occasionally forming eosinophilic microabscesses. Plump endothelial cells are seen.

Cytological features are characterised by the Warthin-Finkeldey type giant cells against a background of a bimodal population of lymphocytes and eosinophils.[97,98] The prominent feature is the presence of significant numbers of eosinophils in a background of lymphoid cells.[99]

Differential diagnosis includes Hodgkin's lymphoma, angioimmunoblastic lymphadenopathy (AILD) and AILD-like T-cell lymphoma, lymphoepithelioid T-cell lymphoma, histiocytosis X, angiolymphoid hyperplasia with eosinophilia, angiofollicular lymph node hyperplasia (Castleman's disease) and other reactive lymphadenopathies.[96,99] Cytologically, Kimura's disease shares some of the morphological and clinical features of all of the above diseases. The cytological features are therefore characteristic but not specific. A primary diagnosis of Kimura's disease may need to be confirmed by a biopsy. FNAC may be valuable in the diagnosis of recurrent lesions and may spare the patient from repeated biopsies.

HODGKIN'S LYMPHOMA

Hodgkin's lymphoma is a clonal proliferation of (in most cases) B-cells. The Rye classification postulated 4 subtypes of Hodgkin's disease and these have remained virtually unchanged up to the present day. The majority of classical Hodgkin's falls into 3 categories plus an additional 'lymphocyte-rich' classical Hodgkin's of the current World Health Organization classification (see Box 4.2). The lymphocyte-predominant type is classified separately.[100]

The *lymphocyte-rich*, *nodular sclerosis*, *mixed cellularity* and *lymphocyte depletion* types of Hodgkin's disease all contain binuclear or multinucleate Reed-Sternberg (RS) cells and mononuclear Hodgkin's cells with a cellular infiltrate of lymphoid cells, eosinophils and other inflammatory cells in various proportions.[101,102] RS cells are typically CD30 and CD15 positive (Table 4.1). The grading system adopted in nodular sclerosis has not been upheld by the World Health Organization classification since it has not shown clinical relevance so far.[103]

The *nodular lymphocyte predominance* type of Hodgkin's disease is, both clinically and immunophenotypically, a distinct entity from lymphocyte-rich Hodgkin's lymphoma. In the nodular lymphocyte predominance type of Hodgkin's disease, scattered neoplastic 'L&H' (lymphocytic and

Table 4.1 Cell phenotype in Hodgkin's disease

	Classical RS cells	L&H cells
CD3/TCR P	Occasionally positive	Negative
CDI5	Usually positive	Usually negative
CD20	Occasionally positive	Usually positive
Other B markers	Rarely positive	Frequently positive
CD30 (Ki-1)	Positive	Sometimes positive
CD45 (LCA)	Usually negative	Often positive
CDw75 (LN 1)	Usually negative	Usually positive
EMA	Usually negative	Often positive
lg	Polytypic or negative	Negative or monotypic
J chain	Negative	Positive
EBV genome	Frequently positive	Infrequently positive

Mason D, Gatter K, Lymphoma Classification. Blackwell Science 1998.

Box 4.2 World Health Organization classification of lymphoid neoplasms[100]

B-cell neoplasms

Precursor B-cell neoplasm

Precursor B-lymphoblastic leukaemia/lymphoma (precursor B-cell acute lymphoblastic leukaemia)

Mature (peripheral) B-cell neoplasms

B-cell chronic lymphocytic leukaemia/small lymphocytic lymphoma
B-cell prolymphocytic leukaemia
Lymphoplasmacytic lymphoma
Splenic marginal zone B-cell lymphoma (+/– villous lymphocytes)
Hairy cell leukaemia
Plasma cell myeloma/plasmacytoma
Extranodal marginal zone B-cell lymphoma of MALT type
Nodal marginal zone B-cell lymphoma (+/– monocytoid B-cells)
Follicular lymphoma
Mantle cell lymphoma
Diffuse large B-cell lymphoma
Mediastinal large B-cell lymphoma
Primary effusion lymphoma
Burkitt lymphoma/Burkitt cell leukaemia

T- and NK-cell neoplasms

Precursor T-cell neoplasm
- Precursor T-lymphoblastic lymphoma/leukaemia (precursor T-cell acute lymphoblastic leukaemia)

Mature (peripheral) T-cell neoplasms
- T-cell prolymphocytic leukaemia
- T-cell granular lymphocytic leukaemia
- Aggressive NK-cell leukaemia
- Adult T-cell lymphoma/leukaemia (HTLV1+)
- Extranodal NK/T-cell lymphoma, nasal type
- Enteropathy-type T-cell lymphoma
- Hepatosplenic $\gamma\delta$ T-cell lymphoma
- Subcutaneous panniculitis-like T-cell lymphoma
- Mycosis fungoides/Sezary syndrome
- Anaplastic large cell lymphoma, T/null cell, primary cutaneous type. Peripheral T-cell lymphoma, not otherwise characterized
- Angioimmunoblastic T-cell lymphoma
- Anaplastic large cell lymphoma, T/null cell, primary systemic type

Hodgkin's lymphoma (Hodgkin's disease)

Nodular lymphocyte predominance Hodgkin's lymphoma
Classical Hodgkin's lymphoma
- Nodular sclerosis Hodgkin's lymphoma (grades 1 and 2)
- Lymphocyte-rich classical Hodgkin's lymphoma
- Mixed cellularity Hodgkin's lymphoma
- Lymphocyte depletion Hodgkin's lymphoma

T, B- and T/NK-cell neoplasms are grouped according to major clinical presentations (predominantly disseminated/leukaemic, primary extranodal, predominantly nodal). Only major categories are included.

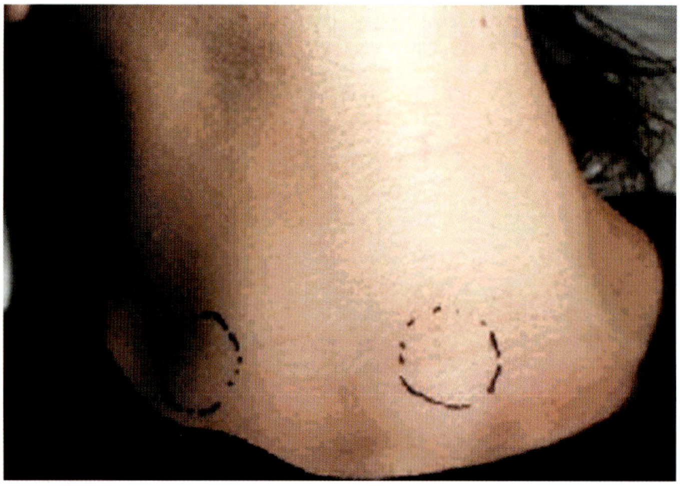

Figure 4.39 Hodgkin's disease. A 34-year-old patient presented with clinically unexplained cervical lymphadenopathy. Nodes were soft, mobile and painless. There was no history of skin itching, temperature or night sweats. FNAC was performed and Hodgkin's disease diagnosed. The patient was referred for biopsy prior to treatment.

histiocytic) or 'popcorn' cells lie within large nodular areas made up of small lymphoid cells. Nodules contain an extensive meshwork of follicular dendritic cells, and lymphoid cells are polyclonal small B-cell lymphocytes expressing both IgM and IgD. T-cells are found around L&H cells and are sparse. This background distinguishes nodular lymphocyte predominance from other types, which have a background rich in T-cells. L&H cells express B-cell markers and J-chain, a protein associated with B-cells but not present in RS cells. Unlike classical RS cells, L&H cells express CD45(LCA), EMA (often) and CDw75 (LN1). CD30 is positive sometimes; CD3 is negative (Table 4.1). Nodular lymphocyte predominance Hodgkin's disease shows male predominance and an indolent course although it may progress to a large B-cell lymphoma.

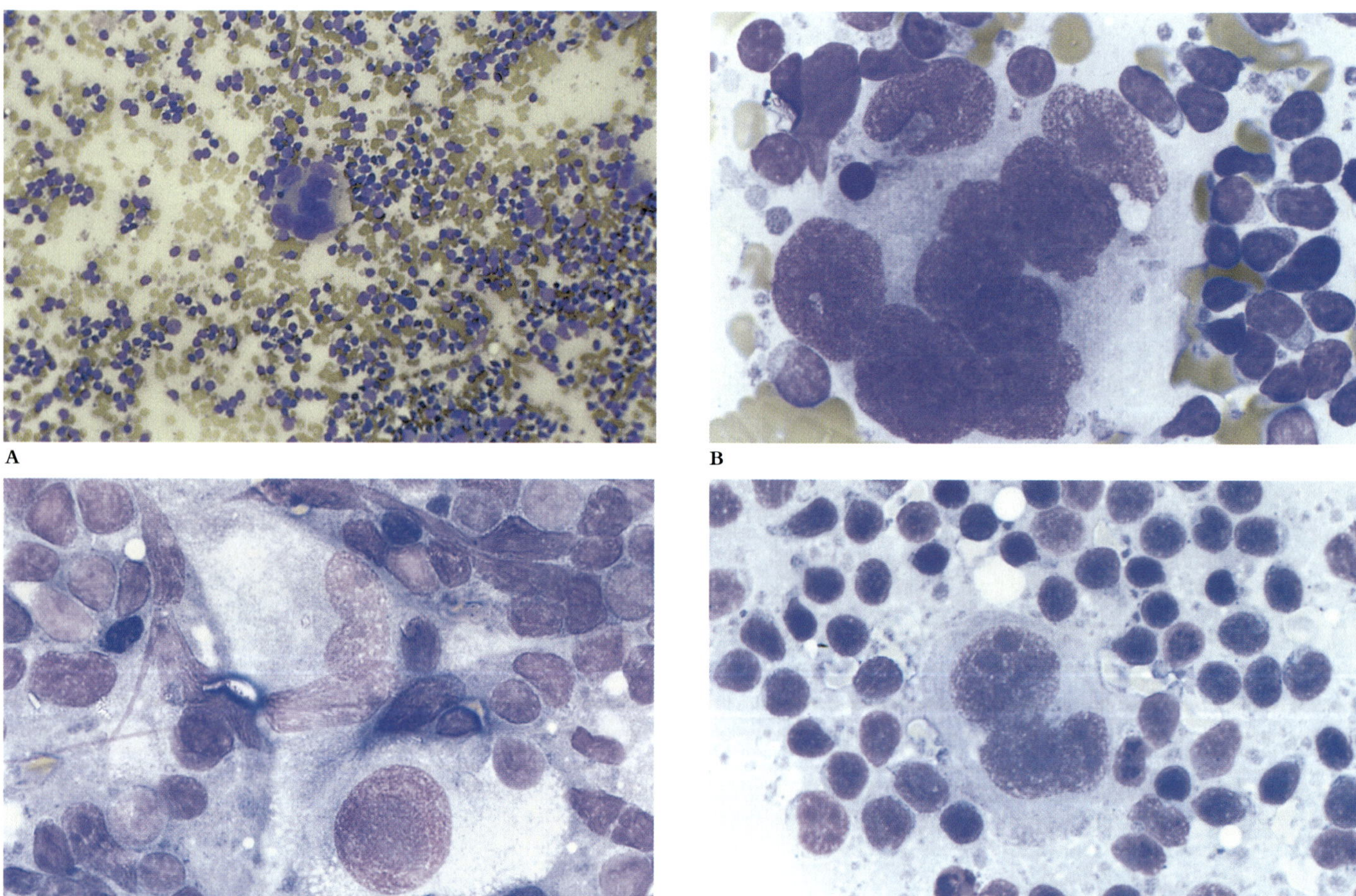

A B C D

Figure 4.40 Hodgkin's disease. **A,B.** Classic RS cells are easily identified in FNAC preparations. They have bilobed or polylobated nuclei with prominent nucleoli and moderately abundant cytoplasm. These cells are scattered among the background of small lymphocytes admixed with other inflammatory cells, particularly eosinophils (MGG ×400, ×1000 oil immersion). **C,D.** Different appearance of mononuclear Hodgkin and RS cells. The prominent basophilic nucleoli with a well-defined nucleolar margin are characteristic. Epithelioid cells, reflecting granulomatous reaction, may be seen (MGG ×1000 oil immersion). ***(continued)***

The **cytological diagnosis** of Hodgkin's disease depends upon demonstration of RS or Hodgkin's cells amongst appropriate reactive cell components. Diagnostic accuracy of FNAC for HD has been invariably high (>85%).[10,104] However, due to the lack of architectural features included in the subtyping, FNAC has limited value in the primary diagnosis and subclassification of Hodgkin's disease but is very useful in diagnosing recurrent disease.[105–111] At present, when Hodgkin's disease is suspected morphologically or immunophenotypically, a biopsy must be performed.

Classic RS cells are easily identified in FNAC preparations. They have bilobed or polylobed nuclei with prominent nucleoli and moderately abundant cytoplasm. These cells are scattered among the background of small lymphocytes admixed with other inflammatory cells, particularly eosinophils (Fig. 4.40).

Hodgkin's cells are CD45 negative, EMA negative, CD30 positive and CD15 positive. Usually they are CD20 and CD3 negative although in 25% of cases they stain with CD20. Cases of EBV-associated Hodgkin's are positive for EBV latent membrane protein.[112]

Pitfalls in diagnosis of Hodgkin's disease include peripheral T-cell lymphoma and anaplastic large cell lymphomas (ALCL). EMA and T-cell antigen activity favours ALCL whereas CD15 positivity favours Hodgkin's disease. In difficult cases T-cell receptor gene rearrangement and t(2;5) translocation can help diagnose peripheral T-cell lymphoma and ALCL respectively. A Hodgkin's-like variant of Richter syndrome is a pitfall[113] (see Chapter 5 Fig. 5.16).

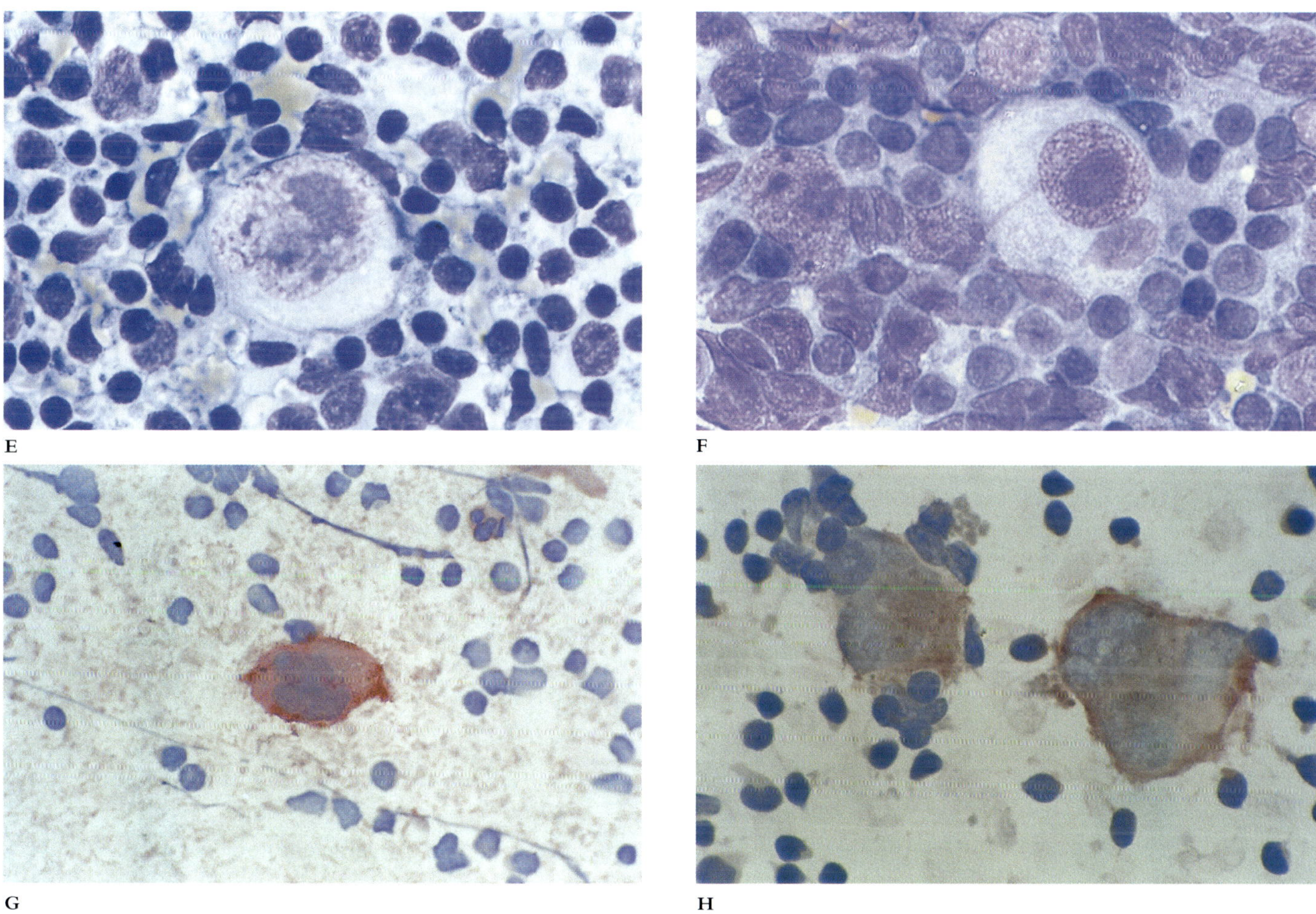

Figure 4.40 ***(continued)*** Hodgkin's disease. **E,F.** Different appearance of mononuclear Hodgkin and RS cells. The prominent basophilic nucleoli with a well-defined nucleolar margin are characteristic. Epithelioid cells, reflecting granulomatous reaction, may be seen (MGG ×1000 oil immersion). **G,H.** CD30 and CD15 positive staining. Hodgkin's cells are CD45 negative, EMA negative, CD20 and CD3 negative although in 25% of cases they stain with CD20.

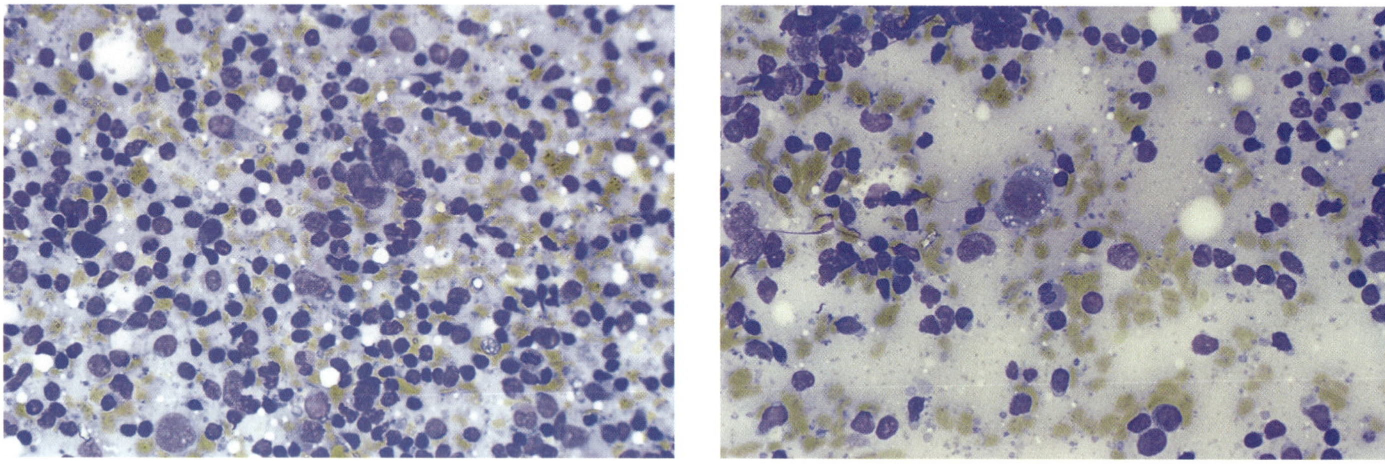

A B

Figure 4.41 Nodular lymphocytic predominance Hodgkin's disease. **A.** Classic RS cells are not present; instead L&H cells may be present in the background of epithelioid cells and mature lymphocytes (MGG ×200). **B.** The L&H cells may be present in the background of epithelioid cells and mature lymphocytes (MGG ×200).

The suppurative type of Hodgkin's disease is another unusual presentation that can be diagnosed on FNAC. Smears are dominated by neutrophils, macrophages and cellular debris. Only a few large, atypical cells of Hodgkin's and RS type are observed.[114–116]

Nodular lymphocyte predominance Hodgkin's disease

As discussed on p. 145, nodular lymphocyte predominance Hodgkin's disease is now recognised as a separate entity from classical Hodgkin's disease and may be closer to peripheral B-cell lymphoma. It involves peripheral lymph nodes sparing the mediastinum.

Cytological features. Classic RS cells are not present; instead L&H cells may be present in the background of epithelioid cells and mature lymphocytes. The L&H cells vary from polypoid cells with large nucleoli to cells with features of RS cells and their variants (Fig. 4.41).

L&H cells are B-cells (CD20 and CD45 positive), Ig negative, CD15 negative CD30+/− and EMA negative. Numerous CD57 T-cells may be present.

Cytological diagnosis may be difficult and the entity has to be borne in mind when encountering FNAC samples from persistent lymphadenopathy without classical RS cells.

NON-HODGKIN'S LYMPHOMA

Diagnosis of malignant lymphoma on FNAC remains a topic of scepticism and controversy.[117] Recent changes in the classification of non-Hodgkin's lymphoma (NHL), in particular the new World Health Organization classification based on the principles of REAL classification, emphasise the diagnostic importance of individual cell cytomorphology, immunophenotyping, genotyping and clinical findings in addition to histology.[100,118] (Box 4.2) These changes have allowed for a greater role of FNAC in the diagnosis of NHL.[112] The FNAC diagnosis of NHL relies on cell morphology as well as the finding of a relatively monotonous population of lymphoid cells in smears.[119] This may sometimes prove difficult, particularly in low-grade NHL with polymorphous cell population. Despite the difficulties, the evidence shows that a large percentage of NHL cases can be recognised and correctly classified using FNAC. This is particularly true of recurrences of lymphoma which amount to up to more than 50% of all lymphomas diagnosed on FNAC (Table 4.2).[120] Diagnostic sensitivity of FNAC is dependent on several factors including the type of NHL and is reported in the literature during the past decade to be 61–100%. Specificity of most studies is >90%.[6,9,21,23,24,38,121–139]

There are recognised difficulties in separating florid reactive hyperplasia and atypical non-neoplastic lymphoid proliferations from low-grade malignant lymphoma on FNAC.[38] The reported cytodiagnostic accuracy of FNAC in diagnosis of follicular lymphomas and nodular sclerosis type of Hodgkin's disease is less compared to other subtypes of NHL and Hodgkin's disease respectively.[10] Similar difficulties exist in diagnosis of marginal zone lymphoma MALT

Table 4.2 Fine needle aspiration cytology of lymph nodes. Experience through the past decade

Author (year)	No. of NHL cases (% primary/ recurrent)	Sensitivity (%)	Specificity (%)	Precise NHL classification (%)	Histological confirmation (%)	Comment
Akhtar (1992)	5 (100/0)	100	100	100	100	All ALCL
Cartagena (1992)	54 (100/0)	82	88	81	100	
Cafferty (1990)	105	66	100	86	57	
Carter (1988)	118 (55/45)	98	91	85	84	
Das (1987)	40 (100/0)	100	100	100	0	All Burkitt's
Daskalopolou (1995)	164 (51/49)	99	98	77	79	
Dunphy (1997)	60 (23/77)	80	100	71	29	
Gagneten (1996)	4 (unknown)	100	100	100	100	All mantle cell
Jacobs (1992)	16 (100/0)	100	100	100	88	All LL
Jeffers (1998)	21 (76/24)	86	100	81	100	
Kardos (1987)	7 (86/14)	100	100	100	14	All LL
Katz (1989)	13 (31/69)	87	100	100	100	All peripheral T-cell
Matsushima (1999)	7 (100/0)	0	0	0	100	All marginal z
Pilloti (1993)	62 (unknown)	71	95	69	100	
Robins (1994)	71(30/70)	100	100	99	100	
Sneige (1990)	145 (unknown)	95	100	86	57	
Sneige (1991)	28 (unknown)	79	100	100	100	
Stasny (1995)	17 (100/0)	100	100	88	82	All Burkitt's
Stewart (1998)	50 (73/27)	78	99	Not done	88	
Tani (1989)	54 (76/24)	93	98	78	59	
Tarantino (1998)	25 (100/0)	82	100	18	Unknown	
Wakeley (1996)	16 (69/31)	100	100	100	6	All LL
Wojcik (1995)	45 (0/100)	100	100	100	100	All mantle cell
Young (1998)	72 (40/60)	80	100	95	10	

Modified from Wakely[117]

(where the helpful lymphoepithelial lesions are absent in the smears), T-cell rich B-cell lymphoma,[140] immunoglobulin-negative malignant lymphoma, composite lymphoma and peripheral T-cell lymphomas. Differential diagnostic problems also include a group of small round cell tumours and non-lymphoid acute leukaemia. These can be overcome by the use of ancillary techniques.

Currently, the role of FNAC in management of lymphomas is evolving.[1,17,40,141–145] While it remains the first line of investigation of most lymphadenopathies, excision biopsy may be required for confirmation only in certain lymphomas, such as follicle centre, mantle zone, MALT/marginal zone lymphoma and Hodgkin's disease. In other disorders, where the diagnosis is not based on architecture and where cytomorphology, immunocytochemistry and molecular techniques complement the clinical setting, excision may not be necessary. These include reactive lymphoid hyperplasia, small lymphocytic lymphoma, anaplastic large cell (Ki-1) lymphoma, diffuse large B-cell lymphoma and Burkitt's lymphoma.[141] Even the subclassification of follicle-derived low-grade NHL (follicle centre and mantle zone) can now be established with high accuracy on FNAC material if cytomorphology is corroborated by a complete immunophenotypic analysis.[143] Biopsy can be avoided also in detecting residual disease, recurrences and progression of low-grade to high-grade lymphoma, and staging of lymphomas. Biopsy of difficult intra-abdominal sites may also be avoided by using FNAC.[27]

With the above management principles in mind, the *ancillary techniques* play an important part of FNAC diagnosis of NHL (see p. 122). Ancillary techniques contribute to the correct distinction between reactive and neoplastic lymphoid proliferation in 97% of cases.[146] A combination of flow cytometry and morphology helps diagnose 80% of NHL (69% of the primary lymphomas and 88% of the recurrent lymphomas) without the need for histological sampling.[23,138,147,148] Similarly, a combination of techniques diagnosed 25 of 26 extranodal lymphomas.[38] In using the ancillary studies, several authors recommend a multiparameter approach ('triple test') i.e. the importance of interpretation of ancillary techniques in conjunction with cytomorphology and clinical information.[16,37,122] While ancillary techniques have made significant contributions to the identification and typing of lymphomas, there is still a requirement for a simple and rapid diagnostic procedure for patients who present with persistent lymphadenopathy. Light microscopic examination of FNAC smears fulfils this role, provided its limitations and pitfalls are recognised.[40]

Obtaining appropriate material

Cytopathologists should be familiar with the possibilities opened to them in handling the FNAC material. With training, it is simple to obtain an average of 20 million cells per procedure without much discomfort for the patient.[141] Use of very fine gauge (25G or higher) heparinised needles, aspiration without suction and rapid movement while within the node, usually produces sufficient cell yield. Less material is needed if a single Feulgen stained slide is used for image analysis for DNA ploidy and proliferation and if marker studies are performed on cytospin preparations instead of flow cytometry. PCR detection of gene rearrangement requires much less cells than Southern blot studies.[36] Recently, a laser scanning cytometer (Compucyte, Cambridge, Massachusetts) has evolved as a hybrid between a flow cytometer and an image analyser that requires only a small quantity of cells (about 50 000). Cells may be placed on a specially configured slide for multiparameter immunophenotyping which can obtain results within 2 hours.[142]

Classification of non-Hodgkin's lymphoma

The history of lymphoma classification has been long and controversial. However, within the last 30 years much has been learned about the biology of lymphoma. The concept of classifying malignant lymphoma according to the (proposed) normal counterpart was developed in the Kiel classification.[149] In 1994, the International Lymphoma Study Group (ILSG) developed a consensus list of lymphoid neoplasms, which was published as the Revised European-American Classification of Lymphoid Neoplasms (REAL) and consisted of clinicopathological entities recognised at the time.[150] These tumours were divided into three major categories: B-cell neoplasms; T-cell and postulated NK-cell neoplasms; and Hodgkin's disease. The classification was based on the principle that a classification is a list of 'real' disease entities, which are defined by a combination of morphology, immunophenotype, genetic features and clinical features. The relative importance of each of these features varies among diseases, and there is no one 'gold standard'. In some tumours morphology is paramount; in others it is immunophenotype, a specific genetic abnormality or clinical features.[100,151] Each distinct disease may have a range of histological grade and clinical aggressiveness. Prognostic factors can be defined within an entity, on a clinical, morphological, immunohistochemical or genetic basis. Although many distinct diseases can now be recognised, 3 of them (follicular lymphoma, diffuse large B-cell lymphoma and Hodgkin's disease) account for the majority of the cases seen in Europe and the USA[152] (Fig. 4.42). Recognition of distinct disease entities is essential in order to develop and test effective therapies.[153] The International Lymphoma Study showed that the REAL classification could be used by pathologists, with inter-observer reproducibility better than for other classifications (>85%).[100] The proposed World Health Organiation classification for lymphomas is similar to the REAL classification for lymphomas, based on the principle of defining disease entities that can be recognised by pathologists and are of clinical relevance (Box 4.2).[100,118,154]

The changes in the classification of NHL emphasise the diagnostic importance of cytomorphology, immunophenotyping and molecular findings in addition to histology.[20] These changes have allowed for a greater role of FNAC in the diagnosis of NHL.[112] The REAL classification of lymphoid neoplasms was reviewed in the context of its adaptability to the cytological diagnosis of lymphoid

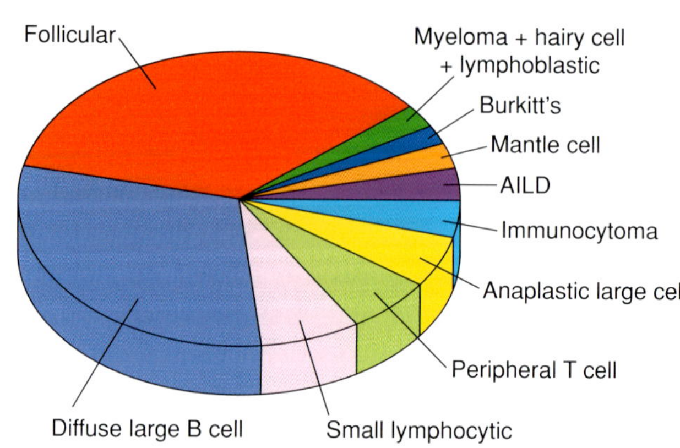

Figure 4.42 Frequency of non-Hodgkin's lymphoma in lymph nodes (from Mason D, Gatter K: Lymphoma Classification, 1998). Follicular and diffuse large cell lymphoma are by far the most frequent non-Hodgkin's lymphoma in the USA and Europe accounting for two-thirds of cases. (With permission from Wiley-Liss, inc.)

neoplasms and it was concluded that FNAC is being used more frequently in the diagnosis, staging and follow-up of lymphoma whenever supportive studies are readily available.[112] Many cases of NHL can be diagnosed and subclassified by FNAC when there is adequate immunophenotypic information.[155]

Precursor lesions

Lymphoblastic leukaemia/lymphoma

Lymphoblastic neoplasms, of B- or T-cell type, present either as localised solid tumours in lymph nodes or, more usually, as a leukaemia (Box 4.2).[100] The disease affects all ages although it is more common in older children and young adults. It usually presents as a symptomatic mediastinal mass with pleural or pericardial effusion and will progress rapidly to involve blood, bone marrow, the central nervous system and the gonads. Lymphoblastic lymphoma/leukaemia is an aggressive but curable disease, particularly in children.[156]

Cytological features. Lymphoblastic lymphomas are composed of medium-sized lymphoid cells, which are oval, rounded or highly convoluted, have pale staining nuclei with fine blast-like chromatin and inconspicuous nucleoli (except in 10% of cases where they are prominent) (Fig. 4.43).[129] The size of the cells and the lack of prominent nucleoli may be misleading into calling the lesion a low-grade lymphoma. Unlike low-grade lymphoma, there are usually many mitoses and blast-like chromatin is apparent. Differentiation from diffuse large cell lymphoma or transformed mantle zone lymphoma and histiocytic lymphoma may be a morphological pitfall that has to be resolved with immunocytochemistry.[134]

Immunophenotypically, lymphoblasts express TdT. All other lymphomas are negative for TdT. CD45 is positive only in 80% of cases. The majority of lymphoblastic lymphomas (85%) are of T-cell lineage and they nearly always express surface or intracytoplasmic CD3. This is important for excluding all other B-cell lymphomas. If lymphoblastic lymphoma is of B-cell lineage it expresses CD10 (CALLA) and CD19. Only about 50% of B-cell lymphoblastic lymphomas express CD20 because of their immaturity. Genotyping for lineage assignment and/or clonality be performed in cases of equivocal markers.[34]

FNAC samples are adequate for accurate characterisation of lymphoblastic lymphomas and may obviate the need for surgical biopsy.[128,134] When combined with immunological phenotyping, definitive initial pathological diagnosis of lymphoblastic lymphoma and recurrent acute lymphocytic leukaemia is possible and preferable using only FNAC. It should be considered as part of the initial evaluation and management whenever a mass lesion appears in a child with a suspected lymphoblastic neoplasm. It can preclude the need for a surgical biopsy in those with a mediastinal mass and the superior mediastinal syndrome.[136]

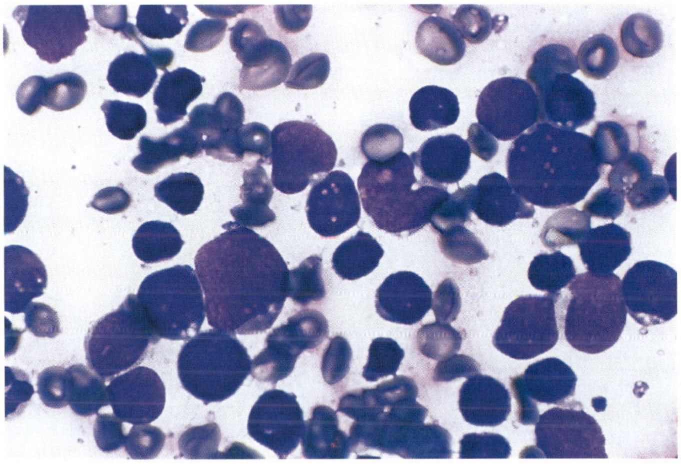

A

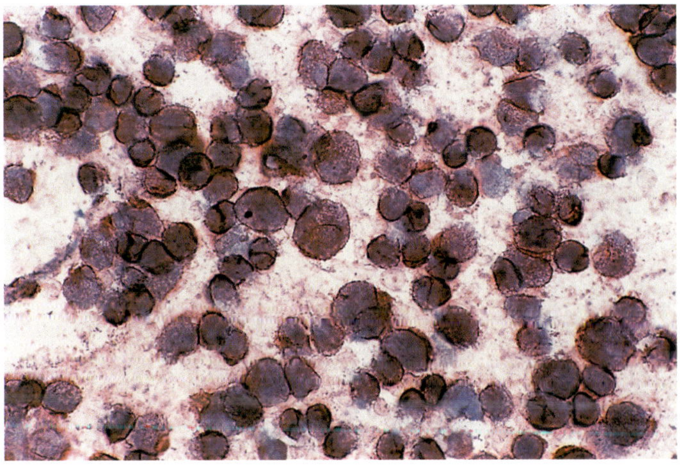

B

Figure 4.43 Lymphoblastic lymphoma. A 16-year-old boy presented with a short history of shortness of breath. Chest X-ray revealed a mediastinal mass. An urgent FNAC result was requested prior to commencement of therapy. **A.** FNAC shows small and medium sized lymphoid cells, with oval or rounded nuclei, pale staining, fine, blast-like chromatin and inconspicuous nucleoli. The size of the cells and lack of prominent nucleoli may be misleading into diagnosis of the lesion as a low-grade lymphoma (MGG ×1000 oil). **B.** CD3 positivity in all cells (APAAP, ×1000 oil).

B-cell lymphomas

B-cell small lymphocytic lymphoma

Lymphocytic lymphoma is a neoplasm composed of small lymphocytes and may present as lymphoma or leukaemia (chronic lymphocytic leukaemia and prolymphocytic leukaemia) (Box 4.2).[100] Histologically, there is an infiltrate of small cells with clusters of larger cells ('proliferation centres'). The disease runs an indolent course but in a percentage of cases may undergo transformation into a high-grade lymphoma (Richter syndrome) (see Chapter 5 Fig. 5.16).

Cytological features. Small lymphocytic lymphoma is composed of small lymphoid cells with round, regular nuclear membranes and coarsely clumped chromatin. Apart from small cells, small lymphocytic lymphoma contains also a population of larger cells, representing prolymphocytes and 'paraimmunoblasts' (Fig. 4.44). These larger cells are observed in aggregates in the proliferation centres that resemble pale areas or pseudofollicles in histological sections. When paraimmunoblasts/prolymphocytes dominate, a paraimmunoblastic variant may be suspected. This has a worse prognosis than small lymphocytic lymphoma but better than diffuse large cell lymphoma (Box 4.3).

The immunophenotype is IgM, CD5 and CD23 positive in addition to 'pan B panel' (CD19, CD20, CD79a, CVd22, CD23) (Table 4.3). Both small lymphocytic lymphoma and

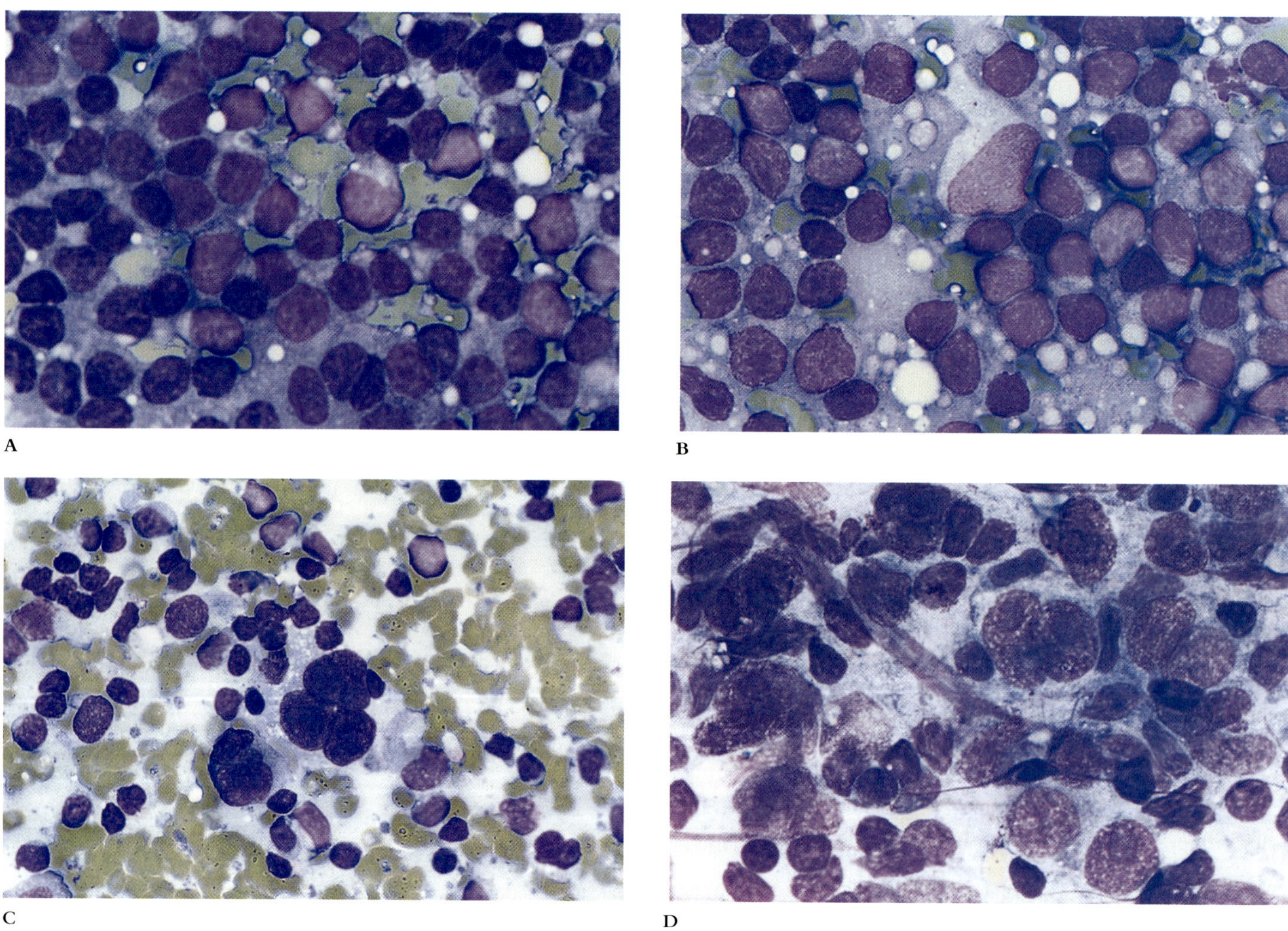

Figure 4.44 Small lymphocytic lymphoma. **A,B.** Small lymphocytic lymphoma is composed of small lymphoid cells with round regular nuclear membranes and coarsely clumped chromatin. Apart from small cells it also shows a population of larger cells representing prolymphocytes and 'paraimmunoblasts'. These larger cells are observed in aggregates reflecting proliferation centres (MGG ×1000 oil immersion). **C.** CLL transformation, sometimes referred to as Richter syndrome. Numerous blasts present, some resembling RS cells (MGG×600). **D.** Same patient, higher magnification shows cellular detail of RS like cells (MGG ×1000, oil immersion).

Box 4.3 Comparative cytomorphology of small cell lymphomas[155]

Follicular:	Mixture of small and large cleaved cells (centrocytes as well as centroblasts)
Mantle cell:	Monomorphic, irregular, small/medium size, clumped chromatin, occasional 'blastoid' cells
Marginal zone/MALT:	Small, round with scattered immunoblast-like nucleolated large cells +/− plasmacytoid
Small lymphocytic/CLL:	Small, round, occasional prolymphocytes and 'paraimmunoblasts', clumped chromatin
Lymphoblastic:	Small, blast-like fine chromatin, inconspicuous nucleoli, mitoses
Burkitt:	Small, round, coarse chromatin, multiple small nucleoli, abundant vacuolated cytoplasm, mitoses, apoptoses, tingible body macrophages

mantle zone lymphoma are CD5 positive and CD10 negative. Small lymphocytic lymphoma is, however, CD23 positive. Small lymphocytic lymphoma shows weak Ig and CD20 positivity while mantle zone lymphoma shows strong positivity. Mantle zone lymphoma is also positive for cyclin D1 (bcl-1) and has a t(11;14). Genetically, small lymphocytic lymphoma shows trisomy 12 or 13Q in some cases.[157]

Lymphoplasmacytic lymphoma (immunocytoma)

Lymphoplasmacytic lymphoma is an uncommon type of NHL comprising only 2–3% of NHL (Fig. 4.42). Lymphocytes in lymphoplasmacytic lymphoma show plasma cell differentiation. Plasmacytoid cells contain IgM, sometimes as intranuclear inclusions (Dutcher bodies). MALT lymphoma and small lymphocytic lymphoma may show plasmacytoid features so the diagnosis should be made by exclusion of other entities.[157] Disease may present as Waldonström's macroglobulinaemia with IgM detectable in the serum, as nodal or extranodal lymphoma.[158] Immunocytoma has generally an indolent course but transformation into large cell lymphoma occurs in approximately 5–10% of cases.

Cytological features. Lymphoplasmacytic lymphoma is composed of a mixed population of small lymphocytes, plasmacytoid lymphocytes, plasma cells and scattered plasmacytoid immunoblasts (Fig. 4.45). Intranuclear inclusions (Dutcher bodies) and intacytoplasmic inclusions (Russell bodies) are usually numerous. If there is predominance of immunoblasts, the disease may be labelled as polymorphous immunocytoma indicating a possible more aggressive course. Epithelioid cells and mast cell infiltration has been reported, the former may cause confusion with T-cell lymphomas (Box 4.3).

The immunophenotype of lymphoplasmocytic lymphoma is, surface IgM, cytoplasmic Ig, CD19,20, 22, 79a positive: CD 5, CD10, CD23 negative. A combination of morphology and immunophenotype is useful in separating the lymphoplasmacytic from small lymphocytic and mantle zone lymphoma (Table 4.3).[157]

Mantle zone lymphoma

Mantle cell lymphoma is a lymphoproliferative disorder derived from a subset of naive pregerminal centre cells characterised by a nodular or diffuse proliferation of atypical lymphoid cells with a monoclonal B-cell phenotype and

Table 4.3 Immunophenotype of low-grade B cell lymphomas[158a]

	B-CLL Small lymphocytic lymphoma	Lymphoplasmacytic lymphoma	Mantle zone lymphoma	Follicular lymphoma
CD20	Pos.	Pos.	Pos.	Pos.
CD79a	Pos.	Pos.	Pos.	Pos.
CD10	Neg.	Neg.	Neg/pos.	Pos/neg.
CD23	Pos.	Neg.	Neg.	Neg/pos.
CD5	Pos.	Neg.	Pos.	Neg.
CD43	Pos.	Pos/neg.	Pos.	Neg.
DBA44	Neg.	Pos/neg.	Pos/neg.	Neg.
TRAP	Neg.	N/A	Neg.	Neg.
bcl-2	Pos.	Pos.	Pos.	Pos.
Cyclin D1	Neg.	Neg.	Pos.	Neg.

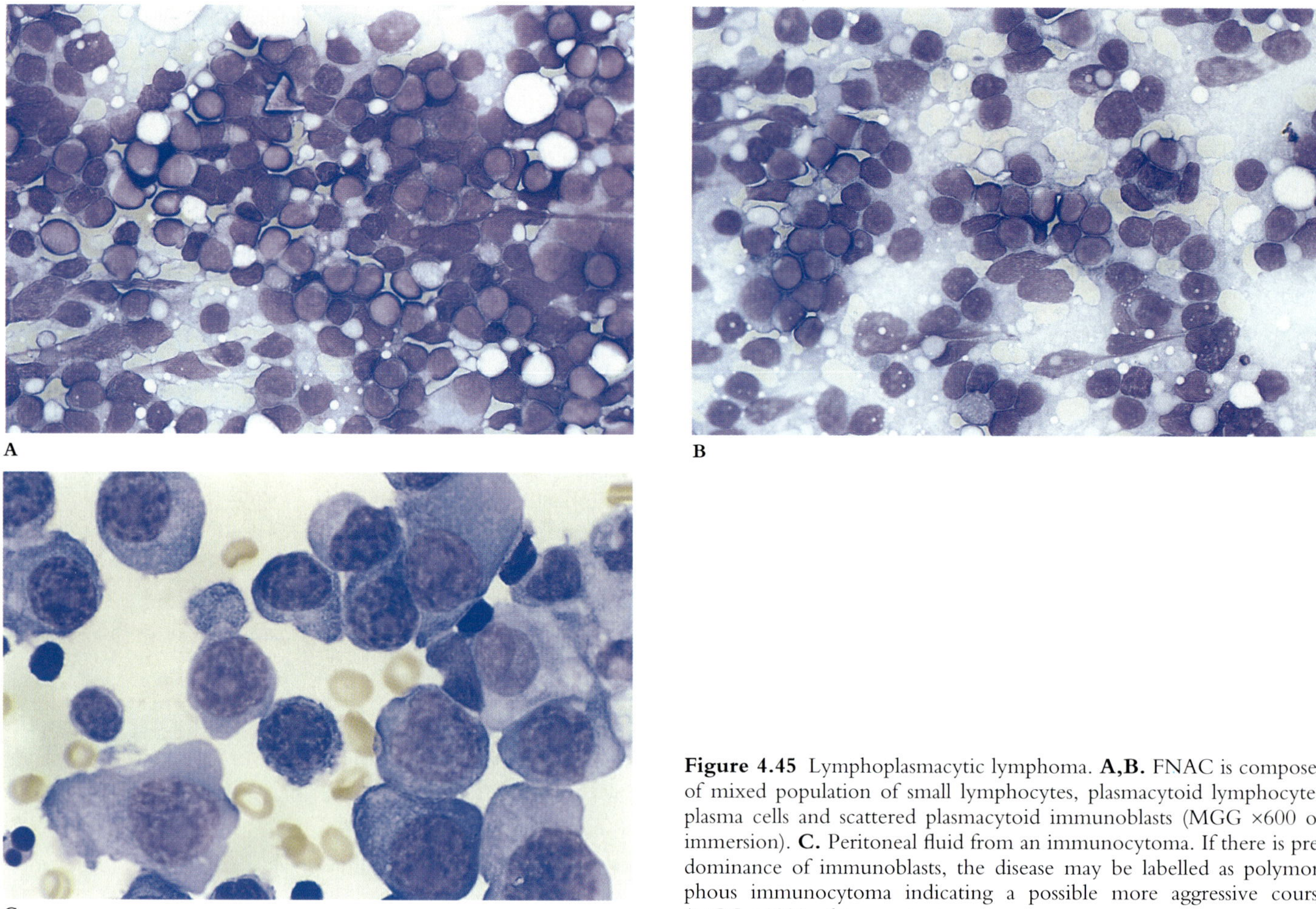

A B C

Figure 4.45 Lymphoplasmacytic lymphoma. **A,B.** FNAC is composed of mixed population of small lymphocytes, plasmacytoid lymphocytes, plasma cells and scattered plasmacytoid immunoblasts (MGG ×600 oil immersion). **C.** Peritoneal fluid from an immunocytoma. If there is predominance of immunoblasts, the disease may be labelled as polymorphous immunocytoma indicating a possible more aggressive course (MGG ×1000 oil immersion).

coexpression of CD5 (Boxes 4.2 and 4.4).[100] Clinically, mantle cell lymphoma presents as advanced disease with frequent extranodal involvement, particularly with involvement of bone marrow, gastrointestinal tract and spleen. The disease usually presents with lymphadenopathy but may be present in extranodal sites, particularly the gastrointestinal tract. Histologically, the growth pattern is often nodular and the cells tend to converge ('home') to the mantle zones of lymphoid follicles. Mantle zone lymphoma has distinct clinical, immunological and genetic characteristics and has been shown to have a worse survival rate than other lymphomas previously grouped as follicle centre derived. The clinical evolution is relatively aggressive, with poor response to conventional therapeutic regimens and a median survival duration of 3–4 years.

Cytological features. Two cytological variants have been identified: typical and blastic. Typical cases show a monotonous population of small to intermediately sized lymphoid cells with irregular nuclei, coarse chromatin, small nucleoli and scarce cytoplasm (centrocytes) (Fig. 4.46) (Box 4.3). Blastic variants include a spectrum of intermediate to large cells with round or irregular nuclei and finely dispersed chromatin. These cases have a higher proliferative activity and a more aggressive clinical evolution.[127,137,159] Chromatin is not clumped as in small lymphocytic lymphoma. There are no larger cells admixed in the tumour as in the marginal zone lymphoma or follicular lymphoma. If present, the large cells represent cells from residual follicles that are overrun by tumour. The blastic variant resembles lymphoblastic lymphoma. The aspirate smears show a monotonous population of intermediate-sized lymphocytes with irregular nuclear contours, finely dispersed nuclear chromatin, and inconspicuous nucleoli.[160] The clinical history and the absence of TdT helps to differentiate mantle zone lymphoma from lymphoblastic lymphoma.

Immunophenotypically, mantle zone lymphoma is surface Ig, CD5, CD19, 20, 22, 79a and cyclin D1 positive, CD23

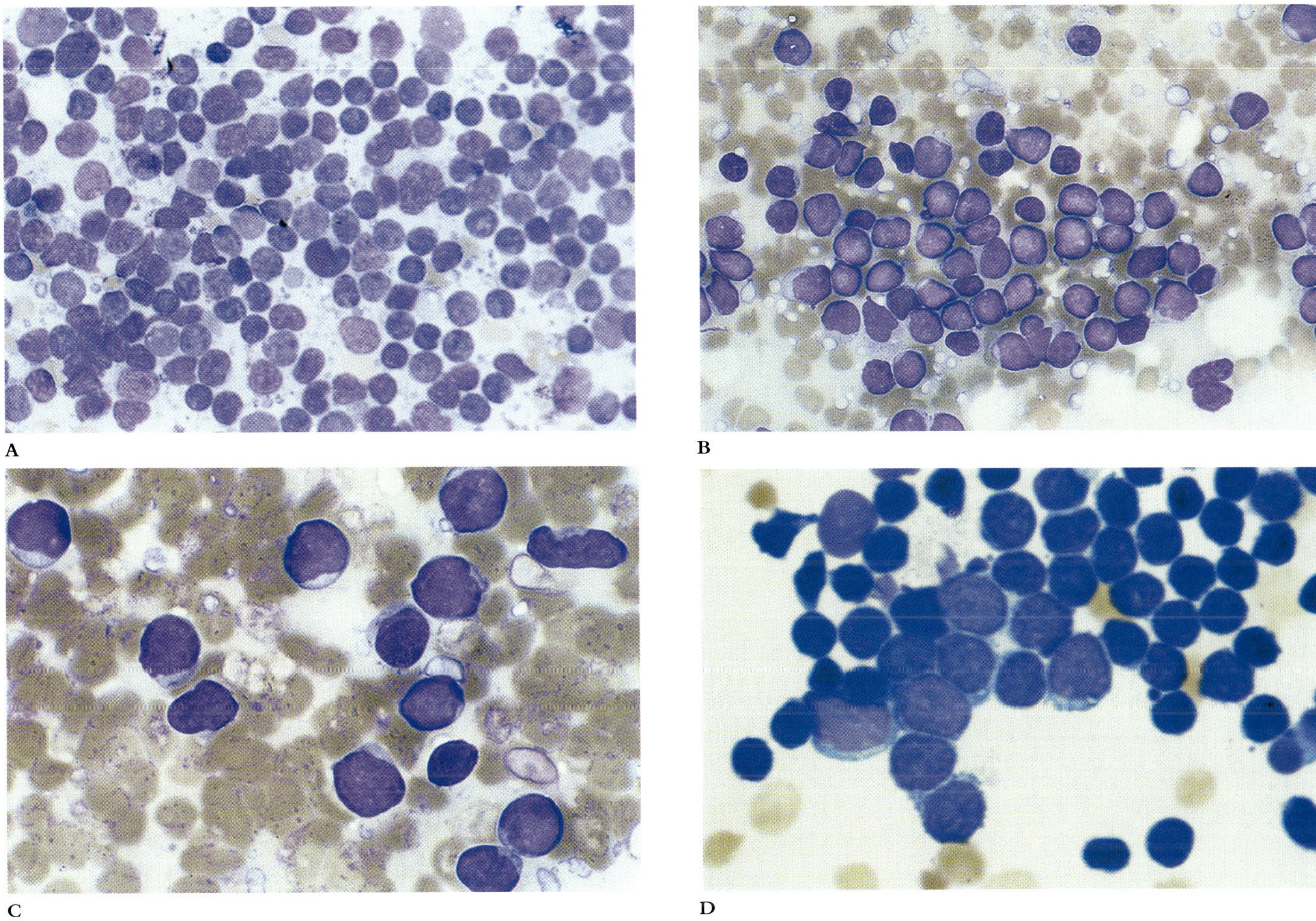

Figure 4.46 Mantle zone lymphoma. **A,B,C.** Monotonous population of small to intermediately sized lymphoid cells with irregular nuclei, coarse chromatin, small nucleoli and scarce cytoplasm (centrocytes). Chromatin is not clumped as in small lymphocytic lymphoma. There are no larger cells admixed in the tumour as in the marginal zone lymphoma or follicular lymphoma (MGG ×600, ×600, ×1000 oil immersion). **D.** Blastic variant includes a spectrum of intermediate to large cells with round or irregular nuclei and finely dispersed chromatin. These cases have a higher proliferative activity and a more aggressive clinical evolution. Features may resemble lymphoblastic lymphoma (MGG ×1000 oil immersion).

Box 4.4 World Health Organization classification of follicular lymphoma and mantle cell lymphoma grading and variants[100]

Follicular lymphoma

Grades
Grade 1: 0–5 centroblasts/hpf
Grade 2: 6–15 centroblasts/hpf
Grade 3: >15 centroblastsl/hpf
- 3a: >15 centroblasts, but centrocytes are still present
- 3b: Centroblasts form solid sheets with no residual centrocytes

Variants
Cutaneous follicle centre lymphoma
Diffuse follicle centre lymphoma
Grade 1: 0–5 centroblasts/hpf
Grade 2: 6–15 centroblasts/hpf

Mantle cell lymphoma
Variant: blastoid

and CD10 negative. Cyclin D1 positivity reflects genetic abnormality t(11;14), reciprocal chromosomal translocation, which causes overexpression of bcl-1 or PRAD-1 gene which encodes cyclin D1. It is present in 50–67% of mantle zone lymphomas. CD5 is commonly present in other lymphomas but it differs from other CD5-positive diseases by being CD23 negative (Table 4.3). Cyclin D1 is present in only a few reported cases of aggressive variants of chronic lymphocytic leukaemia/small lymphocytic lymphoma and a small percentage of cases of multiple myeloma. Aggressive variants of mantle zone lymphoma have additional genetic alterations, including inactivation of p53 and p16INK4a tumour suppressor genes.[159]

Subclassification of follicle-derived low-grade NHL can be established with high accuracy on FNAC material if cytomorphology is corroborated by a complete immunophenotypic analysis, which can be performed on both fresh and frozen material. The currently used criteria can be applied to aspirated cells for a conclusive cytopathological diagnosis of mantle zone lymphoma, which is of great clinical importance.[143,157]

Follicular lymphoma

This is one of the most common lymphomas in Europe and the USA (Fig. 4.42). The cells of origin are centroblasts and centrocytes and their growth pattern is usually follicular ('follicle centre lymphoma', 'centrocytic/centroblastic' and 'follicular centroblastic' lymphoma of previous classifications). Histological grading is proposed according to the number of centroblasts per high power field, e.g. grade 1 (1–5 CB/hpf), grade 2 (6–15 CB/hpf), grade 3 (>15 CB/hpf) (Boxes 4.2 and 4.4).[100]

The disease affects adults and although it has an indolent course with median survival of 7–9 years, so far it is incurable.

Cytological features. The cells of follicular lymphoma are composed of a variable mix of small (small cleaved) and large (large cleaved) lymphoid cells that are commonly found in follicle centre (Fig. 4.47). The small cells (cleaved cells, centrocytes) are slightly larger than mature lymphocytes, have condensed chromatin, irregular nuclear outline and lack prominent nucleoli. The large cells (large cleaved cells) are 2–3 times the size of small cleaved cells. The large noncleaved cells, centroblasts, have round nuclei and prominent nucleoli. CD21, which stains follicular dendritic cells, can be used to outline the nodular, follicular pattern of the lesion. The presence of 'aggregation' of uniform lymphoid cells, probably due to cell adhesions with the support of dendritic reticulum cells, is seen in follicular lymphomas.[161]

The grading of follicular lymphomas proposed in REAL classification and endorsed by the current World Health Organization classification can be applied to cytological preparations but the criteria have not been established yet (Box 4.4). Grade 1 corresponds to predominantly small cleaved cell population, grade 2 to mixed small and large cleaved cells and grade 3 to follicular large cells. Follicular large cell lymphoma is difficult to differentiate from diffuse large cell lymphoma. The distinction is not critical since both lymphomas are treated aggressively. The aggressive lymphomas usually have >20% of centroblasts. Diagnosis of follicular lymphoma without the aid of ancillary techniques may be difficult and the most frequent false-negative diagnoses of non-Hodgkin's lymphoma, prior to the advent of immunocytochemistry and other ancillary techniques, relate to this category.[162]

Immunophenotypically, cells show surface Ig, CD10, CD19, 20, 22, 79a and BCL-2 positivity and are CD5 negative (Table 4.3). The 14;18 translocation is present in the majority of cases (80–90%). This causes expression of bcl-2 protein which is normally not expressed by the follicle centre cells which are bcl-2 negative. Bcl-2 is expressed, even in cases which lack translocation. The expression of bcl-2 is not useful in cytological preparations because of lack of architecture. It is present also in hyperplasia, marginal zone lymphoma and small B-cell follicular lymphoma. Bcl-6 expression is common in low-grade follicular lymphoma but is rare in other indolent B-cell lymphoid disorders, and may be a useful adjunct in classification of indolent lymphomas.[163]

Marginal zone lymphoma (MALT type)

Marginal zone B-cell lymphomas represent a category of non-Hodgkin's lymphoma which may arise in a wide variety of extranodal organs where they are termed low-grade B-cell lymphomas of mucosa-associated lymphoid tissue (MALT) (Chapter 2, Fig. 2.21). Marginal zone lymphomas may involve primarily lymph nodes and/or spleen where they are designated as monocytoid B-cell lymphoma or splenic marginal zone lymphoma respectively. The small cell type of MALT lymphoma derives from B-cells associated with epithelial tissues.[164–166] It tends to remain localised with good prognosis but can undergo blastic transformation to a large B-cell lymphoma. Recent data show that primary large cell lymphomas, of mucosa-associated tissues, differ cytogenetically from low-grade MALT lymphomas. If found, areas of large cell lymphoma within MALT should be diagnosed as diffuse B-cell lymphoma (and not high-grade MALT) so as not to confuse the management of otherwise indolent low-grade MALT lymphomas. The World Health Organization classification proposes grading according to the number of blasts, e.g. > 5%, thought to confer worse prognosis (Box 4.2).

Cytological features. Specimens show a polymorphous proliferation comprising a predominant population of intermediate-sized lymphoid cells with round-to-irregular nuclear outline (centrocyte-like or monocytoid features), chromatin slightly paler and less clumped than in small, mature lymphocytes, small inconspicuous nucleolus and a distinct pale cytoplasm. In addition there are small mature

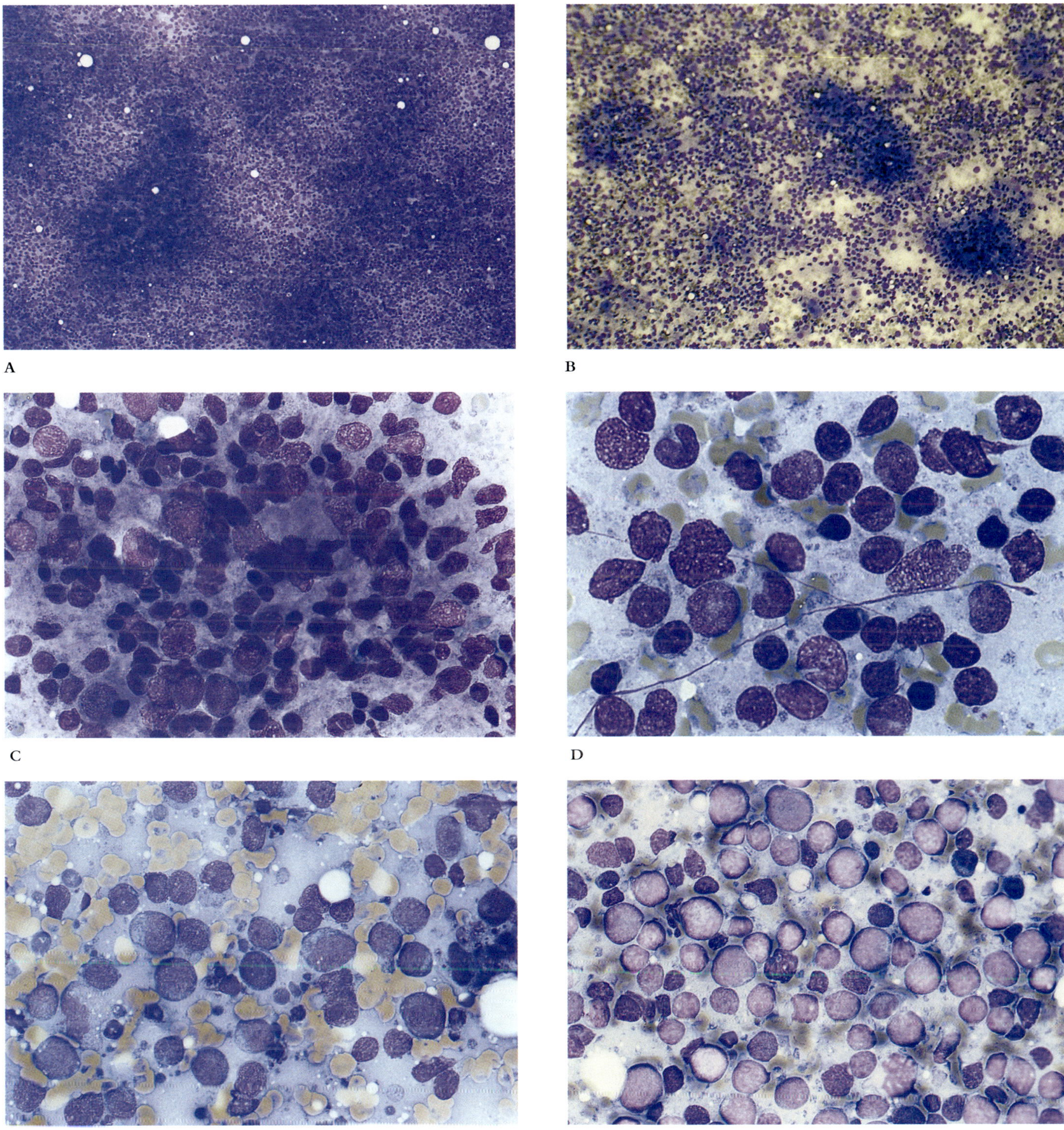

A B C D E F

Figure 4.47 Follicular lymphoma. **A,B.** Cellular aspirates contain numerous lymphoid cells, occasionally presenting as aggregates converging around the follicular dendritic cells (MGG ×100, MGG ×200). **C.** Follicular dendritic cells overrun by lymphoma cells. CD21, which stains follicular dendritic cells, can be used to outline the nodular, follicular pattern, of the lesion (MGG ×600). **D,E.** Cells of follicular lymphoma are composed of variable mix of small (centrocytes) and large (centroblasts) lymphoid cells that are commonly found in the follicle centre. The small cells (cleaved cells, centrocytes) are slightly larger than mature lymphocytes, have condensed chromatin, irregular nuclear outline and lack prominent nucleoli. The large cells (centroblasts) are 2–3 times the size of small cleaved cells. Centroblasts have round nuclei and prominent nucleoli (MGG ×600 oil immersion) (MGG ×600, MGG ×400). **F.** The grading of follicular lymphomas proposed in REAL classification and endorsed by the current World Health Organization classification can be applied to cytological preparations but the criteria have not been established yet. The aggressive lymphomas usually have >20% of centroblasts (MGG ×600, oil immersion).

round lymphocytes, transformed cells and variable numbers of immunoblasts (Fig. 4.48 and Chapter 2, Fig. 2.24).[166] These findings, while highly suggestive of MALT lymphoma in extranodal proliferations, may be more difficult to distinguish from reactive conditions in lymph nodes.[131] In 10% of cases, marginal zone lymphoma transforms into large cell lymphoma. The nuclei of marginal zone lymphoma are usually round or only slightly irregular in contrast to the small-cleaved cells of follicular lymphoma and mantle zone lymphoma. Lymphoid cells may have plasmacytoid features. Mature plasma cells may be seen. Morphologically, follicular lymphomas differ from marginal zone lymphomas in that they have a range of nuclear sizes ranging from small to large. On the other hand, mantle zone lymphoma has

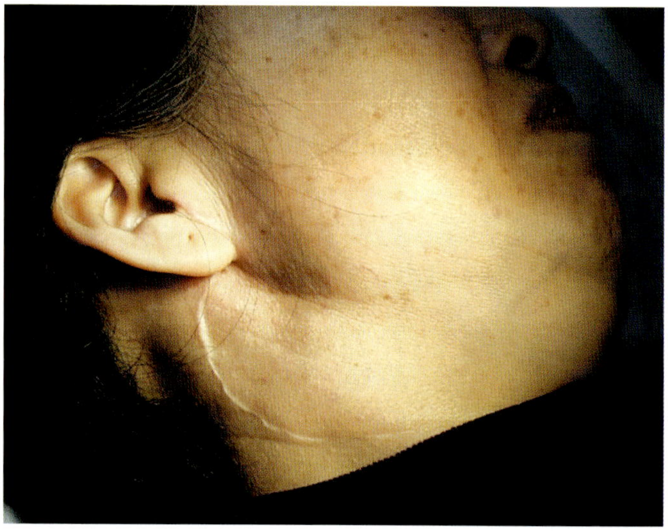

A

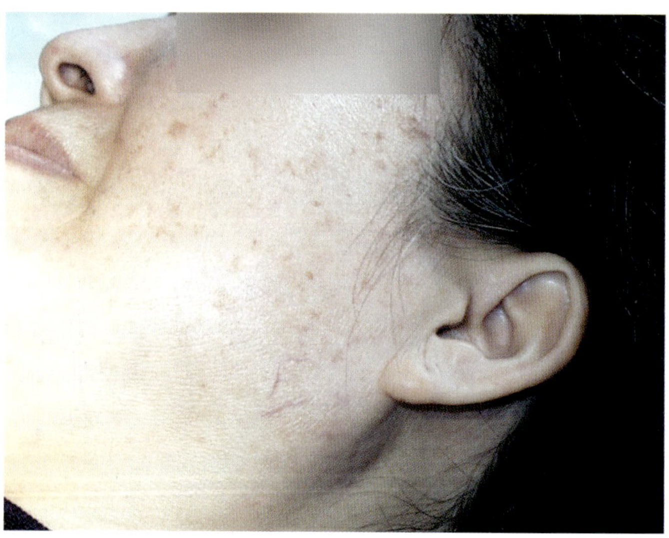

B

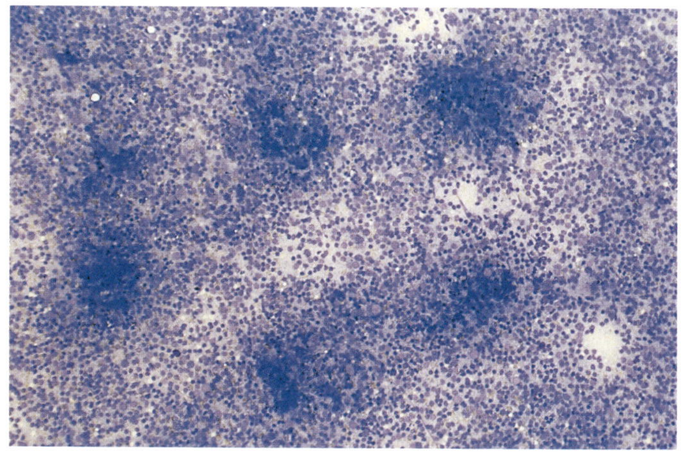

C

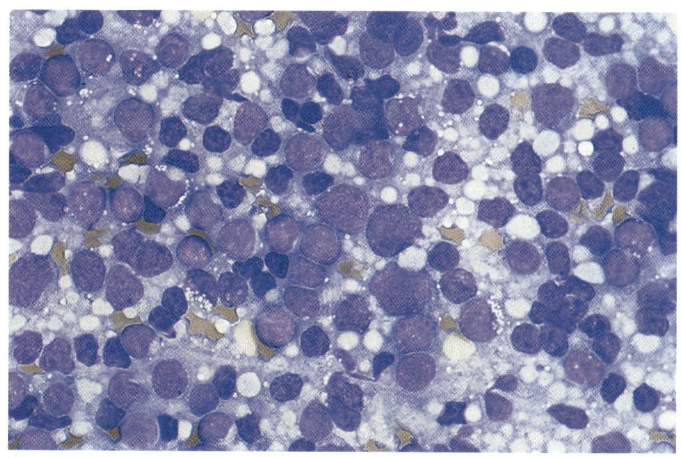

D

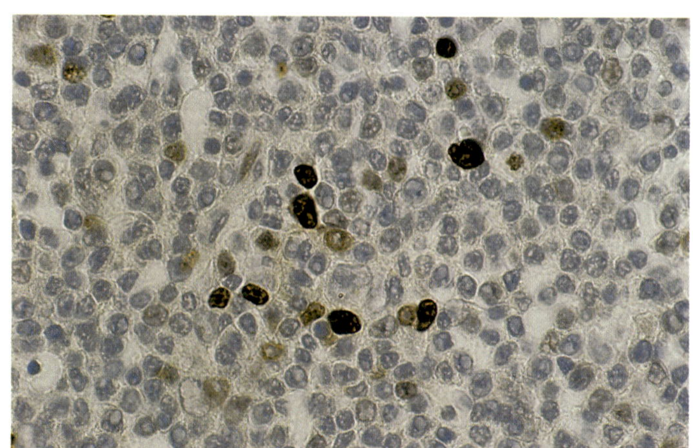

E

Figure 4.48 MALT lymphoma. **A.** A 53-year-old patient who had excision of the MALT lymphoma of the parotid gland 7 years ago. **B.** Now patients presents with a painless diffuse swelling of the left parotid. **C.** Low-power view reveals pseudofollicular aggregates due to preserved follicular dendritic cells (MGG ×200). **D.** Polymorphous proliferation comprising a predominant population of intermediate-sized lymphoid cells with round to irregular nuclear outline (centrocyte-like or monocytoid features)' chromatin slightly paler and less clumped than in small mature lymphocytes, small inconspicuous nucleolus and a distinct pale cytoplasm. In addition there are small mature round lymphocytes, transformed cells and variable numbers of immunoblasts (MGG ×600 oil immersion). **E.** Ki-67 proliferation marker is positive in very few cells (MIB1, IP ×400).

monotonous cell population of irregularly shaped small to medium-sized cells. These contrast with marginal zone lymphoma, which has predominantly small cells with a few large lymphoid cells without transitional forms (Box 4.3).

Nearly all marginal zone lymphomas express surface immunoglobulin. Approximately 50% express intracytoplasmic Ig. CD5, CD10 and CD23 are negative (Table 4.3).

Marginal zone lymphoma usually shows heavy chain and light chain rearrangement. Bcl-1 and bcl-2 are usually not detected.

Diffuse large B-cell lymphoma

This is one of the commonest categories of non-Hodgkin's lymphoma (Fig. 4.42). Previously called 'centroblastic' lymphoma, it was thought to be different from 'immunoblastic' lymphoma and was therefore listed separately. However, there is no evidence as to the validity of this distinction, no survival advantage, specific genetic abnormality or definite morphologic distinction (Box 4.2).[100] Diffuse large cell lymphoma therefore combines characteristics of both of these previously separate entities (Box 4.5). It can arise de novo or can be a result of transformation of other lymphomas. Clinically, there are multiple distinct presentations, e.g. mediastinal/thymic large cell lymphoma, primary central nervous system lymphoma and primary effusion lymphoma (Fig. 4.49).[167] *Cutaneous B-cell lymphoma* is a separate entity, the morphology of which can range from low-grade follicular lymphoma to diffuse large B-cell lymphoma (Fig. 4.50). However, disease has an indolent clinical course and should not be treated aggressively like other systemic large cell lymphomas. Systemic disease requires aggressive treatment and may respond well.[156]

Box 4.5 World Health Organization classification of diffuse large B-cell lymphoma, morphological variants and subtypes[100]

Diffuse large B-cell lymphoma, morphological variants
Centroblastic
Immunoblastic
T cell/histiocyte rich
Lymphomatoid granulomatosis type
Anaplastic large B-cell
Plasmablastic

Diffuse large B-cell lymphoma, subtypes
Mediastinal (thymic) large B-cell lymphoma
Primary effusion lymphoma
Intravascular large B-cell lymphoma

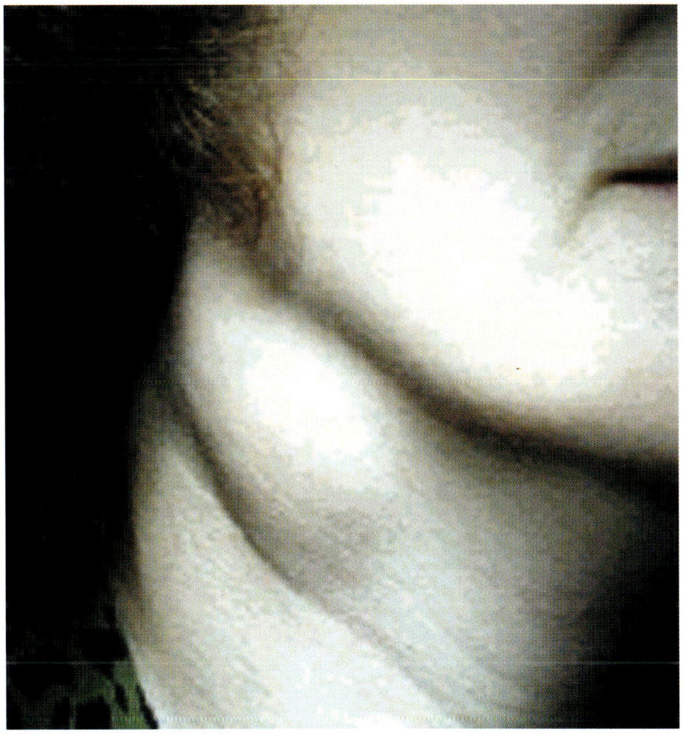

Figure 4.49 Diffuse large B-cell lymphoma. Patient presenting with a lump in the neck 5 years after treatment of carcinoma of the breast.

Cytological features. Diffuse large cell lymphoma has a monomorphous population of large cells with prominent nucleoli and basophilic cytoplasm. Diffuse large B-cell lymphoma represents heterogenous group of entities, all of which have a significant component of large cells (Figs 4.51 and 4.52, also Chapter 1, Fig. 1.9). Immunoblasts are large cells with eccentric nuclei, prominent, usually single, large nucleolus and basophilic cytoplasm. Centroblasts are smaller than immunoblasts, round, with central nucleus, evenly distributed basophilic cytoplasm and usually multiple nucleoli. Pleomorphic polylobed cells, signet ring cells and spindle cells can all be seen in different types of large cell lymphoma.[168]

Immunophenotypically diffuse large B-cell lymphoma is surface Ig +/–, cytoplasmic Ig +/–, CD5, CD10 +/–, CD19, CD20, 22, 79a, CD45 positive, EMA negative. Large B-cell lymphoma may contain a mixture of other cell types, such as T-cell rich B-cell lymphoma or histiocyte-rich B-cell lymphoma.[140] A minority of cases (30%) show t(14–18). Nearly all cases have detectable immunoglobulin light chain or heavy chain rearrangements (Fig. 4.52). Bcl-1 gene rearrangement is generally not found. This helps with distinction from blastic variant of mantle zone lymphoma, which frequently demonstrates this rearrangement.

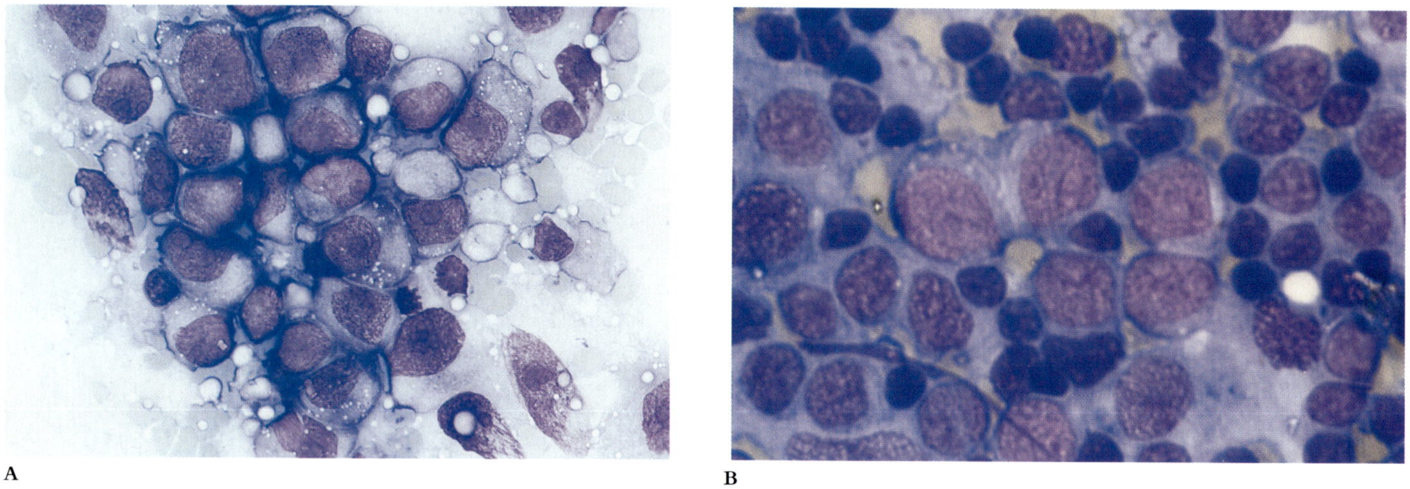

Figure 4.50 Diffuse large cell lymphoma. **A.** Monomorphous population of large cells with prominent nucleoli and basophilic cytoplasm (MGG ×600). **B.** Immunoblasts are large cells with eccentric nuclei, prominent, usually single large nucleolus and basophilic cytoplasm. Centroblasts are smaller than immunoblasts, round, with central nucleus, evenly distributed basophilic cytoplasm and usually multiple nucleoli. Pleomorphic polilobated cells, signet ring cells and spindle cells can all be seen in different types of large cell lymphoma (MGG ×1000 oil immersion).

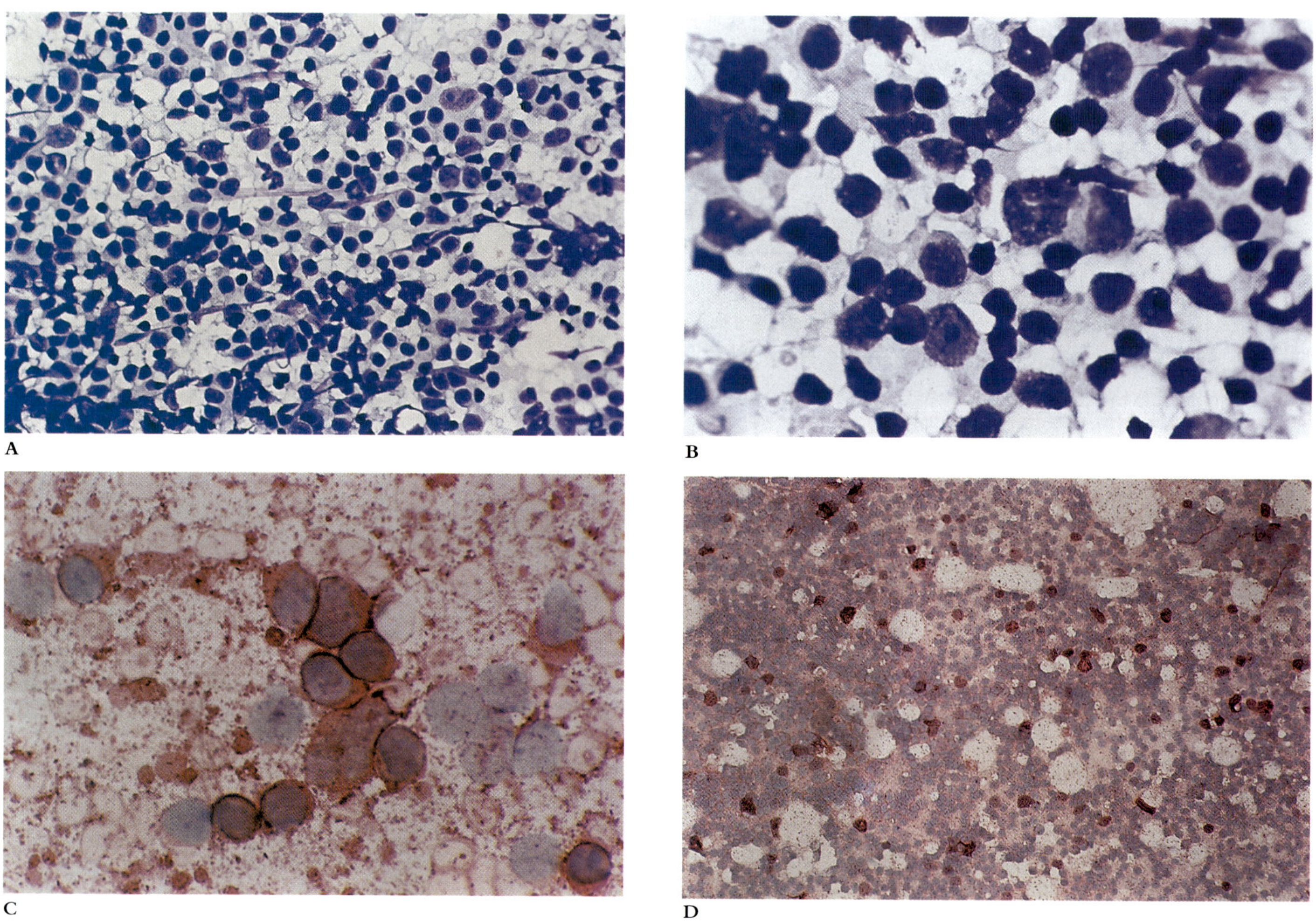

Figure 4.51 Cutaneous B-cell lymphoma. This patient presented with recurrence of cutaneous nodules treated with radiotherapy several years previously. There were no generalised symptoms or lymphadenopathy. **A.** FNAC yielded a monotonous lymphoid cell population (×400). **B.** Cells are predominantly centrocytes with some centroblasts (×600 oil immersion). **C.** B-cell markers are positive (CD20, ×600). **D.** Proliferation fraction is low (MIB-1 ×400).

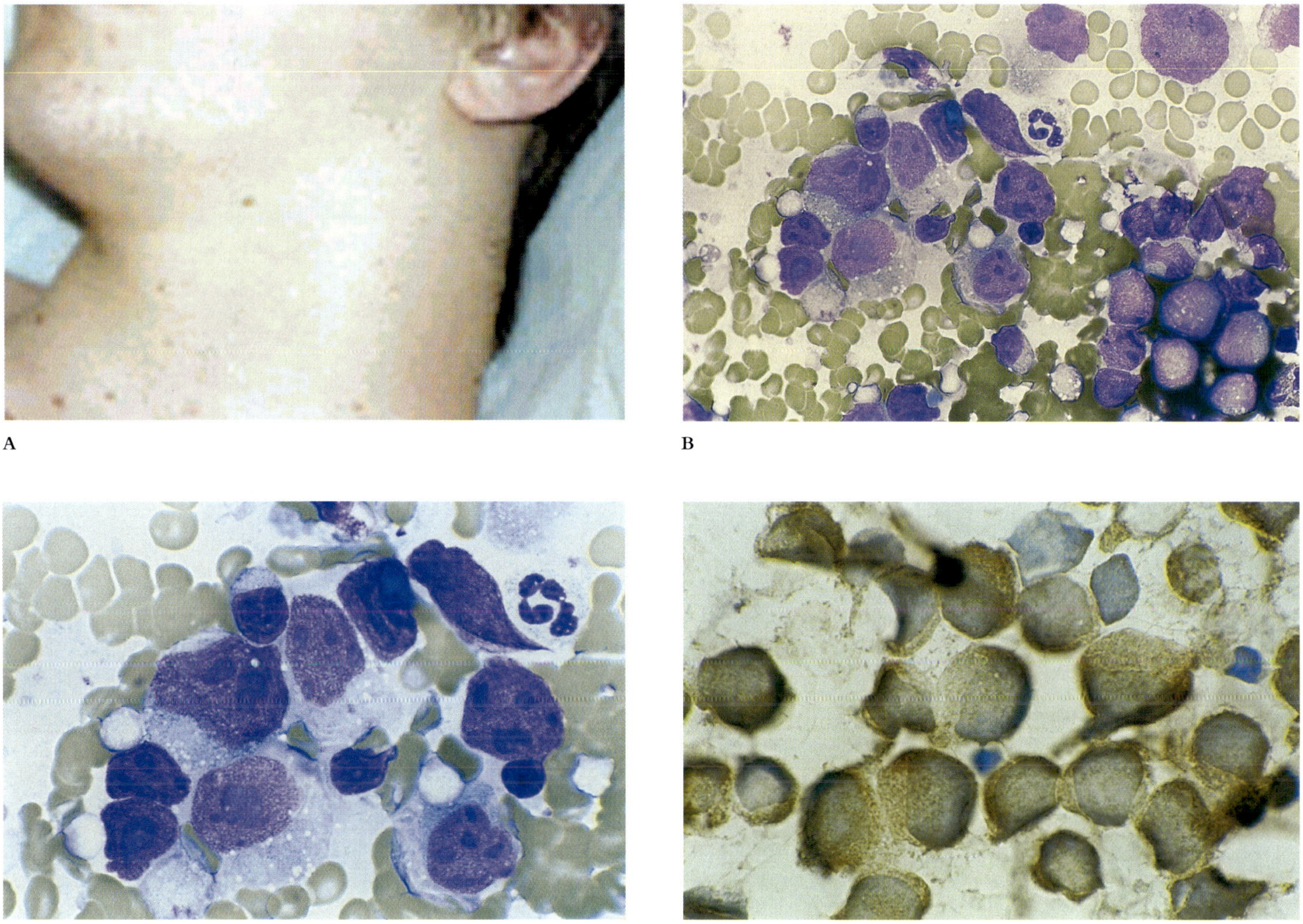

A B C D

Figure 4.52 Diffuse large cell lymphoma. **A.** An adolescent patient presented with a short history of diffuse tender neck swelling. Clinically, an infection was suspected. **B,C.** FNAC shows a lymphoid cell population with predominance of large blasts (MGG ×600, ×1000 oil immersion). **D.** Lymphoid cells are B-marker positive (CD20, Ip ×1000 oil immersion).

Primary effusion lymphoma

Primary effusion lymphoma (PEL) is a subtype of large B cell lymphoma.[100] Since the effusion is often the first and only site of presentation, the disease has special significance for cytopathologists since they are often the first to diagnose the often unsuspected disease. Primary effusion lymphoma, together with Kaposi's sarcoma and multicentric Castleman's disease has been associated with human herpesvirus-8 infection (HHV-8).[169] It arises in a body cavity or space without an associated tumour mass, displays the cytomorphology of anaplastic large cell lymphoma, is a clonal B-cell neoplasm, and contains HHV-8 as well as EBV. Kaposi's sarcoma and multicentric Castleman's disease patients may develop body cavity effusions that, unlike primary effusion lymphoma, are poorly characterised. In the setting of HHV 8 infection, two effusion types may occur. One fulfils the criteria for HHV-8-positive primary effusion lymphoma (lymphoma-morphology, HHV-8-DNA(+), IgH rearrangement). The other seems more reminiscent of an HHV-8-associated non-neoplastic process (monocyte-macrophage morphology, HHV-8-DNA(+/-), germline IgH). A single case of the latter effusion type harboured a B-cell monoclonal proliferation, which suggests the hypothesis that a prelymphomatous effusion may precede overt body cavity lymphoma. Primary effusion lymphoma has been limited almost entirely to the pleural, peritoneal, pericardial cavities and in the subarachnoid space (Fig. 4.53).[170]

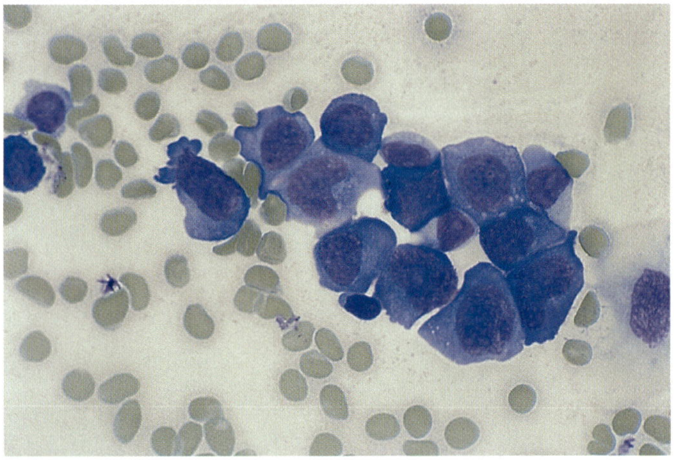

A

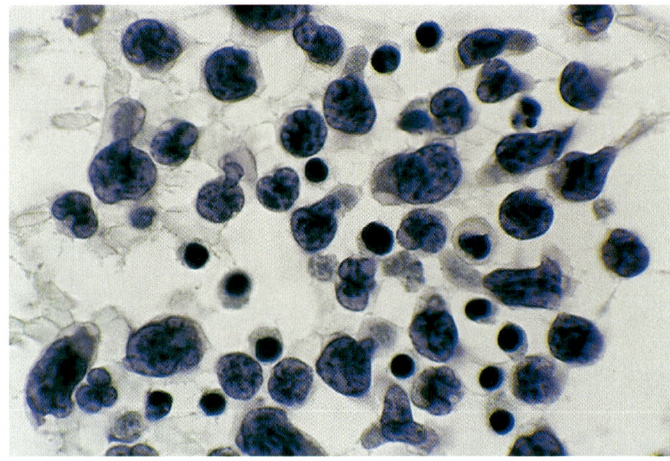

B

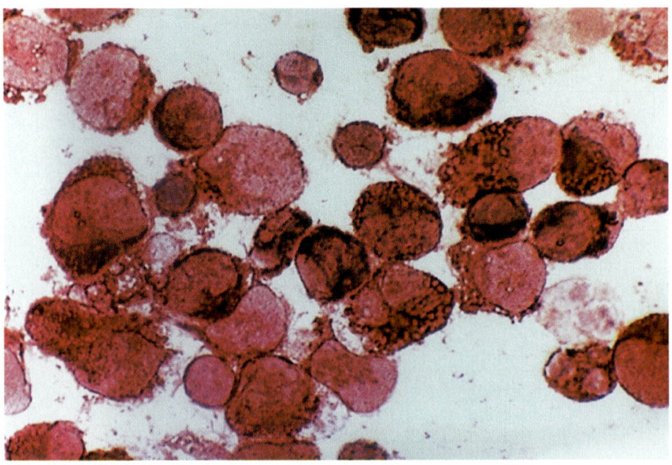

C

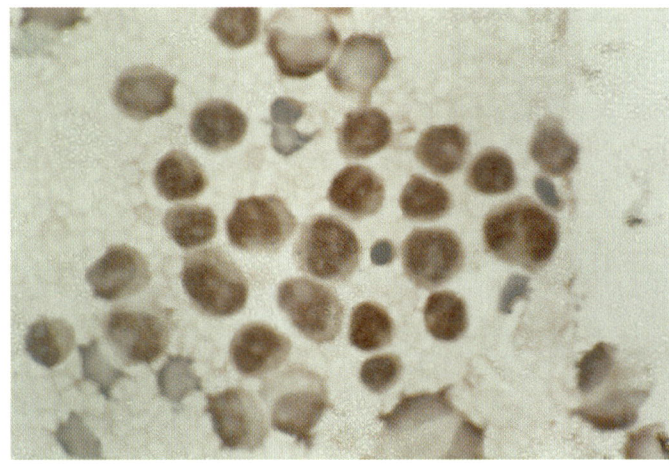

D

Figure 4.53 Primary effusion lymphoma. **A,B.** Pleural effusion containing numerous lymphoid cells with features of high-grade lymphoma. Cells are variably large, immunoblastic or have anaplastic features. They show numerous mitoses (MGG, PAP ×600 oil immersion). **C.** PEL is CD45 positive (APAAP ×600). **D.** EBV positive (APAAP ×600).

Burkitt's lymphoma

For Burkitt's lymphoma, the World Health Organization classification proposes 2 morphological variants, 'Burkitt-like' and 'with plasmacytoid differentiation (AIDS-associated)', and 3 subtypes: 'endemic', 'sporadic' and 'immunodeficiency-associated' (Box 4.4).[100] In most 'endemic' African cases, which affect the jaw or extranodal sites of children, EBV DNA is found in malignant cells. Histologically and phenotypically identical cases are seen in the West. These may be associated with immunosuppression and about half of the cases have EBV detectable. Non-African 'sporadic' cases affect children and adults and present most commonly in the abdomen. They show EBV in about 25% of cases. Histologically, the tumour is made of medium-sized B-cells interspersed with macrophages containing kariorrhectic debris ('starry sky' appearance in sections). The disease affects children more than adults. Treatment is aggressive but successful in children.

Box 4.6 World Health Organization classification of Burkitt's lymphoma, morphological variants and subtypes[100]

Burkitt lymphoma, morphological variants
Burkitt-like
With plasmacytoid differentiation (AIDS-associated)

Burkitt lymphoma, subtypes (clinical and genetic)
Endemic
Sporadic
Immunodeficiency-associated

Cytological features. FNAC smears from Burkitt's lymphoma show high cellularity and an individual cell pattern (Fig. 4.54). Extracellular 'lymphoglandular bodies' are abundant and tingible body macrophages are prominent. Nuclei are intermediate in size (8–25 μm, with an average of 10–12 μm) and round with a finely dispersed chromatin on MGG-stained smears. Cytoplasm is basophilic and scant with prominent vacuoles. Extracellular vacuoles and vacuoles within 'lymphoglandular bodies' are also seen.[133]

Papanicolaou stain shows coarse chromatin and 2–5 prominent nucleoli. 'Burkitt-like' lymphoma represents morphologic appearance with more pleomorphism and large cells than Burkitt's but is probably best managed as a variant of Burkitt's lymphoma, i.e. very high grade tumour with a proliferation fraction greater than 99%, and not as diffuse large B-cell lymphoma. An international panel review of mature B-cell lymphoma/leukaemia in children and adolescents highlighted difficulties in subclassification, particularly with Burkitt-like lymphoma, which is a 'provisional entity' in the REAL classification. Morphology needs to be complemented by other studies, such as molecular genetics and cytogenetics, to discriminate between the B-cell lymphomas.

Immunophenotype is surface IgM positive, CD5, CD23 negative, CD10 positive, CD19, 20, 22, 79a positive, Ki67>85% of cells. Almost all cases show chromosomal

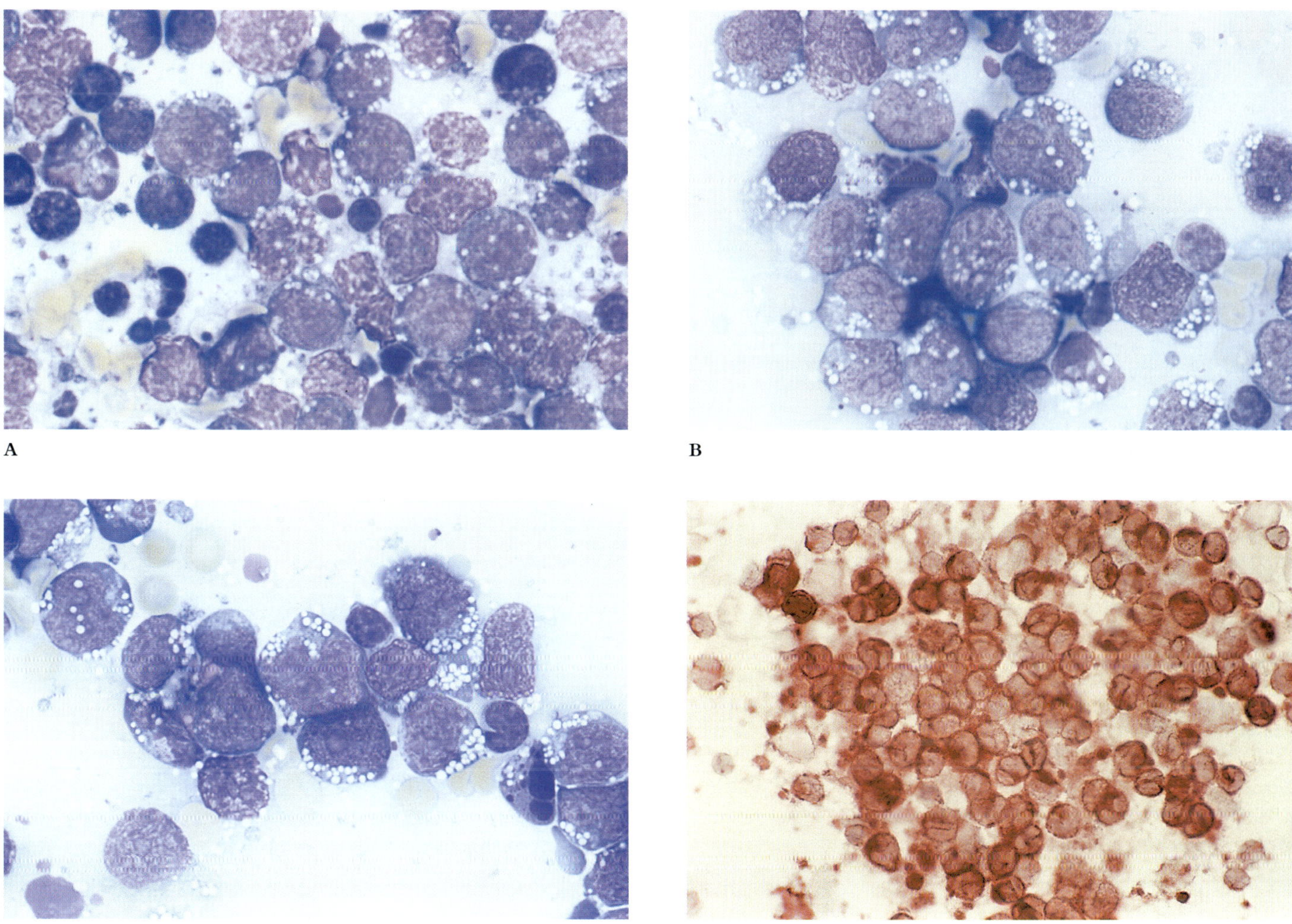

Figure 4.54 Burkitt's lymphoma. **A.** FNAC smears from Burkitt's lymphoma of the jaw show high cellularity and an individual cell pattern. Extracellular 'lymphoglandular bodies' are abundant and tingible body macrophages are prominent (MGG ×600 oil). **B,C.** Burkitt-like disease from the gastrointestinal tract of a HIV positive patients shows similar features. Nuclei are intermediate in size (8–25 μm, with an average of 10–12 μm) and round with finely dispersed chromatin. Cytoplasm is basophilic and scant with prominent vacuoles. Extracellular vacuoles and vacuoles within 'lymphoglandular bodies' are also seen (MGG ×1000 oil). **D.** Ki 67 proliferation marker shows 100% cells positive (MIB 1, APAAP ×600 oil).

translocation involving the cMYC gene on chromosome 8 and the gene for Ig heavy chain or, less commonly, one of the two light chain genes. The gold standard for diagnosis of Burkitt's lymphoma is either cytogenetic analysis or, if not available, proliferation fraction. This should be >99%. In the case of suspected Burkitt's lymphoma, the finding of a translocation (8;14) or associated variant translocation, along with the characteristic cytomorphology and proliferation fraction allows a definitive diagnosis by fine needle aspiration and may alleviate the need for biopsy.[133]

T/NK-cell lymphomas

Peripheral T-cell lymphoma

T-cell lymphomas are rare (10% of all lymphomas) in the Western world although they are more common in the Far East.[171] Peripheral T-cell lymphoma (PTCL) does not have a common cytological composition, immunophenotype or cytogenetic characteristics. Instead, the disease(s) are defined by clinical syndromes and location (nodal vs extranodal and specific extranodal sites) which are important in

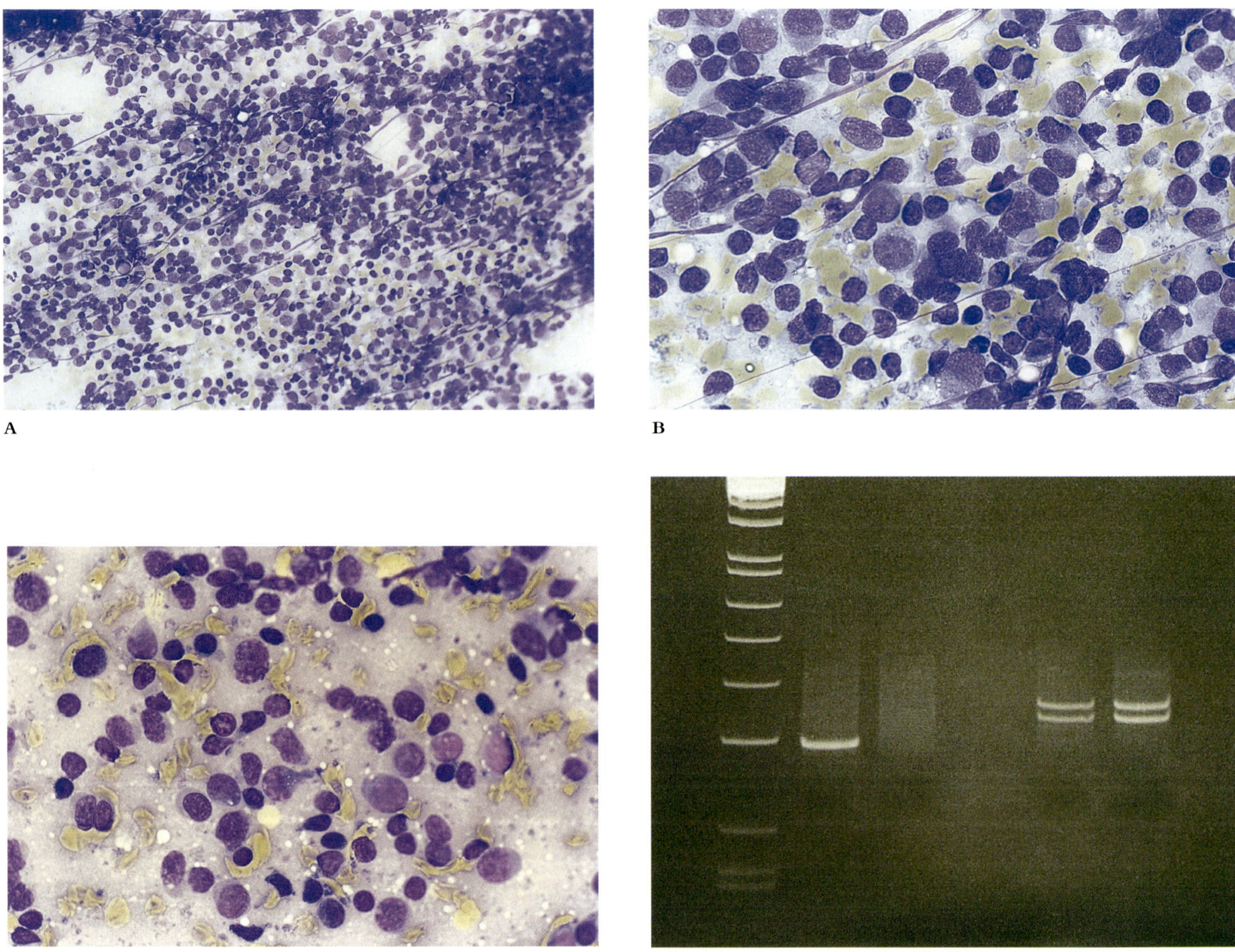

Figure 4.55 Peripheral T-cell lymphoma. FNAC of parotid. **A.** Low-power view reveals a dense lymphoid infiltrate of parotid gland (MGG ×200). **B,C.** Variable combination of small, intermediate and large lymphoid cells with irregular nuclei, epithelioid histiocytes and atypical mononuclear cells (MGG ×600 oil immersion). Diagnosis of lymphoid infiltrate of parotid gland was made. Biopsy revealed a T-cell lymphoma. **D.** Patient with cutaneous lesions (mycosis fungoides), morphologically small lymphocytes ? LN involvement? Peripheral T cell lymphoma. Ten percent polyacrilamide gel of TCR-gamma PCR products. Lane 1. Positive monoclonal control (T-cell lymphoma), 2. Polyclonal control, 3. Negative control, 4. FNAC LN monoclonal (T cell lymphoma), 5. FNAC same patient from 1998, monoclonal (T cell lymphoma) (Courtesy of Mr T Diss).

determining biological behaviour (Box 4.2).[100] Given the difference in clinical behaviour between nodal and extranodal sites, the World Health Organization classification suggests separating the lymphomas into nodal and extranodal types. Cytological subclassification of peripheral T-cell lymphomas is not necessary for clinical purposes.

Cytological features. The most prominent cytological features of PTCL are a variable combination of small, intermediate and large lymphoid cells with irregular nuclei, presence of epithelioid histiocytes and atypical mononuclear cells (Fig. 4.55).[130] The small cells have very irregular nuclei with condensed chromatin. Large cells may have prominent nucleoli and abundant, usually pale cytoplasm. An infiltrate of host cells is common in T-cell lymphomas. This includes small lymphocytes, polymorphs, epithelioid and non-epithelioid histiocytes and plasma cells. The diagnosis of PTCL is difficult. This entity can be misdiagnosed as Hodgkin's disease or a reactive process such as non-necrotising granulomatous lymphadenitis, or it can present a problem in lymphoma classification.[130] Cases of skin and extracutaneous involvement of mycosis fungoides contain atypical small and large lymphocytes with cerebriform appearance (Fig. 4.56).[172–175]

FNAC of high-grade PTCL from human T-lymphotropic virus-1 (HTLV-1)-positive patients show a distinctive cytological pattern with a dominance of rounded cells with irregular nuclei and a moderately basophilic cytoplasm (Fig. 4.57). Irregular cells with a pale abundant cytoplasm are present in varying amounts. Giant cells with cerebriform nuclei, plasma cells and eosinophils are also seen. Epithelioid cells are an inconstant finding. PTCL from HTLV-1-positive patients have cytological patterns which are distinctive enough to allow a conclusive diagnosis of high-grade T-cell lymphoma.[176]

Unless there is history or a suspicion of T-cell lymphoma, the first line of investigation will be to exclude B-cell lymphoma, which is more common. To establish a diagnosis of T-cell lymphoma, all B-cell markers must be negative and at least one of the pan T-cell markers positive (Figs 4.55–4.59). T-cell panel includes CD1a, CD2, CD3, CD4, CD5, CD7 and CD8. Detection of T-cell gene rearrangement may be helpful in diagnosis of difficult cases (Fig. 4.55d). The failure to demonstrate this rearrangement does not rule out diagnosis of T-cell lymphoma. Many of the cases of T cell lymphoma are mixed small and large cell, and in Korea, where the incidence of extranodal and T-cell lymphoma is high, the usefulness of FNAC for the initial diagnosis of malignant lymphoma is limited. For a definitive diagnosis, biopsy is required.[171]

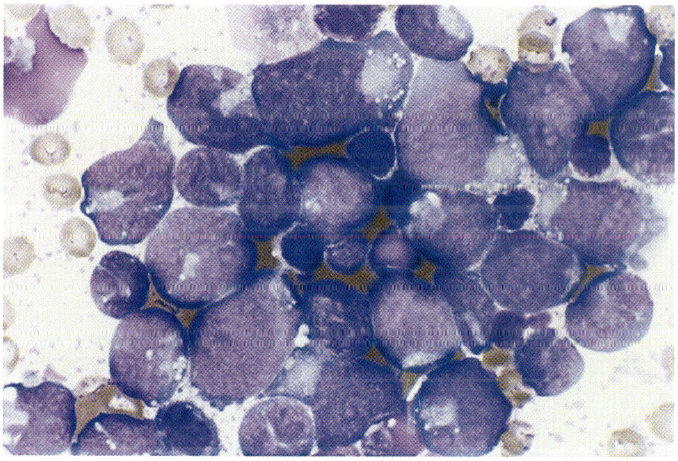

A

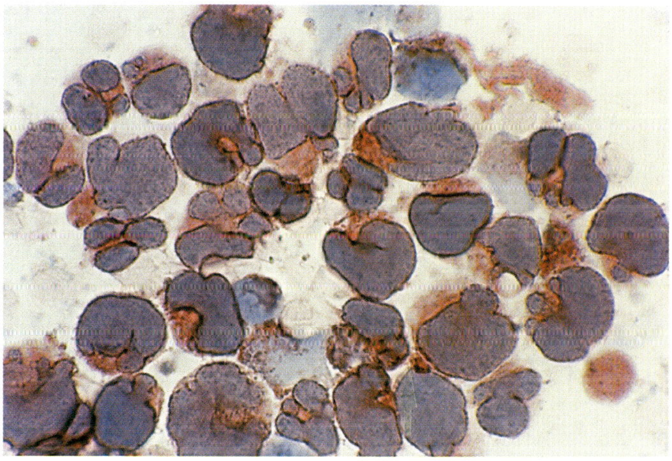

B

Figure 4.56 High-grade peripheral T-cell lymphoma. **A.** FNAC of a skin nodule contains atypical small and large lymphocytes with cerebriform appearance (MGG ×1000 oil). **B.** Cells are strongly CD3 positive. Note cerebriform outline of the nucleus (CD3, APAAp ×1000 oil immersion).

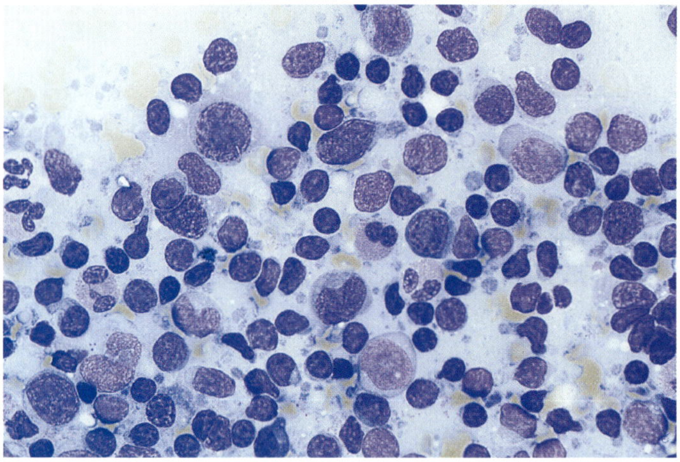

A

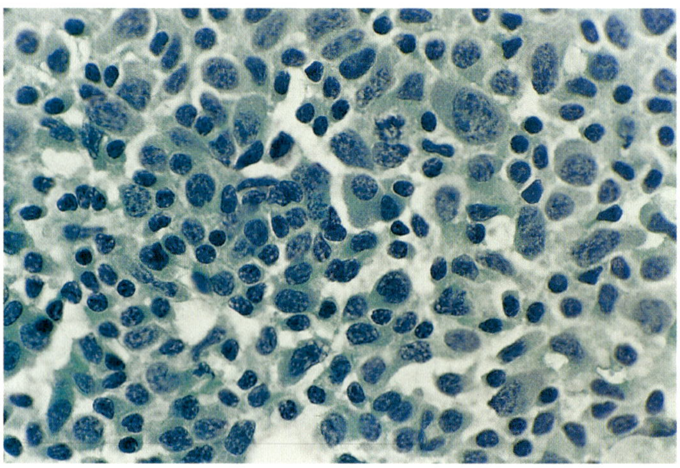

B

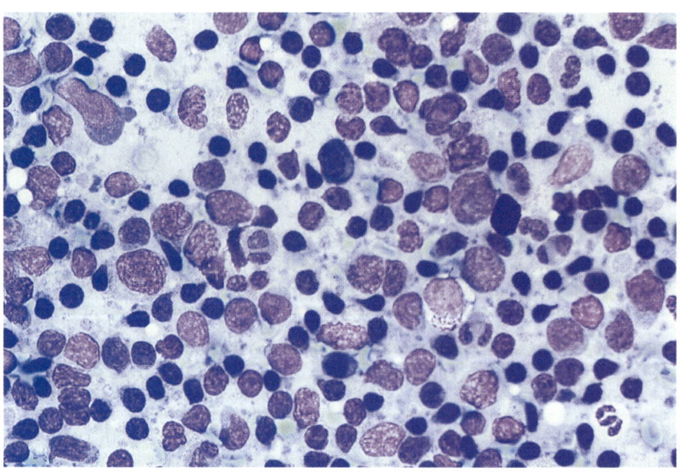

C

Figure 4.57 HTLV1-associated T-cell lymphoma. **A,B,C.** Rounded cells with irregular nuclei and a moderately basophilic cytoplasm. Irregular cells with a pale abundant cytoplasm are present in varying amounts. Giant cells with cerebriform nuclei, plasma cells and eosinophils may be seen. Epithelioid cells are an inconstant finding. This case was misdiagnosed as reactive node. Diagnosis of T-cell lymphoma may be difficult (MGG, PAP, MGG ×600 oil immersion).

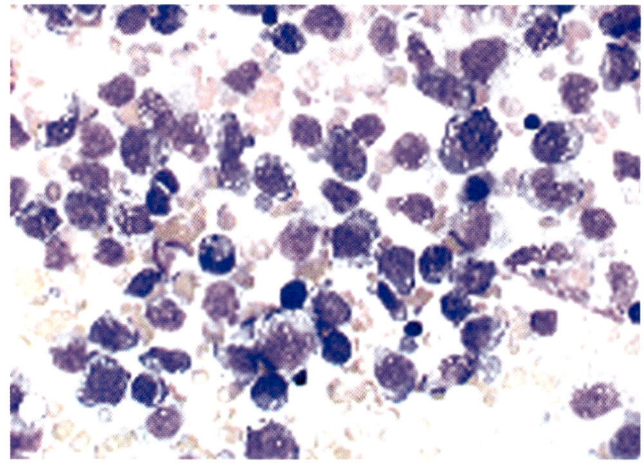

A

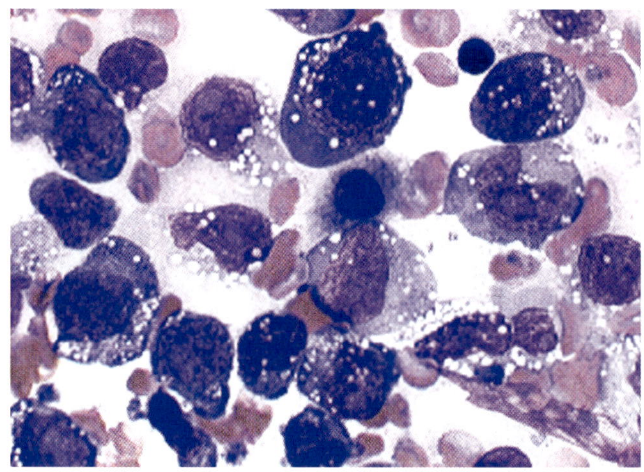

B

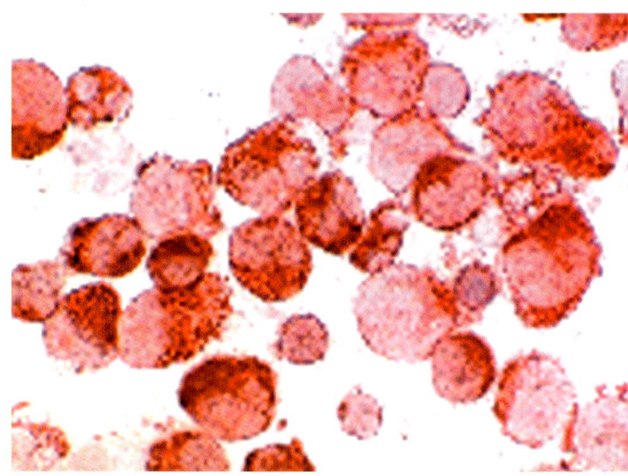

C

Figure 4.58 Large cell T-cell lymphoma. **A.** FNAC smears show high-grade lymphoma with immunoblastic features (MGG ×400). **B.** Individual cells show pleomorphism (MGG ×1000 oil immersion). **C.** CD3 positive staining confirms the lymphoma to be T-cell (CD3, APAAP ×600 oil immersion).

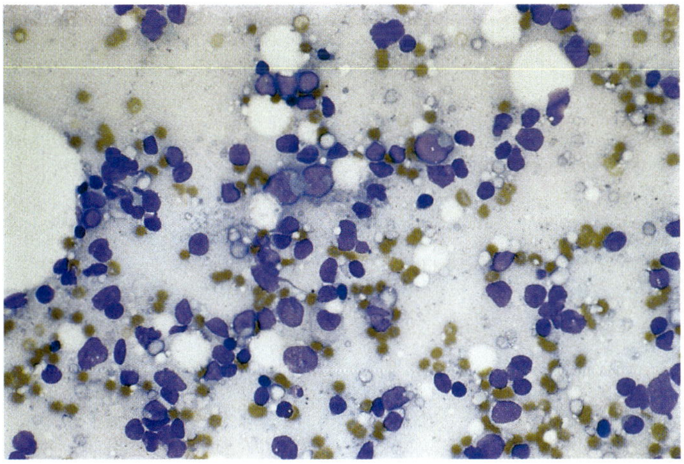

Figure 4.59 Cutaneous T-cell lymphoma. This is a separate entity from the cutaneous variant of ALCL and lymphomatoid papulosis. Cells are mixed, small and medium sized, some with cerebriform nuclei.

Anaplastic large cell lymphoma

Anaplastic large cell lymphoma (ALCL) was first recognised as a neoplasm which was positive for the Ki-1 or CD30 antigen, also found on RS cells. The tumour presents in children or young adults and can have two different patterns of presentation: a systemic type with widespread involvement of lymph nodes; or a localised form that is confined to the skin (Figs 4.61 and 4.62). The two types have very different prognoses: the cutaneous type is usually indolent but resistant to cure while the systemic type is aggressive but potentially curable.[156] The cutaneous type also lacks t(2;5)(p23;q35) and is ALK protein negative. This entity should be regarded as separate from the systemic type. Cutaneous ALCL is part of the 'CD30-positive lymphoproliferative skin conditions' which also include lymphomatoid papulosis and CD30 + cutanous T-cell lymphomas that do not have typical 'anaplastic' morphology (Fig. 4.60).[100]

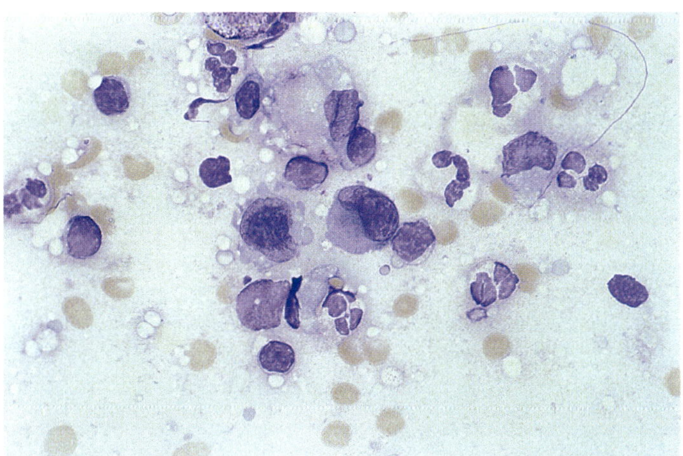

A

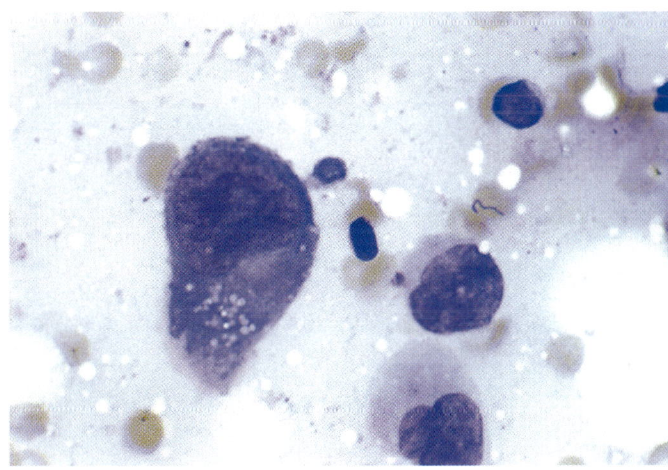

B

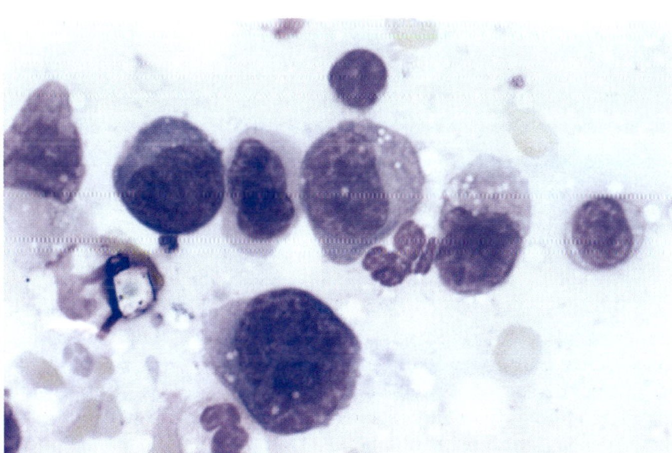

C

Figure 4.60 CD30-positive lymphoproliferative conditions of the skin. **A.** Lymphomatoid papulosis is a lymphoid infiltrate of the skin containing a mixture of large atypical lymphoid cells, histiocytes and inflammatory cells. **B,C.** Some of the cells have bizarre features tempting a diagnosis of malignancy. The disease is self-limiting and morphologically difficult to distinguish from the cutaneous variant of ALCL (MGG ×1000 oil immersion).

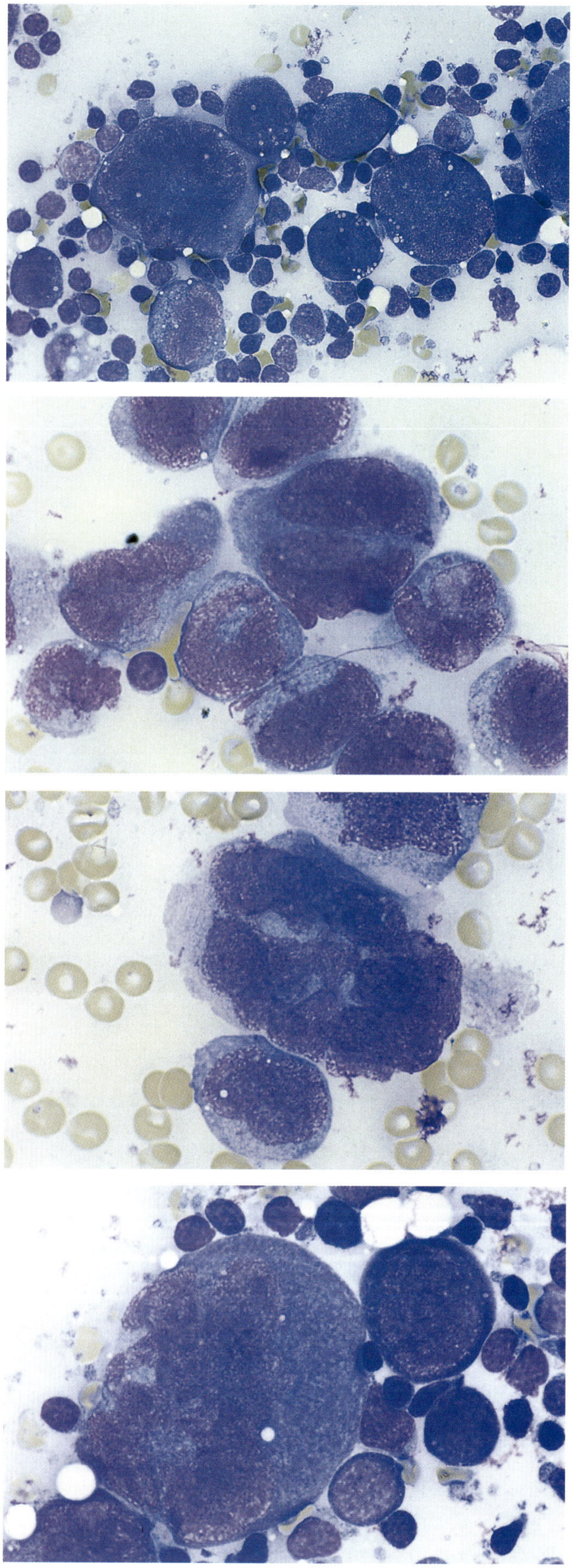

A B C D

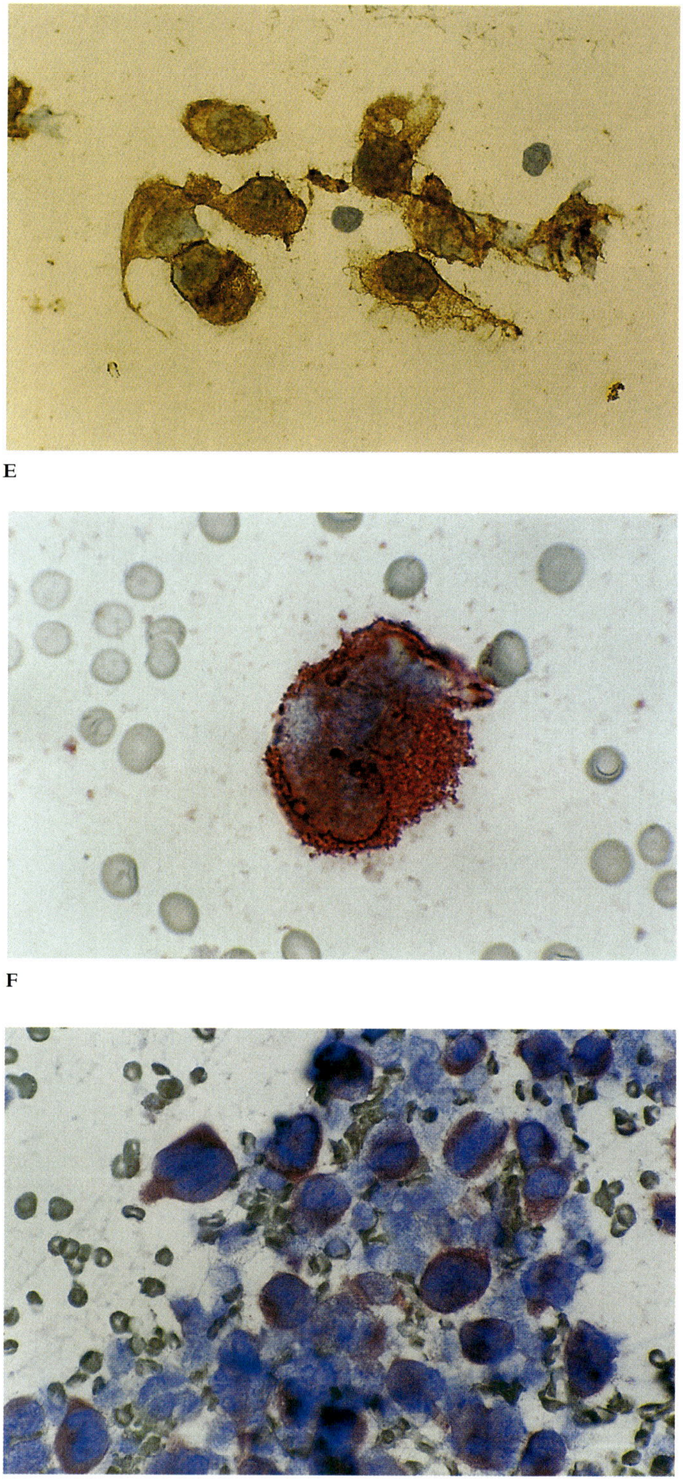

E F G

Figure 4.61 Anaplastic large cell lymphoma. A 25-year-old patient was referred for suprasternal swelling thought to be thyroid gland. **A.** FNAC shows a population of large bizarre cells against a background of mature lymphocytes (MGG ×400). **B,C,D.** A high power view shows cells with large, pleomorphic nuclei, many containing prominent nucleoli, and a moderate amount of cytoplasm. Many binucleate and multinucleate tumour cells are present (average size 42 μm), some with a 'wreath-like' arrangement of nuclei. **D**. Cells have a coarse chromatin pattern and deeply basophilic, variably vacuolated cytoplasm (MGG ×1000 oil immersion). **E.** CD30 positivity (IP ×600 oil immersion). **F.** CD30 positivity (APAAP ×600 oil immersion). **G** ALK 1 positivity (see text) (APPAP ×400).

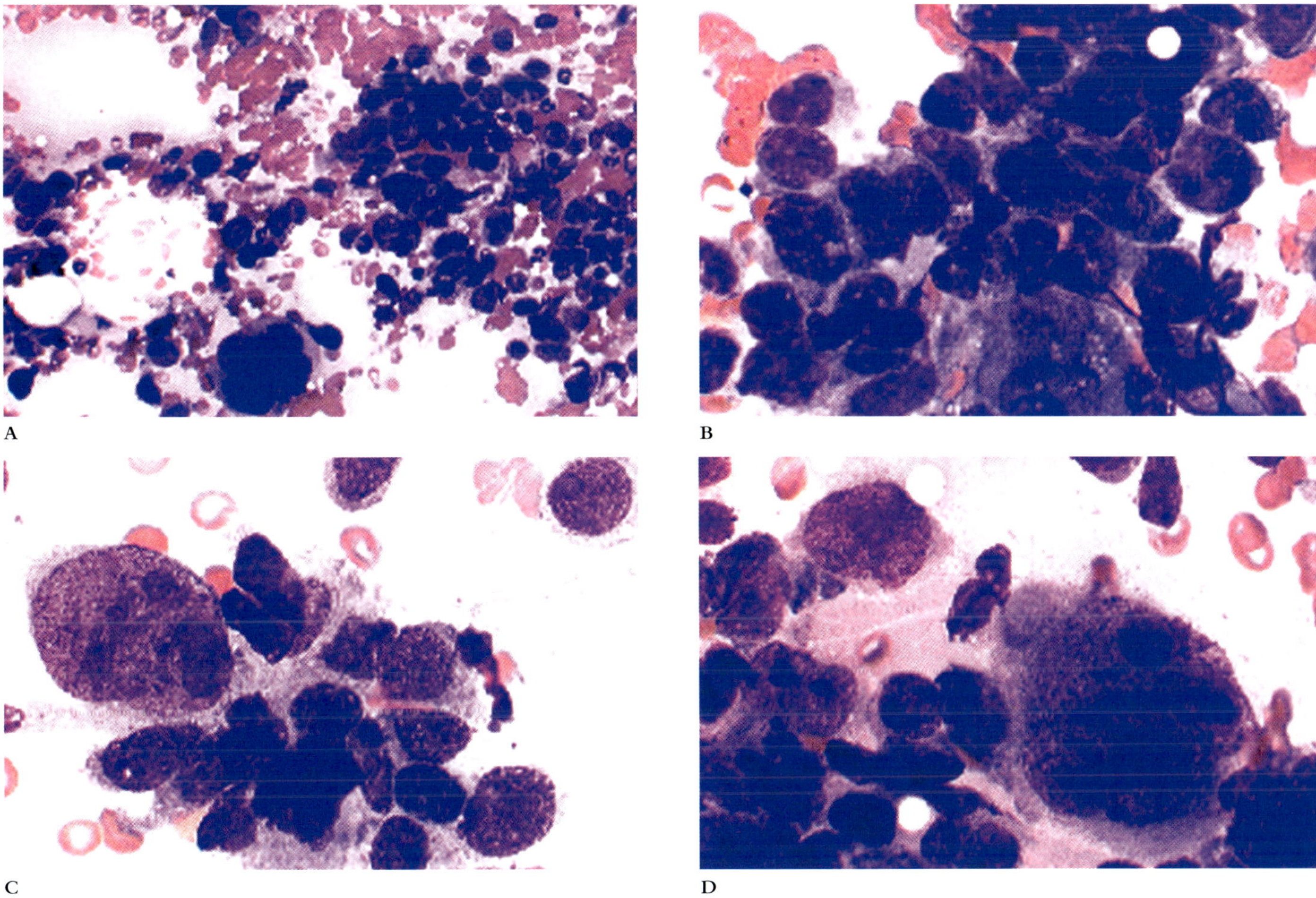

Figure 4.62 The cutaneous type of ALCL. Cutaneous form of ALCL is a defined clinical entity (see text) which cytopathologists should be aware of, because its anaplastic features are indistinguishable from the systemic type of ALCL (Figure 4.61), and yet its management and prognosis are different (MGG ×200, ×600, ×1000 oil immersion). Cells are CD30 positive.

Systemic ALCL has neoplastic cells larger than any other type of lymphoma and can be misdiagnosed as malignant histiocytosis or Hodgkin's lymphoma. The most common phenotype is that of pleomorphic cells with multilobated and multinucleated cells, although a monomorphic variant exists.

Cytological features. ALCL is a cytologically undifferentiated malignant lymphoma that needs to be distinguished from a variety of other neoplasms using immunohistochemistry. It is composed of single cells and poorly cohesive groups of cells with large, pleomorphic nuclei, many containing prominent nucleoli, and a moderate amount of cytoplasm (Figs 4.61 and 4.62). Many binucleate and multinucleate tumour cells are present (average size 42 mm), some with a 'wreath-like' arrangement of nuclei.[177] Cells have a 'ropy' chromatin pattern and deeply basophilic, variably vacuolated cytoplasm. Necrosis is frequent. A proteinaceous background is prominent in cellular samples. Lymphoglandular bodies and lymphoid tangles are not prominent.[178] Cytological features may suggest metastatic anaplastic carcinoma since anaplastic cells may be admixed with mature lymphocytes and follicle centre cells, reflecting the histological features of malignant cells in ALCL often being confined to subcapsular and medullary sinuses resembling metastatic carcinoma.[179]

Immunocytochemistry is essential in distinguishing these tumours from metastatic carcinoma, melanoma and Hodgkin's disease. ALCL is positive for CD45 (LCA) in only 67% of cases. It is nearly always negative for cytokeratin but positive for EMA in systemic cases (75%).[178] Nearly all malignant cells express CD30 positivity (surface membrane and cytoplasmic paranuclear dot-like staining)[180] (Fig. 4.61E, F). CD15 is usually negative in ALCL. When cell lineage markers are present, they show T-cell origins.

The cytogenetic abnormality in ALCL, t(2;5)(p23;q35), can be successfully detected with antibodies against ALK protein in 65% of classical nodal ALCL[181] (Fig. 4.61G). The ALK-positive group seems to have a good prognosis. Given the importance of ALK protein, the World Health Organization classification recommends that all ALCL be classified as ALK positive or ALK negative.

HHV-8 can associate with solid lymphomas and take anaplastic large cell morphology. The recently described HHV-8-associated lymphomas in HIV-positive patients may exhibit anaplastic large cell morphology and express CD30. However, the chromosomal translocation t(2;5)-associated chimaeric protein p80NPM/ALK is not observed in any of these cases.[181,182] This suggests that ALCL is not pathogenetically related to the majority of other types of aggressive T-NHL. Those lymphomas should be distinguished from the classical ALCL as were defined by the REAL and World Health Organization classifications of lymphoid neoplasms even though morphology and a part of immunophenotype mimic that of classical ALCL. Lymphomas developing as a sequel to post-transplant lymphadenopathy may exceptionally also have ALCL phenotype.[183]

The FNAC diagnosis of ALCL should be considered in the cytological differential diagnosis of anaplastic tumour within a lymph node or extranodal sites.[180,184,185] The differential diagnosis may include anaplastic carcinoma, malignant melanoma, sarcoma, Hodgkin's disease and histiocytic lymphoma (Fig. 4.68).[186] Immunostaining of FNAC is necessary for confirmation of the diagnosis. ALCL has a distinct cytomorphologic appearances and immunocytochemical staining pattern such that a reliable diagnosis can be made on cytological material.[178,179,187,188]

METASTATIC CARCINOMA

The neck lymph nodes are one of the most common palpable masses bearing cancer metastases. Metastatic carcinoma represents the most commonly diagnosed condition in the FNAC of lymph nodes in our practice (Fig. 4.2).

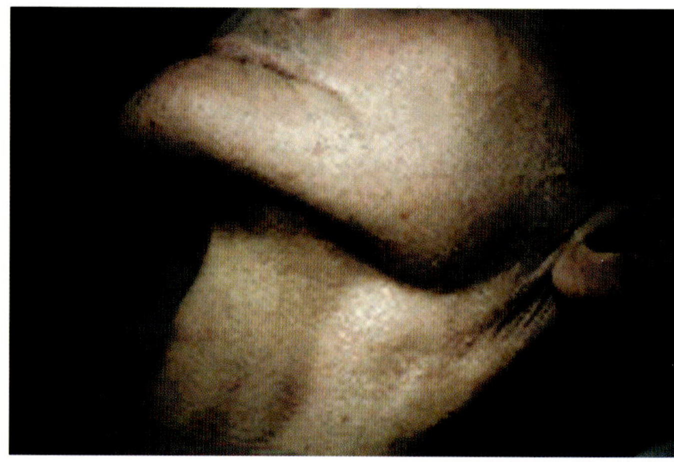

Figure 4.63 This 63-year-old patient was referred to the FNAC clinic for enlarged cervical lymph node. He had a history of squamous cell carcinoma in the oropharynx. FNAC revealed reactive changes only. There was no evidence of metastases.

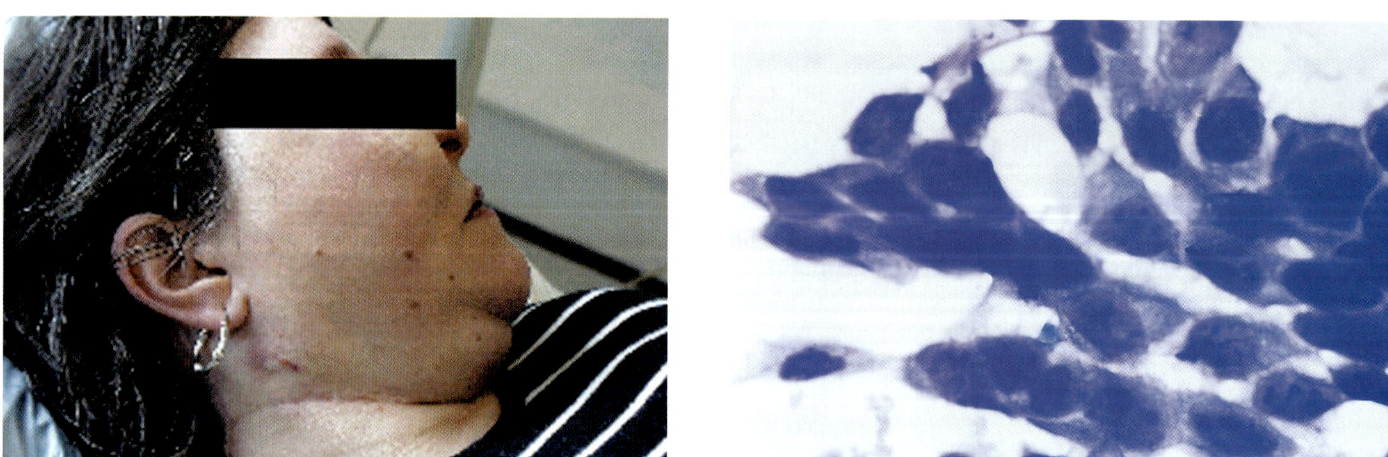

A B

Figure 4.64 Metastatic squamous cell carcinoma. **A.** This 33-year-old patient has had squamous carcinoma treated and skin grafted. She was referred for investigation of enlarged lymph node at the angle of the mandible. **B.** Regional lymph node contained mature squamous epithelium consistent with metastatic carcinoma (MGG ×1000 oil).

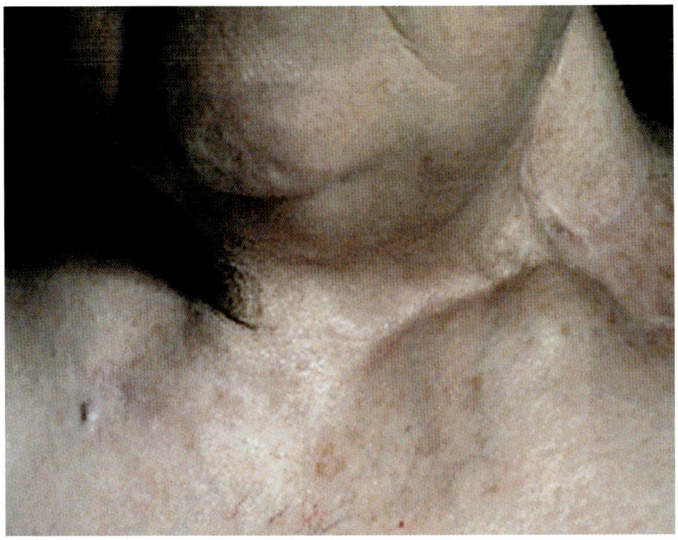

A

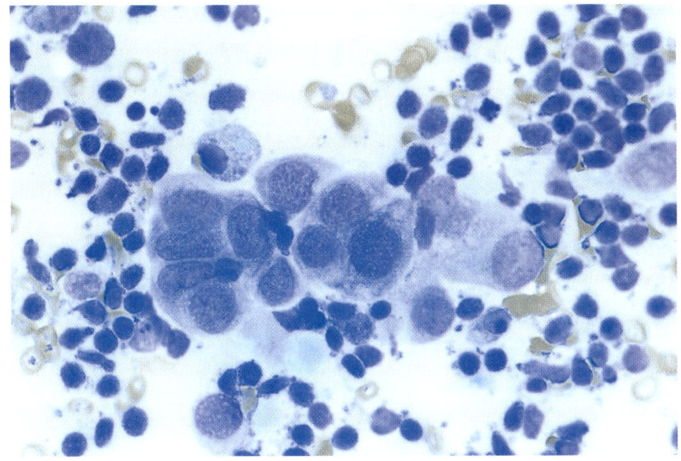

B

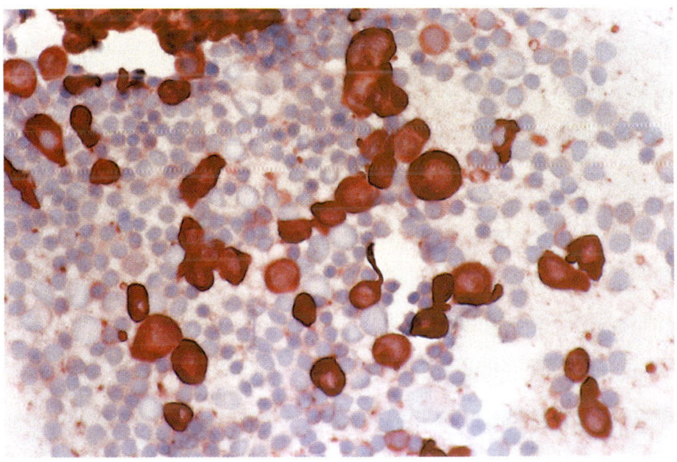

C

Figure 4.65 Metastatic carcinoma. **A.** This 75-year-old woman was referred to FNAC clinic for a swelling in the left supraclavicular fossa near the SC joint. There was no previous history. **B.** Metastatic carcinoma. Clusters and single epithelial cells with features of malignancy against a background of lymphoid cells (MGG ×600). **C.** Cytokeratin marker highlights the epithelial cells and confirms the diagnosis. Primary site was found in the breast (MNF 116, APAAP ×600 oil immersion).

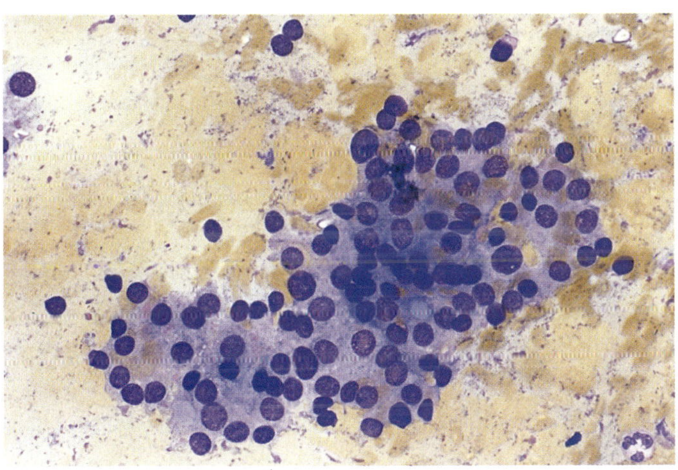

A

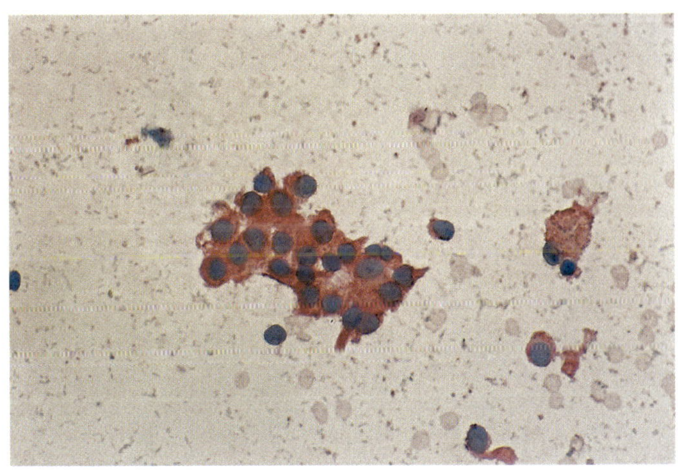

B

Figure 4.66 Metastatic papillary carcinoma of the thyroid. **A.** FNAC of cervical lymph node yielded a small amount of cystic fluid. Microscopy reveals scanty papillary clusters of monotonous-looking epithelium-forming follicles. A suspicion of an endocrine pathology was raised (MGG ×600). **B.** Antithyroglobulin positivity in the cells confirms the cells to be of thyroid origin. The patient was investigated and a primary papillary carcinoma was found in the thyroid. The tumour was resected together with regional metastases (antithyroglobulin, APAAP ×600).

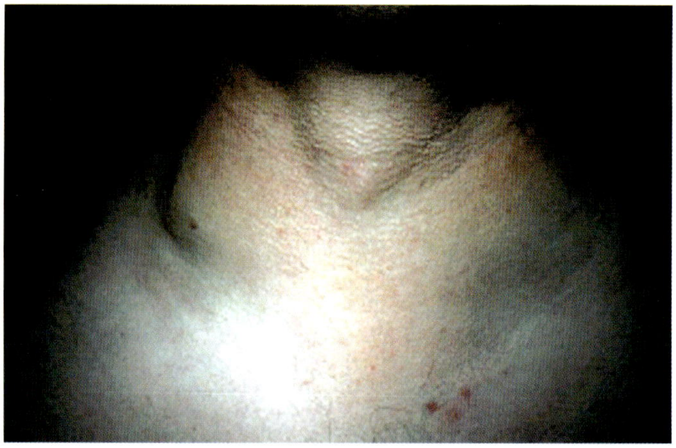
A

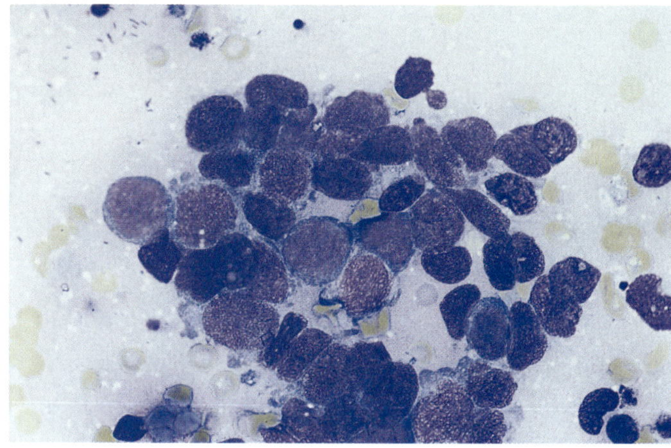
B

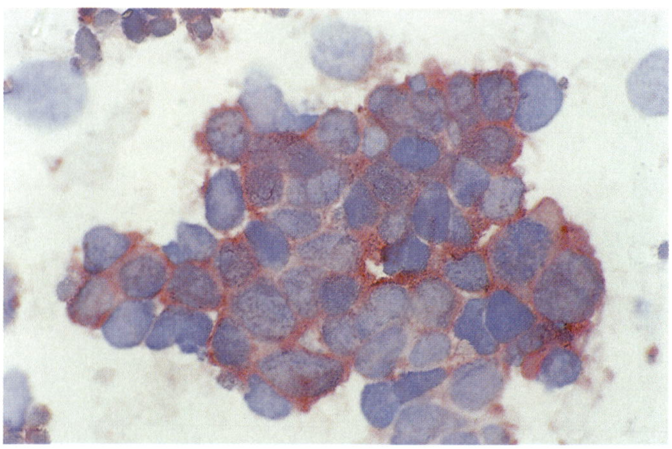
C

Figure 4.67 Metastatic small cell carcinoma of the lung. **A.** This 70-year-old man with SVC obstruction was referred for urgent FNAC of his bilateral supraclavicular swellings. **B.** FNAC smear shows a cluster of small to medium-sized cells with fine granular chromatin pattern, inconspicuous nucleoli and scant basophilic cytoplasm. Cells show nuclear moulding (MGG ×600 oil immersion). **C.** Neuroendocrine and epithelial marker positivity confirms the tumour to be metastasis of a small cell anaplastic carcinoma of the lung. Chemotherapy was commenced immediately (UJ13A ×600, oil immersion).

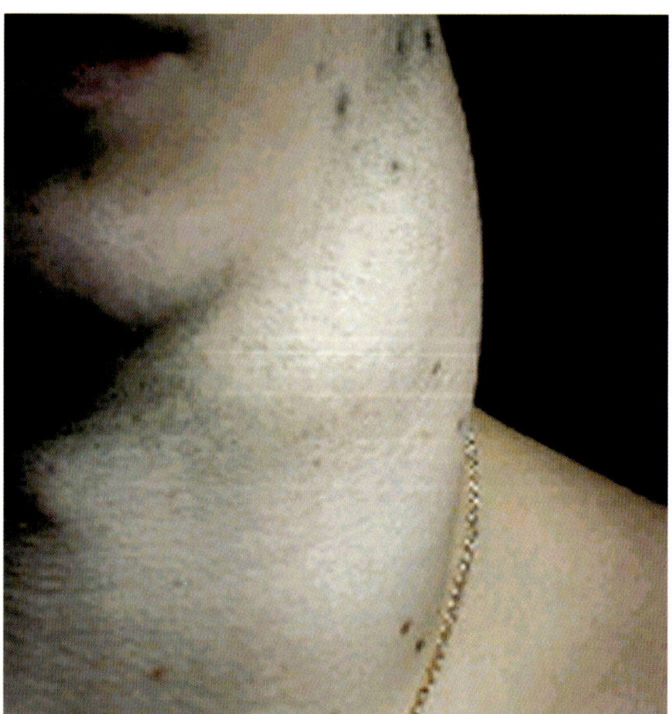
A

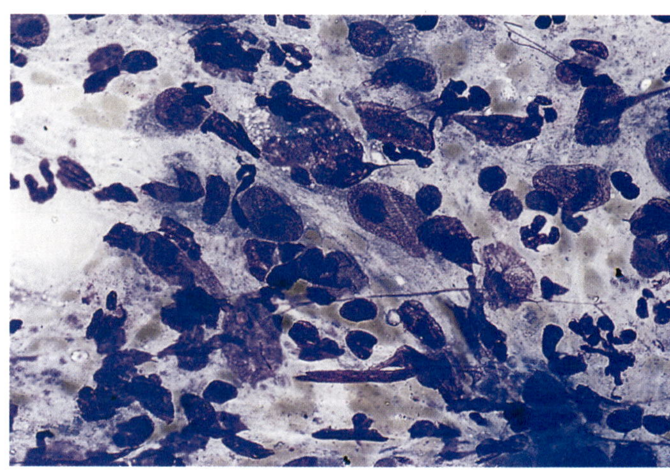
B

Figure 4.68 Metastatic nasopharyngeal carcinoma. **A.** A 19-year-old Caucasian patient was referred to the FNAC clinic for unilateral, diffuse, tender swelling of the neck preventing the patient from being able to turn the head. On examination, the mass was hard and fixed with no definite edge to it. Clinically it was hard and fixed with no definite edge to it. Clinically it was thought to be an infection. **B.** FNAC smears reveal a malignant tumour with large anaplastic nuclei and prominent nucleoli (MGG ×600, oil immersion). ***(continued)***

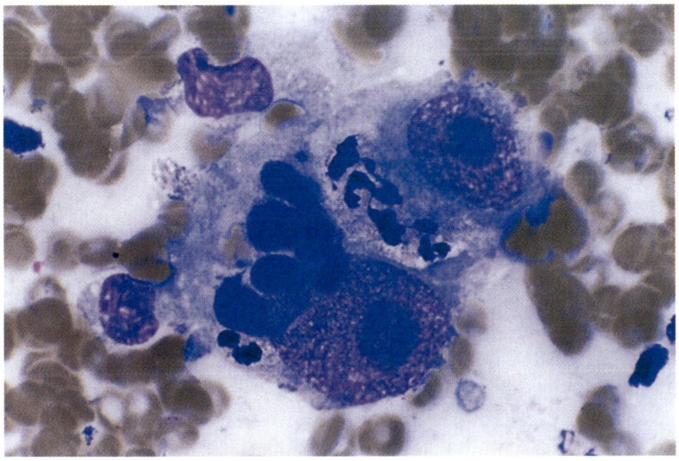

C

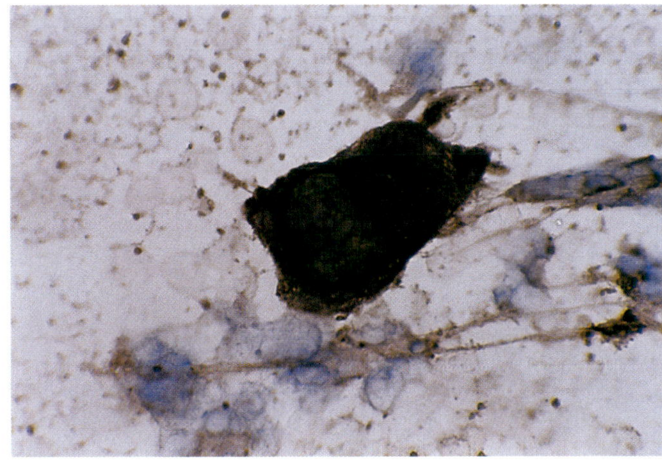

D

Figure 4.68 ***(continued)*** Metastatic nasopharyngeal carcinoma. **C.** Some bizarre Hodgkin's cells were noted. Morphologically, the tumour was thought to be a lymphoma (Hodgkin's or ALCL) (MGG ×1000, oil immersion). **D.** Immunocytochemistry shows positive staining for cytokeratin (MNF 116). CD 30 was weakly positive. LMP EBV positivity on histological sections of the biopsy contributed to the correct diagnosis (MNF 116, IP ×1000 oil).

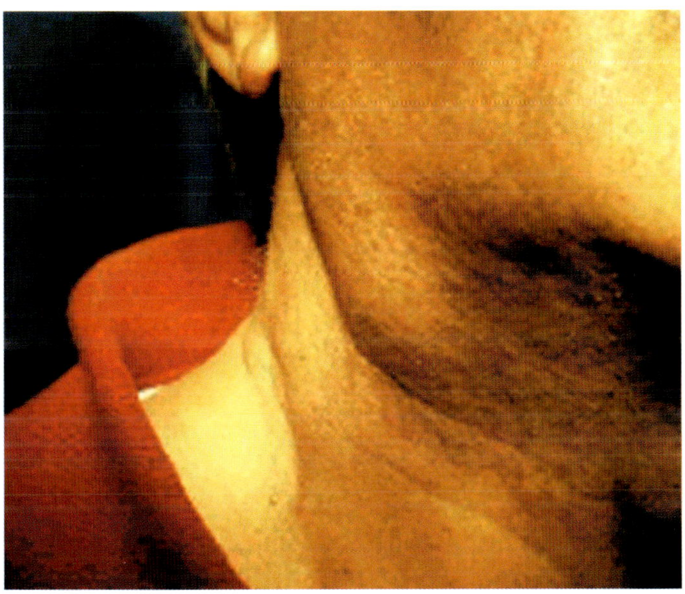

A

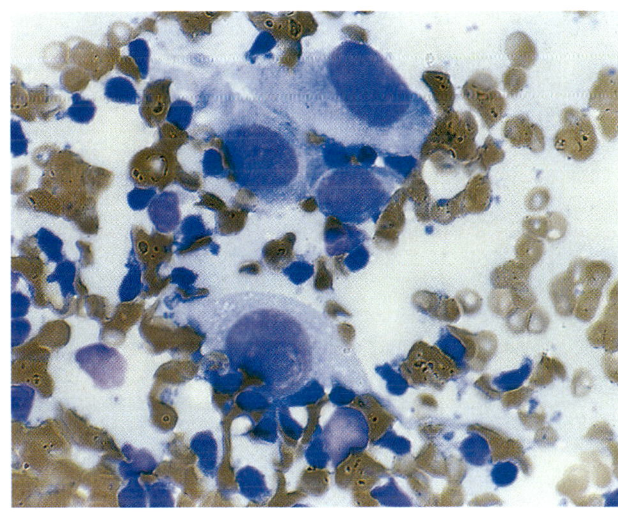

B

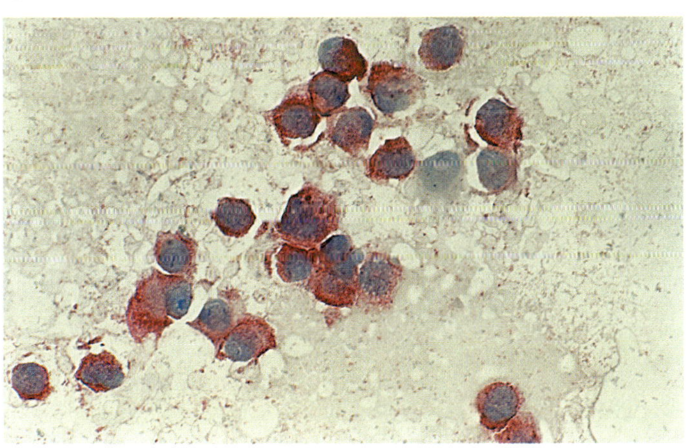

C

Figureure 4.69 Metastatic malignant melanoma. **A.** The patient presented with cervical lymphadenopathy. Clinical history revealed previous melanoma of the facial skin. **B.** Large, mainly single cells with eccentric round or oval nuclei, prominent nucleoli and grey, finely vacuolated cytoplasm. No pigment was seen (MGG ×66 oil immersion). **C.** HMB-45, melanoma marker positivity confirms the diagnosis (APAAP ×600 oil immersion).

Sometimes, neck node enlargement is the first manifestation of an occult cancer. The location of the lymph node may be helpful in determining the nature of the lesion and the origin of malignancy. FNAC is usually used to confirm malignancy, identify the histological type of tumour and possibly establish the primary site of the carcinoma (Figs 4.63–4.71).

The most common primary sites of metastatic carcinoma in the neck nodes are from the perioral area. They include

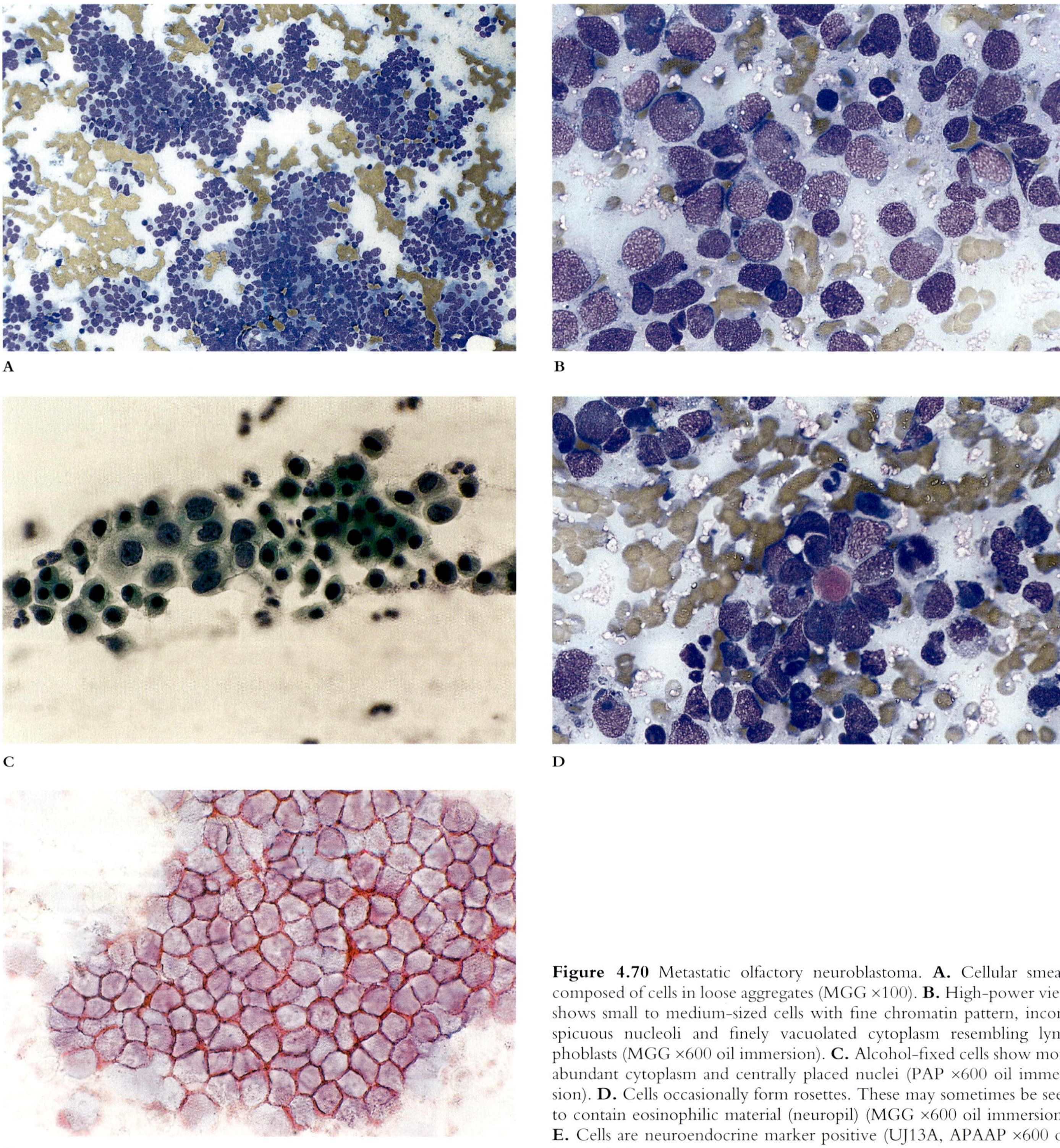

Figure 4.70 Metastatic olfactory neuroblastoma. **A.** Cellular smears composed of cells in loose aggregates (MGG ×100). **B.** High-power view shows small to medium-sized cells with fine chromatin pattern, inconspicuous nucleoli and finely vacuolated cytoplasm resembling lymphoblasts (MGG ×600 oil immersion). **C.** Alcohol-fixed cells show more abundant cytoplasm and centrally placed nuclei (PAP ×600 oil immersion). **D.** Cells occasionally form rosettes. These may sometimes be seen to contain eosinophilic material (neuropil) (MGG ×600 oil immersion). **E.** Cells are neuroendocrine marker positive (UJ13A, APAAP ×600 oil immersion).

cancers of the lip, buccal mucosa, tongue, larynx, nasopharynx and hypopharynx. These are followed by the metastases from the lung, breast, gastrointestinal tract, urinary bladder, cervix and thyroid. Some cytomorphological characteristics are useful for presumption of primary sites, such as: monolayered papillary fronds with intranuclear cytoplasmic inclusions in thyroid papillary carcinoma; large, polygonal, keratinised cells with a low nuclear:cytoplasmic ratio and anucleate squames in perioral cancers; and numerous naked nuclei, destroyed nuclei and marked lymphocytic infiltrates in nasopharyngeal carcinoma. The accuracy rate of presumption of primary sites is 100% in thyroid papillary carcinoma, 83% in perioral cancer and 77% in nasopharyngeal carcinoma but low in other malignancies.[189] The occurrence of both carcinoma and lymphoma in the same lymph node is extremely rare and may be diagnosed on FNAC.[190]

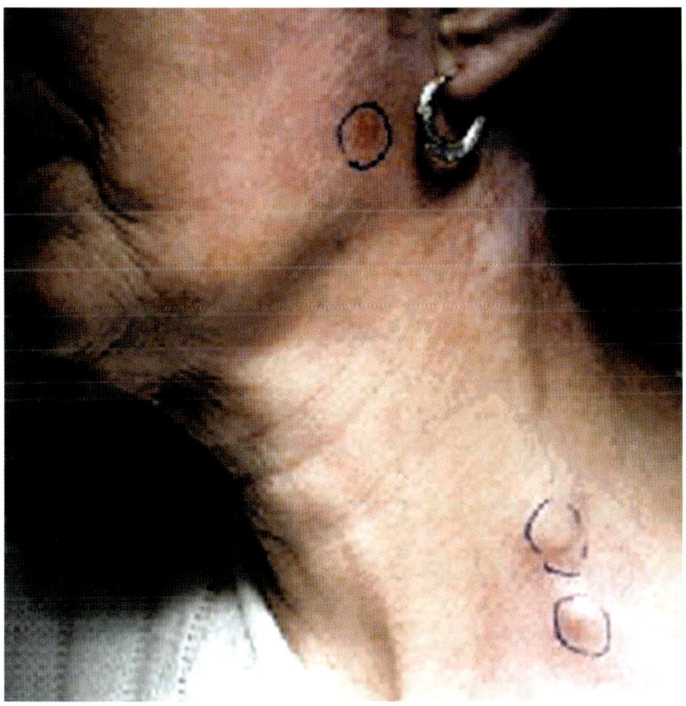

A

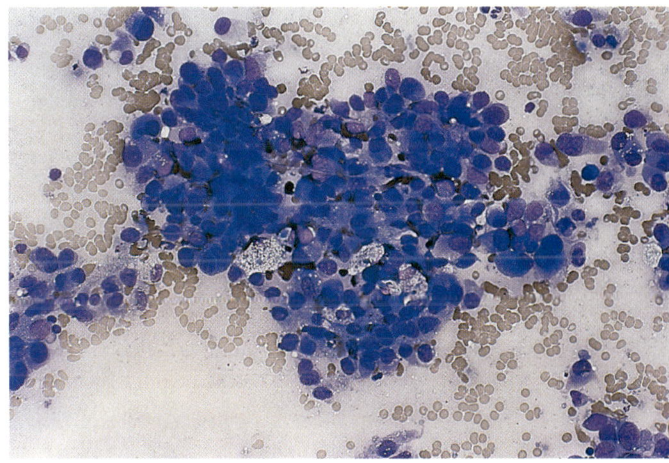

B

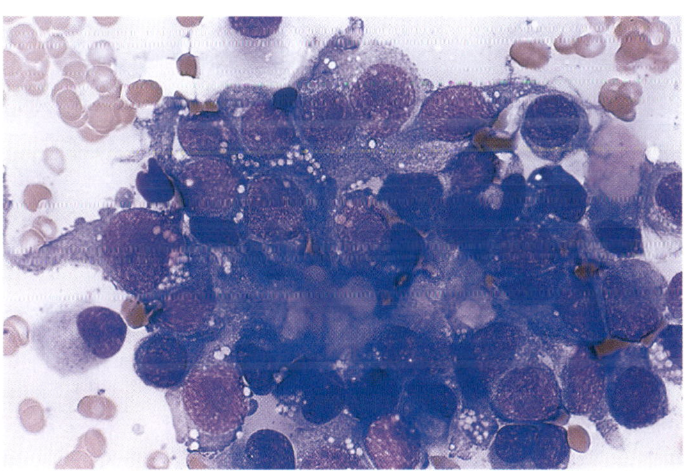

C

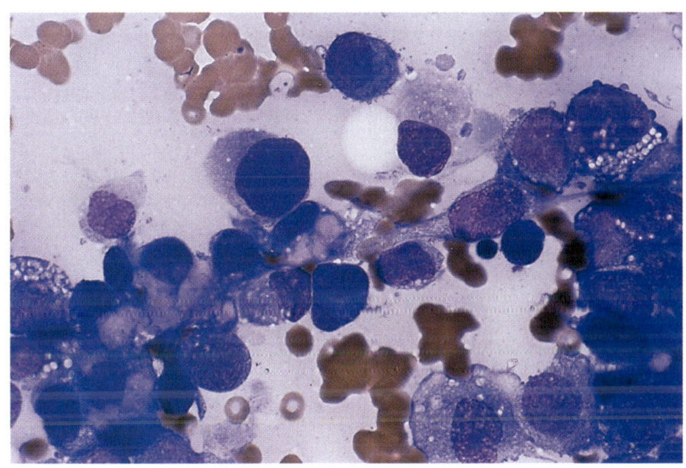

D

Figure 4.71 Metastatic angiosarcoma. **A.** This patient had radiotherapy for angiosarcoma of the scalp. She presented to the FNAC clinic with two enlarged lymph nodes in the posterior triangle. There was also a hardening of the preauricular area outside the radiation field. **B.** FNAC of lymph nodes was cellular, composed of clusters forming occasional acini (MGG ×400). **C.** Individual cells were oval, round or spindle with eccentric nuclei, visible nucleoli and moderate to abundant amount of pale blue grey, vacuolated cytoplasm. The cells were 2–9 times the size of red cells (MGG ×600 oil immersion). **D.** Intracytoplasmic lumina with red cells are characteristic (MGG ×600).

REFERENCES

1. Lopes Cardozo P. The significance of fine needle aspiration cytology for the diagnosis and treatment of malignant lymphomas. *Folia Haematol (Leipz)* 1980; 107(4): 601–20.

2. Layfield LJ. Fine-needle aspiration of the head and neck. *Pathology (Phila)* 1996; 4(2): 409–38.

3. Nasuti JF, Yu G, Boudousquie A, Gupta P. Diagnostic value of lymph node fine needle aspiration cytology: an institutional experience of 387 cases observed over a 5-year period. *Cytopathology* 2000; 11(1): 18–31.

4. Kocjan G. The role of FNAC in diagnosis of lymph node enlargements. *Cytopathology* 1997; 8(suppl): 2–3.

5. Thomas JO, Adeyi D, Amanguno H. Fine-needle aspiration in the management of peripheral lymphadenopathy in a developing country. *Diagn Cytopathol* 1999; 21(3): 159–62.

6. Pilotti S, Di Palma S, Alasio L, Bartoli C, Rilke F. Diagnostic assessment of enlarged superficial lymph nodes by fine needle aspiration. *Acta Cytol* 1993; 37(6): 853–66.

7. Steel BL, Schwartz MR, Ramzy I. Fine needle aspiration biopsy in the diagnosis of lymphadenopathy in 1,103 patients. Role, limitations and analysis of diagnostic pitfalls. *Acta Cytol* 1995; 39(1): 76–81.

8. Schoengen A, Binder T, Fembacher P, Zeelen U. The fine-needle aspiration cytology of lymph nodes suspected of malignancy. Its diagnostic value and capacity to predict the histogenesis. *Dtsch Med Wochenschr* 1995; 120(16): 549–54.

9. Sneige N, Dekmezian RH, Katz RL et al. Morphologic and immunocytochemical evaluation of 220 fine needle aspirates of malignant lymphoma and lymphoid hyperplasia. *Acta Cytol* 1990; 34(3): 311–22.

10. Das DK. Value and limitations of fine-needle aspiration cytology in diagnosis and classification of lymphomas: a review. *Diagn Cytopathol* 1999; 21(4): 240–9.

11. Lioe TF, Elliott H, Allen DC, Spence RA. The role of fine needle aspiration cytology (FNAC) in the investigation of superficial lymphadenopathy; uses and limitations of the technique. *Cytopathology* 1999; 10(5): 291–7.

12. Katz RL. Pitfalls in the diagnosis of fine-needle aspiration of lymph nodes. *Monogr Pathol* 1997; (39): 118–33.

13. Tani EM, Christensson B, Porwit A, Skoog L. Immunocytochemical analysis and cytomorphologic diagnosis on fine needle aspirates of lymphoproliferative disease. *Acta Cytol* 1988; 32(2): 209–15.

14. Katz RL, Wojcik EM, el-Naggar AK, Ordonez NG, Johnston DA. Proliferation markers in non-Hodgkin's lymphoma. A comparative study between cytophotometric quantitation of Ki-67 and flow cytometric proliferation index on fine needle aspirates. *Anal Quant Cytol Histol* 1993; 15(3): 179–86.

15. Brown DC, Gatter KC, Mason DY. Proliferation in non-Hodgkin's lymphoma: a comparison of Ki-67 staining on fine needle aspiration and cryostat sections. *J Clin Pathol* 1990; 43(4): 325–8.

16. Reid MM. Fine needle aspiration and the diagnosis of non-Hodgkin's lymphoma [letter, comment]. *J Clin Pathol* 1998; 51(9): 712.

17. Simsir A, Fetsch P, Stetler-Stevenson M, Abati A. Immunophenotypic analysis of non-Hodgkin's lymphomas in cytologic specimens: a correlative study of immunocytochemical and flow cytometric techniques. *Diagn Cytopathol* 1999; 20(5): 278–84.

18. Cha I, Goates JJ. Fine-needle aspiration of lymph nodes: use of flow cytometry immunophenotyping. *Pathology (Phila)* 1996; 4(2): 337–64.

19. Ravinsky E, Morales C, Kutryk E, Chrobak A, Paraskevas F. Cytodiagnosis of lymphoid proliferations by fine needle aspiration biopsy. Adjunctive value of flow cytometry. *Acta Cytol* 1999; 43(6): 1070–8.

20. Henrique RM, Sousa ME, Godinho MI, Costa I, Barbosa IL, Lopes CA. Immunophenotyping by flow cytometry of fine needle aspirates in the diagnosis of lymphoproliferative disorders: A retrospective study. *J Clin Lab Anal* 1999; 13(5): 224–8.

21. Jeffers MD, Milton J, Herriot R, McKean M. Fine needle aspiration cytology in the investigation on non-Hodgkin's lymphoma. *J Clin Pathol* 1998; 51(3): 189–96.

22. Chernoff WG, Lampe HB, Cramer H, Banerjee D. The potential clinical impact of the fine needle aspiration/flow cytometric diagnosis of malignant lymphoma. *J Otolaryngol* 1992; 21(suppl 1): 1–15.

23. Dunphy CH, Ramos R. Combining fine-needle aspiration and flow cytometric immunophenotyping in evaluation of nodal and extranodal sites for possible lymphoma: a retrospective review. *Diagn Cytopathol* 1997; 16(3): 200–6.

24. Robins DB, Katz RL, Swan F Jr, Atkinson EN, Ordonez NG, Huh YO. Immunotyping of lymphoma by fine-needle aspiration. A comparative study of cytospin preparations and flow cytometry. *Am J Clin Pathol* 1994; 101(5): 569–76.

25. Lima CE, Mizushima Y, Masuda S, Kitagawa M. Comparison of DNA flow cytometric analysis of body cavity fluids with conventional cytology. *In Vivo* 1994; 8(3): 359–62.

26. Saikia UN, Dey P, Vohra H, Gupta SK. DNA flow cytometry of non-Hodgkin's lymphomas: correlation with cytologic grade and clinical relapse. *Diagn Cytopathol* 2000; 22(3): 152–6.

27. Liu K, Mann KP, Vitellas KM et al. Fine-needle aspiration with flow cytometric immunophenotyping for primary diagnosis of intra-abdominal lymphomas. *Diagn Cytopathol* 1999; 21(2): 98–104.

28. Jeffers MD, McCorriston J, Farquharson MA, Stewart CJ, Mutch AF. Analysis of clonality in cytologic material using the polymerase chain reaction (PCR). *Cytopathology* 1997; 8(2): 114–21.

29. Alkan S, Lehman C, Sarago C, Sidawy MK, Karcher DS, Garrett CT. Polymerase chain reaction detection of immunoglobulin gene rearrangement and bcl-2 translocation in archival glass slides of cytologic material. *Diagn Mol Pathol* 1995; 4(1): 25–31.

30. Shivnarain D, Ladanyi M, Zakowski MF. Detection of BCL2 rearrangement in archival cytological smears of B-cell lymphomas. *Mod Pathol* 1994; 7(9): 915–9.

31. Kube MJ, McDonald DA, Quin JW, Greenberg ML. Use of archival and fresh cytologic material for the polymerase chain reaction. Detection of the bcl-2 oncogene in lymphoid tissue obtained by fine needle biopsy. *Anal Quant Cytol Histol* 1994; 16(3): 174–82.

32. Aiello A, Delia D, Giardini R et al. PCR analysis of IgH and BCL2 gene rearrangement in the diagnosis of follicular lymphoma in lymph node fine-needle aspiration. A critical appraisal. *Diagn Mol Pathol* 1997; 6(3): 154–60.

33. Grosso LE, Collins BT. DNA polymerase chain reaction using fine needle aspiration biopsy smears to evaluate non-Hodgkin's lymphoma. *Acta Cytol* 1999; 43(5): 837–41.

34. Katz RL, Hirsch-Ginsberg C, Childs C et al. The role of gene rearrangements for antigen receptors in the diagnosis of lymphoma obtained by fine-needle aspiration. A study of 63 cases with concomitant immunophenotyping. *Am J Clin Pathol* 1991; 96(4): 479–90.

35. Alkan S, Eltoum IA, Tabbara S, Day E, Karcher DS. Usefulness of molecular detection of human herpesvirus-8 in the diagnosis of Kaposi sarcoma by fine-needle aspiration. *Am J Clin Pathol* 1999; 111(1): 91–6.

36. Williams ME, Frierson HF Jr, Tabbarah S, Ennis PS. Fine-needle aspiration of non-Hodgkin's lymphoma. Southern blot analysis for antigen receptor, bcl-2, and c-myc gene rearrangements. *Am J Clin Pathol* 1990; 93(6): 754–9.

37. Stewart CJ, Farquharson MA, Kerr T, McCorriston J. Immunoglobulin light chain mRNA detected by in situ hybridisation in diagnostic fine needle aspiration cytology specimens. *J Clin Pathol* 1996; 49(9): 749–54.

38. Stewart CJ, Duncan JA, Farquharson M, Richmond J. Fine needle aspiration cytology diagnosis of malignant lymphoma and reactive lymphoid hyperplasia. *J Clin Pathol* 1998; 51(3): 197–203.

39. Vianello F, Tison T, Radossi P et al. Detection of B-cell monoclonality in fine needle aspiration by PCR analysis. *Leuk Lymphoma* 1998; 29(1–2): 179–85.

40. Leong AS, Stevens M. Fine-needle aspiration biopsy for the diagnosis of lymphoma: a perspective. *Diagn Cytopathol* 1996; 15(4): 352–7.

41. Pontifex AH, Haley L. Fine-needle aspiration cytology in lymphomas and related disorders. *Diagn Cytopathol* 1989; 5(1): 132–5.

42. Layfield LJ. Fine needle aspiration cytologic findings in a case of sinus histiocytosis with massive lymphadenopathy (Rosai-Dorfman syndrome). *Acta Cytol* 1990; 34(6): 767–70.

43. Gupta S, Gupta DC. Cytologic appearance of sinus histiocytosis with massive lymphadenopathy: a case report. *Acta Cytol* 1996; 40(3): 595–8.

44. Trautman BC, Stanley MW, Goding GS, Rosai J. Sinus histiocytosis with massive lymphadenopathy (Rosai-Dorfman disease): diagnosis by fine-needle aspiration. *Diagn Cytopathol* 1991; 7(5): 513–6.

45. Schmitt FC. Sinus histiocytosis with massive lymphadenopathy (Rosai-Dorfman disease): cytomorphologic analysis on fine-needle aspirates. *Diagn Cytopathol* 1992; 8(6): 596–9.

46. Alvarez Alegret R, Martinez Tello A, Ramirez T, Gallego P, Martinez D, Garcia Julian G. Sinus histiocytosis with massive lymphadenopathy (Rosai-Dorfman disease): diagnosis with fine-needle aspiration in a case with nodal and nasal involvement [see comments]. *Diagn Cytopathol* 1995; 13(4): 333–5.

47. Chang YW. Sinus histiocytosis with massive lymphadenopathy. Report of a case with fine needle aspiration cytology. *Acta Cytol* 1993; 37(2): 186–90.

48. Stastny JF, Wilkerson ML, Hamati HF, Kornstein MJ. Cytologic features of sinus histiocytosis with massive lymphadenopathy. A report of three cases. *Acta Cytol* 1997; 41(3): 871–6.

49. Viguer JM, Jimenez-Heffernan JA, Lopez-Ferrer P, Vicandi B. Importance of Papanicolaou-stained smears and immunocytochemistry in the diagnosis of Rosai-Dorfman disease [letter]. *Acta Cytol* 1999; 43(2): 328–30.

50. Pettinato G, Manivel JC, d'Amore ES, Petrella G. Fine needle aspiration cytology and immunocytochemical characterization of the histiocytes in sinus histiocytosis with massive lymphadenopathy (Rosai-Dorfman syndrome). *Acta Cytol* 1990; 34(6): 771–7.

51. Deshpande V, Verma K. Fine needle aspiration (FNA) cytology of Rosai Dorfman disease. *Cytopathology* 1998; 9(5): 329–35.

52. Suh KW, Park CS, Lee JT, Lee KG. Diagnosis of cervical tuberculous lymphadenitis with fine needle aspiration biopsy and cytologic examination under ultrasonographic guides. *Yonsei Med J* 1993; 34(4): 328–33.

53. Lapuerta P, Martin SE, Ellison E. Fine-needle aspiration of peripheral lymph nodes in patients with tuberculosis and HIV. *Am J Clin Pathol* 1997; 107(3): 317–20.

54. Donnelly A, Hendricks G, Martens S, Strovers C, Wiemerslage S, Thomas PA. Cytologic diagnosis of cat scratch disease (CSD) by fine-needle aspiration. *Diagn Cytopathol* 1995; 13(2): 103–6.

55. Kojima M, Nakamura S, Koshikawa T et al. Imprint cytology of cat scratch disease. A report of eight cases. *Apmis* 1996; 104(5): 389–94.

56. Silverman JF. Fine needle aspiration cytology of cat scratch disease. *Acta Cytol* 1985; 29(4): 542–7.

57. Christ ML, Feltes-Kennedy M. Fine needle aspiration cytology of toxoplasmic lymphadenitis. *Acta Cytol* 1982; 26(4): 425–8.

58. Macey-Dare LV, Kocjan G, Goodman JR. Acquired toxoplasmosis of a submandibular lymph node in a 9-year-old boy diagnosed by fine-needle aspiration cytology. *Int J Paediatr Dent* 1996; 6(4): 265–9.

59. Zaharopoulos P. Demonstration of parasites in toxoplasma lymphadenitis by fine-needle aspiration cytology: report of two cases. *Diagn Cytopathol* 2000; 22(1): 11–5.

60. al-Jitawi SA, Farraj SE, Ramahi SA. Conventional scraping versus fine needle aspiration cytology in the diagnosis of cutaneous leishmaniasis. *Acta Cytol* 1995; 39(1): 82–4.

61. Perez-Guillermo M, Hernandez-Gil A, Bonmati C. Diagnosis of cutaneous leishmaniasis by fine needle aspiration cytology. Report of a case. *Acta Cytol* 1988; 32(4): 485–8.

62. Tallada N, Raventos A, Martinez S, Compano C, Almirante B. Leishmania lymphadenitis diagnosed by fine-needle aspiration biopsy. *Diagn Cytopathol* 1993; 9(6): 673–6.

63. Tsang WY, Chan JK. Fine-needle aspiration cytologic diagnosis of

Kikuchi's lymphadenitis. A report of 27 cases. *Am J Clin Pathol* 1994; 102(4): 454–8.

64. Mannara GM, Boccato P, Rinaldo A, La Rosa F, Ferlito A. Histiocytic necrotizing lymphadenitis (Kikuchi-Fujimoto disease) diagnosed by fine needle aspiration biopsy. *ORL J Otorhinolaryngol Relat Spec* 1999; 61(6): 367–371.

65. Stanley MW, Steeper TA, Horwitz CA, Burton LG, Strickler JG, Borken S. Fine-needle aspiration of lymph nodes in patients with acute infectious mononucleosis. *Diagn Cytopathol* 1990; 6(5): 323–9.

66. Hanks D, Bhargava V. Fine-needle aspiration diagnosis of HIV-related conditions. *Pathology (Phila)* 1996; 4(2): 221–52.

67. Reid AJ, Miller RF, Kocjan GI. Diagnostic utility of fine needle aspiration (FNA) cytology in HIV-infected patients with lymphadenopathy [see comments]. *Cytopathology* 1998; 9(4): 230–9.

68. Strigle SM, Rarick MU, Cosgrove MM, Martin SE. A review of the fine-needle aspiration cytology findings in human immunodeficiency virus infection. *Diagn Cytopathol* 1992; 8(1): 41–52.

69. Ellison E, Lapuerta P, Martin SE. Fine needle aspiration (FNA) in HIV+ patients: results from a series of 655 aspirates. *Cytopathology* 1998; 9(4): 222–9.

70. Shapiro AL, Pincus RL. Fine-needle aspiration of diffuse cervical lymphadenopathy in patients with acquired immunodeficiency syndrome. *Otolaryngol Head Neck Surg* 1991; 105(3): 419–21.

71. Burton F, Patete ML, Goodwin WJ, Jr. Indications for open cervical node biopsy in HIV-positive patients. *Otolaryngol Head Neck Surg* 1992; 107(3): 367–9.

72. Nathan DL, Belsito DV. Carbamazepine-induced pseudolymphoma with CD-30 positive cells. *J Am Acad Dermatol* 1998; 38(5 pt 2): 806–9.

73. Abbondazo SL, Irey NS, Frizzera G. Dilantin-associated lymphadenopathy. Spectrum of histopathologic patterns. *Am J Surg Pathol* 1995; 19(6): 675–86.

74. Meyer L, Gibbons D, Ashfaq R, Vuitch F, Saboorian MH. Fine-needle aspiration findings in Castleman's disease. *Diagn Cytopathol* 1999; 21(1): 57–60.

75. Kirchgraber PR, Weaver MG, Arafah BM, Abdul-Karim FW. Fine needle aspiration cytology of Langerhans cell histiocytosis involving the thyroid. A case report. *Acta Cytol* 1994; 38(1): 101–6.

76. Dey P, Luthra UK, Sheikh ZA. Fine needle aspiration cytology of Langerhans cell histiocytosis of the thyroid. A case report. *Acta Cytol* 1999; 43(3): 429–31.

77. Sahoo M, Karak AK, Bhatnagar D, Bal CS. Fine-needle aspiration cytology in a case of isolated involvement of thyroid with Langerhans cell histiocytosis. *Diagn Cytopathol* 1998; 19(1): 33–7.

78. Nagaoka S, Maruyama R, Koike M et al. Cytology of Langerhans cell histiocytosis in effusions: a case report. *Acta Cytol* 1996; 40(3): 563–6.

79. Elsheikh T, Silverman JF, Wakely PE Jr, Holbrook CT, Joshi VV. Fine-needle aspiration cytology of Langerhans' cell histiocytosis (eosinophilic granuloma) of bone in children. *Diagn Cytopathol* 1991; 7(3): 261–6.

80. Shabb N, Fanning CV, Carrasco CH et al. Diagnosis of eosinophilic granuloma of bone by fine-needle aspiration with concurrent institution of therapy: a cytologic, histologic, clinical, and radiologic study of 27 cases. *Diagn Cytopathol* 1993; 9(1): 3–12.

81. Katz RL, Silva EG, deSantos LA, Lukeman JM. Diagnosis of eosinophilic granuloma of bone by cytology, histology, and electron microscopy of transcutaneous bone-aspiration biopsy. *J Bone Joint Surg [Am]* 1980; 62(8): 1284–90.

82. Musy JP, Ruf L, Ernerup I, Baltisser-Bielecka I. Cytopathologic diagnosis of an eosinophilic granuloma of bone by needle aspiration biopsy [letter]. *Acta Cytol* 1989; 33(5): 683–5.

83. Yasko AW, Fanning CV, Ayala AG, Carrasco CH, Murray JA. Percutaneous techniques for the diagnosis and treatment of localized Langerhans-cell histiocytosis (eosinophilic granuloma of bone). *J Bone Joint Surg [Am]* 1998; 80(2): 219–28.

84. Lee JS, Lee MC, Park CS, Juhng SW. Fine needle aspiration cytology of Langerhans cell histiocytosis confined to lymph nodes. A case report. *Acta Cytol* 1997; 41(6): 1793–6.

85. Das DK, Nayak NC. Diagnosis of Langerhans cell histiocytosis by fine needle aspiration cytology [letter]. *Acta Cytol* 1995; 39(6): 1260–3.

86. Van Heerde P, Maarten Egeler R. The cytology of Langerhans cell histiocytosis (histiocytosis X). *Cytopathology* 1991; 2(3): 149–58.

87. Layfield LJ, Bhuta S. Fine-needle aspiration cytology of histiocytosis X: a case report. *Diagn Cytopathol* 1988; 4(2): 140–3.

88. Akhtar M, Ali MA, Bakry M, Sackey K, Sabbah R. Fine-needle aspiration biopsy of Langerhans histiocytosis (histiocytosis-X). *Diagn Cytopathol* 1993; 9(5): 527–33.

89. Pohar-Marinsek Z, Us-Krasovec M. Cytomorphology of Langerhans cell histiocytosis. *Acta Cytol* 1996; 40(6): 1257–64.

90. Dusenbery D, Nalesnik MA, Locker J, Swerdlow SH. Cytologic features of post-transplant lymphoproliferative disorder. *Diagn Cytopathol* 1997; 16(6): 489–96.

91. Gattuso P, Castelli MJ, Peng Y, Reddy VB. Posttransplant lymphoproliferative disorders: a fine-needle aspiration biopsy study. *Diagn Cytopathol* 1997; 16(5): 392–5.

92. Davey DD, Gulley ML, Walker WP, Zaleski S. Cytologic findings in posttransplant lymphoproliferative disease. *Acta Cytol* 1990; 34(3): 304–10.

93. Reyes CV, Jensen JA, Chinoy M. Pulmonary lymphoma in cardiac transplant patients treated with OKT3 for rejection: diagnosis by fine-needle aspiration. *Diagn Cytopathol* 1995; 12(1): 32–6.

94. Collins BT, Ramos RR, Grosso LE. Combined fine needle aspiration biopsy, and immunophenotypic and genotypic approach to posttransplantation lymphoproliferative disorders. *Acta Cytol* 1998; 42(4): 869–74.

95. Haddad MG, Silverman JF, Joshi VV, Geisinger KR. Effusion cytology in Burkitt's lymphoma. *Diagn Cytopathol* 1995; 12(1): 3–7.

96. Gumbs MA, Pai NB, Saraiya RJ, Rubinstein J, Vythilingam L, Choi YJ. Kimura's disease: a case report and literature review. *J Surg Oncol* 1999; 70(3): 190–3.

97. Kini U, Shariff S. Cytodiagnosis of Kimura's disease. *Indian J Pathol Microbiol* 1998; 41(4): 473–7.

98. Jayaram G, Peh KB. Fine-needle aspiration cytology in Kimura's disease. *Diagn Cytopathol* 1995; 13(4): 295–9.

99. Chow LT, Yuen RW, Tsui WM, Ma TK, Chow WH, Chan SK. Cytologic features of Kimura's disease in fine-needle aspirates. A study of eight cases. *Am J Clin Pathol* 1994; 102(3): 316–21.

100. Harris NL, Jaffe ES, Diebold J et al. The World Health Organization classification of neoplastic diseases of the haematopoietic and lymphoid tissues: report of the clinical advisory committee meeting, Airlie House, Virginia, November 1997. *Histopathology* 2000; 36(1): 69–86.

101. Grosso LE, Collins BT, Dunphy CH, Ramos RR. Lymphocyte-depleted Hodgkin's disease: diagnostic challenges by fine-needle aspiration. *Diagn Cytopathol* 1998; 19(1): 66–9.

102. Das DK, Gupta SK. Fine needle aspiration cytodiagnosis of Hodgkin's disease and its subtypes. II. Subtyping by differential cell counts. *Acta Cytol* 1990; 34(3): 337–41.

103. Stanley MW, Powers CN. Syncytial variant of nodular sclerosing Hodgkin's disease: fine-needle aspiration findings in two cases. *Diagn Cytopathol* 1997; 17(6): 477–9.

104. Kardos TF, Vinson JH, Behm FG, Frable WJ, O'Dowd GJ. Hodgkin's disease: diagnosis by fine-needle aspiration biopsy. Analysis of cytologic criteria from a selected series. *Am J Clin Pathol* 1986; 86(3): 286–91.

105. Das DK, Gupta SK, Datta BN, Sharma SC. Fine needle aspiration cytodiagnosis of Hodgkin's disease and its subtypes. I. Scope and limitations. *Acta Cytol* 1990; 34(3): 329–36.

106. Daskalopoulou D, Tamiolakis D, Tsousis S, Apostolikas N, Markidou S. Sources of discrepancies in the diagnosis of Hodgkin's disease by fine needle aspiration. *Arch Anat Cytol Pathol* 1996; 44(4): 166–73.

107. Fulciniti F, Vetrani A, Zeppa P et al. Hodgkin's disease: diagnostic accuracy of fine needle aspiration; a report based on 62 consecutive cases. *Cytopathology* 1994; 5(4): 226–33.

108. Krasne DL, Naritoku WY, Cosgrove MM. Diagnosis of syncytial (lacunar cell-predominant) nodular sclerosing Hodgkin's disease by fine needle aspiration. A case report. *Acta Cytol* 1993; 37(3): 418–22.

109. Spina M, Sandri S, Tirelli U. Hodgkin's disease in HIV-infected individuals. *Curr Opin Oncol* 1999; 11(6): 522–6.

110. Stephen MR, Mallon EA. An unusual presentation of fine needle aspiration (FNA) cytology from the syncytial variant of nodular sclerosing Hodgkin's disease. *Cytopathology* 1998; 9(4): 271–6.

111. Boudjerra N, Hamladji R, Abdennebi A, Colonna P. [Value and limits of fine needle aspiration biopsy in Hodgkin disease. Usefulness in developing countries]. *Bull Cancer* 1993; 80(4): 339–44.

112. Young NA, Al-Saleem T. Diagnosis of lymphoma by fine-needle aspiration cytology using the revised European-American classification of lymphoid neoplasms [see comments]. *Cancer* 1999; 87(6): 325–45.

113. Simpson JL, Moriarty AT, Earls J, Snyder W, McCloskey DW. Hodgkin's disease variant of Richter's syndrome. Report of a case with diagnosis by fine needle biopsy. *Acta Cytol* 1997; 41(3): 823–9.

114. Tani E, Ersoz C, Svedmyr E, Skoog L. Fine-needle aspiration cytology and immunocytochemistry of Hodgkin's disease, suppurative type. *Diagn Cytopathol* 1998; 18(6): 437–40.

115. Fulciniti F, Zeppa P, Vetrani A, Troncone G, Palombini L. Hodgkin's disease mimicking suppurative lymphadenitis: a possible pitfall in fine-needle aspiration biopsy cytology. *Diagn Cytopathol* 1989; 5(3): 282–5.

116. Vicandi B, Jimenez-Heffernan JA, Lopez-Ferrer P, Gamallo C, Viguer JM. Hodgkin's disease mimicking suppurative lymphadenitis: a fine-needle aspiration report of five cases. *Diagn Cytopathol* 1999; 20(5): 302–6.

117. Wakely PE Jr. Fine-needle aspiration cytopathology in diagnosis and classification of malignant lymphoma: accurate and reliable? *Diagn Cytopathol* 2000; 22(2): 120–5.

118. Jaffe ES, Harris NL, Diebold J, Muller-Hermelink HK. World Health Organization classification of neoplastic diseases of the hematopoietic and lymphoid tissues. A progress report. *Am J Clin Pathol* 1999; 111(1 suppl 1): S8–12.

119. Suhrland MJ, Wieczorek R. Fine needle aspiration biopsy in the diagnosis of lymphoma. *Cancer Invest* 1991; 9(1): 61–8.

120. Carrasco CH, Richli WR, Lawrence D, Katz RL, Wallace S. Fine needle aspiration biopsy in lymphoma. *Radiol Clin North Am* 1990; 28(4). 879–83.

121. Akhtar M, Ali MA, Haider A, Antonius J, Hainau B, al Dayel F. Fine-needle aspiration biopsy of Ki-1-positive anaplastic large-cell lymphoma. *Diagn Cytopathol* 1992; 8(3): 242–7.

122. Cartagena N, Jr., Katz RL, Hirsch-Ginsberg C, Childs CC, Ordonez NG, Cabanillas F. Accuracy of diagnosis of malignant lymphoma by combining fine-needle aspiration cytomorphology with immunocytochemistry and in selected cases, Southern blotting of aspirated cells: a tissue-controlled study of 86 patients. *Diagn Cytopathol* 1992; 8(5): 456–64.

123. Cafferty LL, Katz RL, Ordonez NG, Carrasco CH, Cabanillas FR. Fine needle aspiration diagnosis of intraabdominal and retroperitoneal lymphomas by a morphologic and immunocytochemical approach. *Cancer* 1990; 65(1): 72–7.

124. Carter TR, Feldman PS, Innes DJ Jr, Frierson HF Jr, Frigy AF. The role of fine needle aspiration cytology in the diagnosis of lymphoma [published erratum appears in Acta Cytol 1989; 33(6): 951]. *Acta Cytol* 1988; 32(6): 848–53.

125. Das DK, Gupta SK, Pathak IC, Sharma SC, Datta BN. Burkitt-type lymphoma. Diagnosis by fine needle aspiration cytology. *Acta Cytol* 1987; 31(1): 1–7.

126. Daskalopoulou D, Harhalakis N, Maouni N, Markidou SG. Fine needle aspiration cytology of non-Hodgkin's lymphomas. A morphologic and immunophenotypic study. *Acta Cytol* 1995; 39(2): 180–6.

127. Gagneten D, Hijazi YM, Jaffe ES, Solomon D. Mantle cell lymphoma: a cytopathological and immunocytochemical study. *Diagn Cytopathol* 1996; 14(1): 32–7.

128. Jacobs JC, Katz RL, Shabb N, el-Naggar A, Ordonez NG, Pugh W. Fine needle aspiration of lymphoblastic lymphoma. A multiparameter diagnostic approach. *Acta Cytol* 1992; 36(6): 887–94.

129. Kardos TF, Sprague RI, Wakely PE Jr, Frable WJ. Fine-needle aspiration biopsy of lymphoblastic lymphoma and leukemia. A clinical, cytologic, and immunologic study. *Cancer* 1987; 60(10): 2448–53.

130. Katz RL, Gritsman A, Cabanillas F et al. Fine-needle aspiration cytology of peripheral T-cell lymphoma. A cytologic, immunologic, and cytometric study. *Am J Clin Pathol* 1989; 91(2): 120–31.

131. Matsushima AY, Hamele-Bena D, Osborne BM. Fine-needle aspiration biopsy findings in marginal zone B cell lymphoma. *Diagn Cytopathol* 1999; 20(4): 190–8.

132. Sneige N, Dekmezian R, el-Naggar A, Manning J. Cytomorphologic, immunocytochemical, and nucleic acid flow cytometric study of 50 lymph nodes by fine-needle aspiration. Comparison with results obtained by subsequent excisional biopsy. *Cancer* 1991; 67(4): 1003–7.

133. Stastny JF, Almeida MM, Wakely PE Jr, Kornstein MJ, Frable WJ. Fine-needle aspiration biopsy and imprint cytology of small non-cleaved cell (Burkitt's) lymphoma. *Diagn Cytopathol* 1995; 12(3): 201–7.

134. Tani E, Liliemark J, Svedmyr E, Mellstedt H, Biberfeld P, Skoog L. Cytomorphology and immunocytochemistry of fine needle aspirates from blastic non-Hodgkin's lymphomas. *Acta Cytol* 1989; 33(3): 363–71.

135. Tarantino DR, McHenry CR, Strickland T, Khiyami A. The role of fine-needle aspiration biopsy and flow cytometry in the evaluation of persistent neck adenopathy. *Am J Surg* 1998; 176(5): 413–7.

136. Wakely PE Jr, Kornstein MJ. Aspiration cytopathology of lymphoblastic lymphoma and leukemia: the MCV experience. *Pediatr Pathol Lab Med* 1996; 16(2): 243–52.

137. Wojcik EM, Katz RL, Fanning TV, el-Naggar A, Ordonez NG, Johnston D. Diagnosis of mantle cell lymphoma on tissue acquired by fine needle aspiration in conjunction with immunocytochemistry and cytokinetic studies. Possibilities and limitations. *Acta Cytol* 1995; 39(5): 909–15.

138. Young NA, Al-Saleem TI, Ehya H, Smith MR. Utilization of fine-needle aspiration cytology and flow cytometry in the diagnosis and subclassification of primary and recurrent lymphoma. *Cancer* 1998; 84(4): 252–61.

139. Liliemark J, Tani E, Mellstedt H, Skoog L. Fine-needle aspiration cytology and immunocytochemistry of malignant non-Hodgkin's lymphoma in the oral cavity. *Oral Surg Oral Med Oral Pathol* 1989; 68(5): 599–603.

140. Galindo LM, Havlioglu N, Grosso LE. Cytologic findings in a case of T-cell rich B-cell lymphoma: potential diagnostic pitfall in FNA of lymph nodes. *Diagn Cytopathol* 1996; 14(3): 253–7, discussion 257–8.

141. Katz RL, Caraway NP. FNA lymphoproliferative diseases: myths and legends [editorial]. *Diagn Cytopathol* 1995; 12(2): 99–100.

142. Katz RL. Controversy in fine-needle aspiration of lymph nodes. A territorial imperative? [editorial]. *Am J Clin Pathol* 1997; 108(4 suppl 1): S3–5.

143. Rassidakis GZ, Tani E, Svedmyr E, Porwit A, Skoog L. Diagnosis and subclassification of follicle center and mantle cell lymphomas on fine-needle aspirates: A cytologic and immunocytochemical approach based on the Revised European-American Lymphoma (REAL) classification. *Cancer* 1999; 87(4): 216–23.

144. Wakely PE Jr. Fine needle aspiration cytopathology of malignant lymphoma. *Clin Lab Med* 1998; 18(3): 541–59, vi-vii.

145. Wakely PE Jr. Aspiration cytopathology of malignant lymphoma: coming of age [editorial, comment]. *Cancer* 1999; 87(6): 322–4.

146. Stewart CJ, Jackson R, Farquharson M, Richmond J. Fine-needle aspiration cytology of extranodal lymphoma. *Diagn Cytopathol* 1998; 19(4): 260–6.

147. Sapia S, Sanchez Avalos JC, Monreal M et al. Fine needle aspiration for flow cytometry immunophenotyping of non Hodgkin lymphoma. *Medicina (B Aires)* 1995; 55(6): 675–80.

148. Zander DS, Iturraspe JA, Everett ET, Massey JK, Braylan RC. Flow cytometry. In vitro assessment of its potential application for diagnosis and classification of lymphoid processes in cytologic preparations from fine-needle aspirates. *Am J Clin Pathol* 1994; 101(5): 577–86.

149. Muller-Hermelink HK. [Worldwide consensus: the way from the KIEL classification to the REAL classification to the WHO classification]. *Verh Dtsch Ges Pathol* 1999; 83: 155–61.

150. Chan JK, Banks PM, Cleary ML et al. A proposal for classification of lymphoid neoplasms (by the International Lymphoma Study Group). *Histopathology* 1994; 25(6): 517–36.

151. Harris NL, Jaffe ES, Diebold J, Flandrin G, Muller-Hermelink HK, Vardiman J. Lymphoma classification – from controversy to consensus: the R.E.A.L. and WHO Classification of lymphoid neoplasms. *Ann Oncol* 2000; 11(suppl 1): 3–10.

152. Siebert JD, Mulvaney DA, Potter KL, Fishkin PA, Geoffroy FJ. Relative frequencies and sites of presentation of lymphoid neoplasms in a community hospital according to the revised European-American classification. *Am J Clin Pathol* 1999; 111(3): 379–86.

153. Harris NL. Principles of the revised European-American Lymphoma Classification (from the International Lymphoma Study Group). *Ann Oncol* 1997; 8(suppl 2): 11–6.

154. Harris NL, Jaffe ES, Diebold J et al. World Health Organization classification of neoplastic diseases of the hematopoietic and lymphoid tissues: report of the clinical advisory committee meeting, Airlie House, Virginia, November 1997. *J Neurooncol* 1999; 43(3): 203–8.

155. Young NA, Al-Saleem T. Hematopathologists and cytopathologists: enemies or allies? [editorial]. *Diagn Cytopathol* 1999; 21(5): 305–6.

156. Coiffier B. Treatment of aggressive non-Hodgkin's lymphoma. *Semin Oncol* 1999; 26(5 suppl 14): 12–20.

157. Tworek JA, Singleton TP, Schnitzer B, Hsi ED, Ross CW. Flow cytometric and immunohistochemical analysis of small lymphocytic lymphoma, mantle cell lymphoma, and plasmacytoid small lymphocytic lymphoma. *Am J Clin Pathol* 1998; 110(5): 582–9.

158. Kuruvilla S, Gomathy DV, Shanthi AV, Thanasekharaan V, Deivanayagam CN. Primary pulmonary lymphoma. Report of a case diagnosed by fine needle aspiration cytology. *Acta Cytol* 1994; 38(4): 601–4.

158a. Wotherspoon A. Immunocytochemistry of low grade B-cell lymphomas. *CPD Bulletin Cellular Pathology* 1999; 1: 158–161.

159. Campo E, Raffeld M, Jaffe ES. Mantle-cell lymphoma. *Semin Hematol* 1999; 36(2): 115–27.

160. Hughes JH, Caraway NP, Katz RL. Blastic variant of mantle-cell lymphoma: cytomorphologic, immunocytochemical, and molecular genetic features of tissue obtained by fine-needle aspiration biopsy. *Diagn Cytopathol* 1998; 19(1): 59–62.

161. Suh YK, Shabaik A, Meurer WT, Shin SS. Lymphoid cell aggregates: a useful clue in the fine-needle aspiration diagnosis of follicular lymphomas. *Diagn Cytopathol* 1997; 17(6): 467–71.

162. McNeely TB. Diagnosis of follicular lymphoma by fine needle aspiration biopsy. *Acta Cytol* 1992; 36(6): 866–8.

163. Raible MD, Hsi ED, Alkan S. Bcl-6 protein expression by follicle center lymphomas. A marker for differentiating follicle center lymphomas from other low-grade lymphoproliferative disorders. *Am J Clin Pathol* 1999; 112(1): 101–7.

164. Allen EA, Ali SZ, Mathew S. Lymphoid lesions of the parotid. *Diagn Cytopathol* 1999; 21(3): 170–3.

165. MacCallum PL, Lampe HB, Cramer H, Matthews TW. Fine-needle aspiration cytology of lymphoid lesions of the salivary gland: a review of 35 cases. *J Otolaryngol* 1996; 25(5): 300–4.

166. Cha I, Long SR, Ljung BM, Miller TR. Low-grade lymphoma of mucosa associated tissue in the parotid gland: a case report of fine-needle aspiration cytology diagnosis using flow cytometric immunophenotyping. *Diagn Cytopathol* 1997; 16(4): 345–9.

167. Hughes JH, Katz RL, Fonseca GA, Cabanillas FF. Fine-needle aspiration cytology of mediastinal non-Hodgkin's nonlymphoblastic lymphoma. *Cancer* 1998; 84(1): 26–35.

168. Yu GH, Shin HJ, Santos-Ocampo R, Katz RL. Fine-needle aspiration of a case of non-Hodgkin's lymphoma containing signet ring cells [letter]. *Diagn Cytopathol* 1995; 13(2): 183–5.

169. Ascoli V, Sirianni MC, Mezzaroma I et al. Human herpesvirus-8 in lymphomatous and nonlymphomatous body cavity effusions developing in Kaposi's sarcoma and multicentric Castleman's disease. *Ann Diagn Pathol* 1999; 3(6): 357–63.

170. Ely SA, Powers J, Lewis D, Chang S et al. Kaposi's sarcoma-associated herpesvirus-positive primary effusion lymphoma arising in the subarachnoid space. *Hum Pathol* 1999; 30(8): 981–4.

171. Park IA, Kim CW. FNAC of malignant lymphoma in an area with a high incidence of T-cell lymphoma. Correlation of accuracy of cytologic diagnosis with histologic subtype and immunophenotype. *Acta Cytol* 1999; 43(6): 1059–69.

172. Laforga JB, Chorda D, Sevilla F. Intramammary lymph node involvement by mycosis fungoides diagnosed by fine-needle aspiration biopsy. *Diagn Cytopathol* 1998; 19(2): 124–6.

173. Ludwig RA, Balachandran I. Mycosis fungoides. The importance of pulmonary cytology in the diagnosis of a case with systemic involvement. *Acta Cytol* 1983; 27(2): 198–201.

174. Rosen SE, Koprowska I, Vonderheid EC. Skin imprint cytology in the diagnosis of cutaneous T-cell lymphomas. A preliminary report. *Acta Cytol* 1982; 26(6): 819–22.

175. Rosen SE, Vonderheid EC, Koprowska I. Mycosis fungoides with pulmonary involvement. Cytopathologic findings. *Acta Cytol* 1984; 28(1): 51–7.

176. Oshima K, Tani E, Masuda Y, Skoog L, Kikuchi M. Fine needle aspiration cytology of high grade T-cell lymphomas in human T-lymphotropic virus type 1 carriers. *Cytopathology* 1992; 3(6): 365–72.

177. Jayaram G, Abdul Rahman N. Cytology of Ki-1-positive anaplastic large cell lymphoma. A report of two cases. *Acta Cytol* 1997; 41(4 suppl): 1253–60.

178. Sgrignoli A, Abati A. Cytologic diagnosis of anaplastic large cell lymphoma. *Acta Cytol* 1997; 41(4): 1048–52.

179. McCluggage WG, Anderson N, Herron B, Caughley L. Fine needle aspiration cytology, histology and immunohistochemistry of anaplastic large cell Ki-1-positive lymphoma. A report of three cases. *Acta Cytol* 1996; 40(4): 779–85.

180. Zakowski MF, Feiner H, Finfer M, Thomas P, Wollner N, Filippa DA. Cytology of extranodal Ki-1 anaplastic large cell lymphoma. *Diagn Cytopathol* 1996; 14(2): 155–61.

181. Wellmann A, Otsuki T, Vogelbruch M, Clark HM, Jaffe ES, Raffeld M. Analysis of the t(2; 5)(p23; q35) translocation by reverse transcription-polymerase chain reaction in CD30+ anaplastic large-cell lymphomas, in other non-Hodgkin's lymphomas of T-cell phenotype, and in Hodgkin's disease. *Blood* 1995; 86(6): 2321–8.

182. Katano H, Suda T, Morishita Y et al. Human herpesvirus 8-associated solid lymphomas that occur in AIDS patients take anaplastic large cell morphology. *Mod Pathol* 2000; 13(1): 77–85.

183. Jimenez-Heffernan JA, Viguer JM, Vicandi B et al. Posttransplant CD30 (Ki-1)-positive anaplastic large cell lymphoma. Report of a case with presentation as a pleural effusion. *Acta Cytol* 1997; 41(5): 1519–24.

184. Das DK, Chowdhury V, Kishore B, Chachra K, Bhatt NC, Kakar AK. CD-30(Ki-1)-positive anaplastic large cell lymphoma in a pleural effusion. A case report with diagnosis by cytomorphologic and immunocytochemical studies. *Acta Cytol* 1999; 43(3): 498–502.

185. Liu K, Dodd LG, Osborne BM, Martinez S, Olatdioye BA, Madden JF. Diagnosis of anaplastic large-cell lymphoma, including multifocal osseous KI-1 lymphoma, by fine-needle aspiration biopsy. *Diagn Cytopathol* 1999; 21(3): 174–9.

186. Bizjak-Schwarzbartl M. Large cell anaplastic Ki-1+ non-Hodgkin's lymphoma vs. Hodgkin's disease in fine needle aspiration biopsy samples. *Acta Cytol* 1997; 41(2): 351–6.

187. Aljajeh IA, Das DK, Krajci D. Ki-1-positive anaplastic large cell lymphoma initially diagnosed as Hodgkin's disease by fine needle aspiration (FNA) cytology. *Cytopathology* 1995; 6(4): 226–35.

188. Yazdi HM, Burns BF. Fine needle aspiration biopsy of Ki-1-positive large-cell 'anaplastic' lymphoma. *Acta Cytol* 1991; 35(3): 306–10.

189. Liu YJ, Lee YT, Hsieh SW, Kuo SH. Presumption of primary sites of neck lymph node metastases on fine needle aspiration cytology. *Acta Cytol* 1997; 41(5): 1477–82.

190. Caraway NP, Wojcik EM, Saboorian HM, Katz RL. Concomitant lymphoma and metastatic carcinoma in a lymph node: diagnosis by fine-needle aspiration biopsy in two cases. *Diagn Cytopathol* 1997; 17(4): 287–91.

5

Miscellaneous lesions of the head and neck

Introduction
Benign soft tissue lesions
Lipoma

INTRODUCTION

In addition to having specific pathology, head and neck swellings are often a presenting site for more general conditions. In this chapter, we describe pathological and clinical entities encountered in our own practice. As a result, this is not a comprehensive account of all conditions that can be seen in the head and neck, but a selection of clinical cases which illustrate different lesions and groups of lesions. For clarity, these have been grouped into the following categories:

- Benign soft tissue lesions
- Cysts of the head and neck
- Small round cell tumours
- Locally arising miscellaneous tumours.

Benign soft tissue lesions

Lipoma

Cytological diagnosis of lipoma is one of exclusion. Patients usually present with a soft, mobile swelling that has been present for some time and usually does not cause any concern to the patient. Referral for FNAC is mainly in order to exclude other pathology (Figs 5.1–5.4).

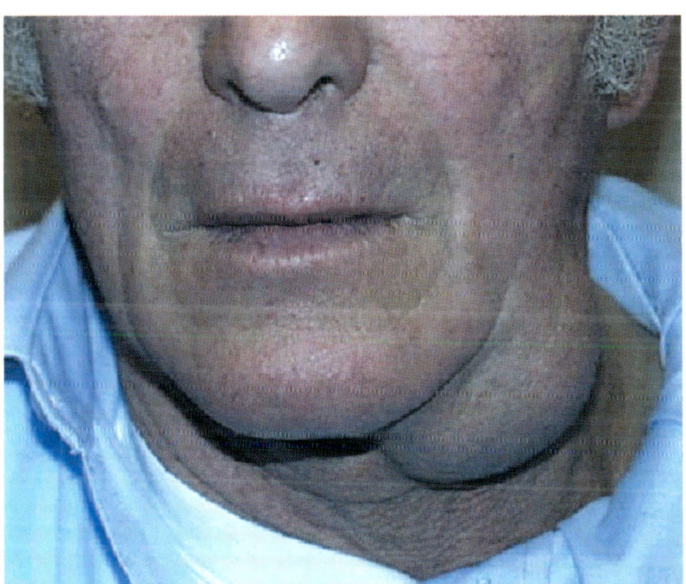

Figure 5.1 Submandibular swelling in a 70-year-old man: soft, fluctuant, present for several years and slow growing. Patient was referred to the FNAC clinic to elucidate the nature of swelling although it was believed to be benign.

Cytological features of lipoma include sparse microbiopsy fragments of adipose tissue composed of a meshwork of delicate capillaries surrounding aggregates of fat cells. These are univacuolated with nuclei that are small and inconspicuous. There are often bare nuclei in the background. Capillary endothelium may be seen sometimes.

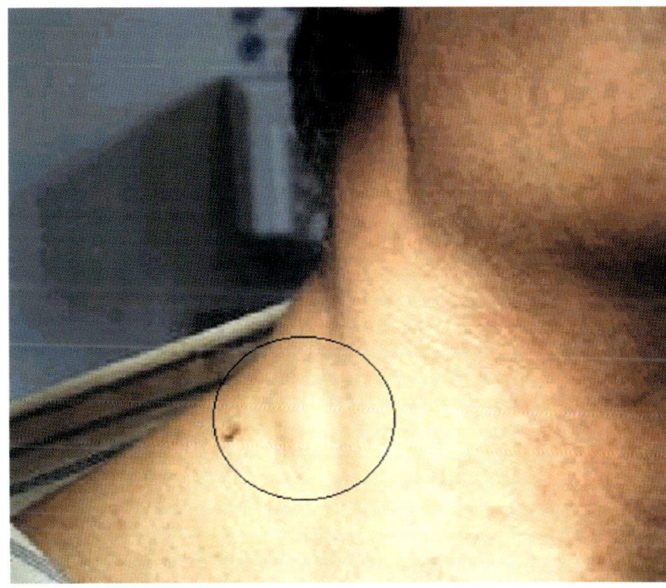

Figure 5.2 Patient with a clinical history of tuberculosis presented with a soft swelling in the posterior triangle which was thought to be a lymph node. FNAC revealed adipose tissue only, consistent with lipoma.

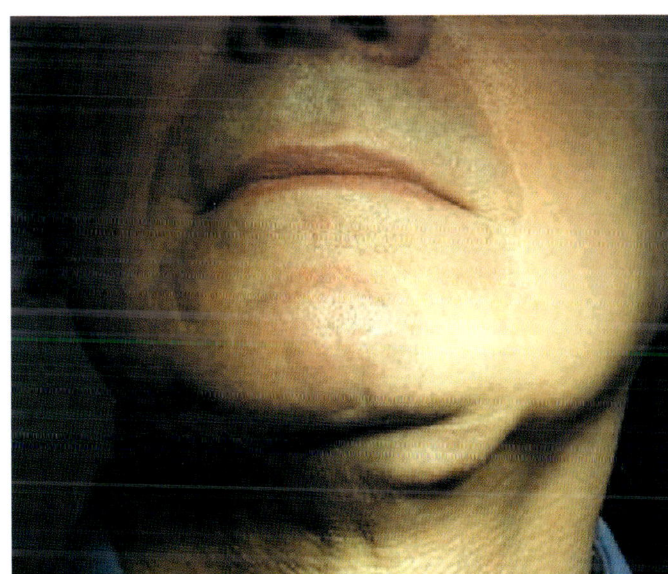

Figure 5.3 Patient with a soft painless submandibular swelling which he had noticed after losing some weight. Clinically, it was thought to be an enlarged submental lymph node; FNAC showed adipose tissue only, consistent with lipoma.

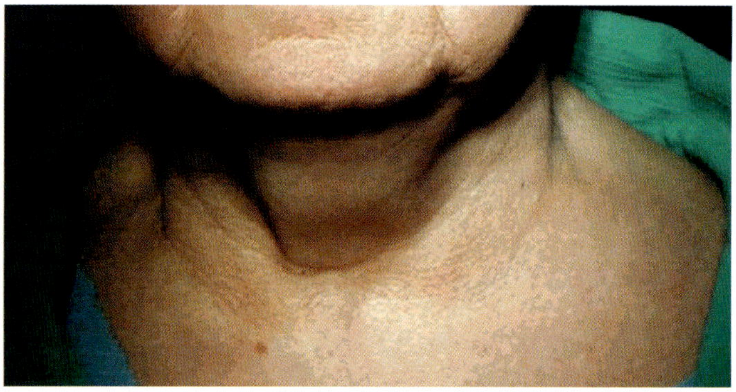

Figure 5.4 Elderly patient with diffuse unilateral soft swelling in the left supraclavicular fossa. She was referred for FNAC to exclude lymphadenopathy. FNAC yielded fatty material, consistent with lipoma.

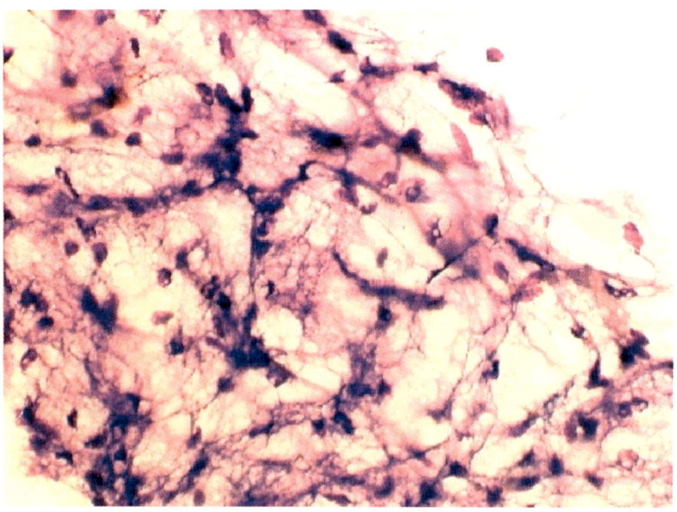

Figure 5.5 Lipoma. Sparse microbiopsy fragments of adipose tissue composed of fat cells in a meshwork of delicate capillaries. Fat cells are univacuolated with nuclei that are small and inconspicuous. It is not possible to distinguish between lipoma and fat tissue on FNAC. It is therefore important that the FNAC is taken from representative area under standard conditions, if any conclusions are to be drawn from the material containing fat cells only (MGG ×600).

Depending on the type of lipoma, cellular components may be varied, e.g. hybernoma, angiolipoma or intramuscular lipoma. Since it is not possible to distinguish adipose tissue from a lipoma on FNAC, the diagnosis is made according to clinical circumstances. Provided the FNAC is representative, the diagnosis is made by exclusion of other significant pathology (Fig. 5.5). In atypical lipoma there are large cells with abundant cytoplasm and hyperchromatic, irregular nuclei, singly and in clusters. Atypical lypoma may be impossible to distinguish from a well-differentiated liposarcoma.[1]

Fibromatosis colli

Fibromatoses form a spectrum of clinicopathological entities characterised by the infiltrative proliferation of fibroblasts that lack malignant cytological features. Fibromatoses present as nodular soft tissue masses almost anywhere in the body including the shoulder and the sternocleidomastoid muscle (fibromatosis colli). Clinical presentation may be of a rapidly growing mass.

Cytological features. FNAC aspirates consist of groups of loosely cohesive, bland-appearing, spindle-shaped cells having oval to elongated nuclei and cytoplasmic tags. Individual spindle cells and rare inflammatory cells are also present. The aspirate may also contain degenerating skeletal muscle cells. FNAC is a useful procedure for the initial and recurrent diagnosis of fibromatoses and in the separation of fibromatoses from other benign and malignant soft tissue lesions. In the initial diagnosis, histological confirmation is recommended.[2]

Proliferative fasciitis

Proliferative fasciitis is defined histologically as a spindle cell lesion containing basophilic giant cells that resemble ganglion cells; the FNAC smears from this lesion are cellular and contain spindle cells as well as numerous large cells with abundant cytoplasm, 1–2 eccentric nuclei and macronucleoli. The large cells seen on the aspiration smears correspond well with the classic ganglion-like cells seen on histological sections. Care must be taken so that this distinctive lesion is not misdiagnosed as a malignant soft tissue neoplasm.[3]

Nodular fasciitis

Nodular fasciitis, the most common pseudosarcomatous proliferative lesion of the soft tissues, is well-defined histologically but not cytomorphologically. Nodular fasciitis is characterised histologically by proliferating fibroblast-like cells that vary from thin, elongated and spindle shaped with elongated nuclei to plump with one or more large oval nuclei.

Cytological features. There is myxoid background substance and tufts of fibrillary myxoid material[1] (Fig. 5.6). As a rule, the smears are hypercellular and composed of fibroblast-like cells which vary widely from spindle shaped with long cytoplasmic processes to more plump with one or

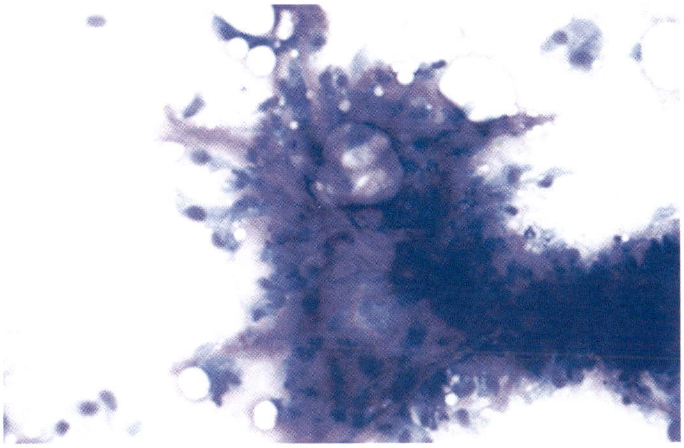

A

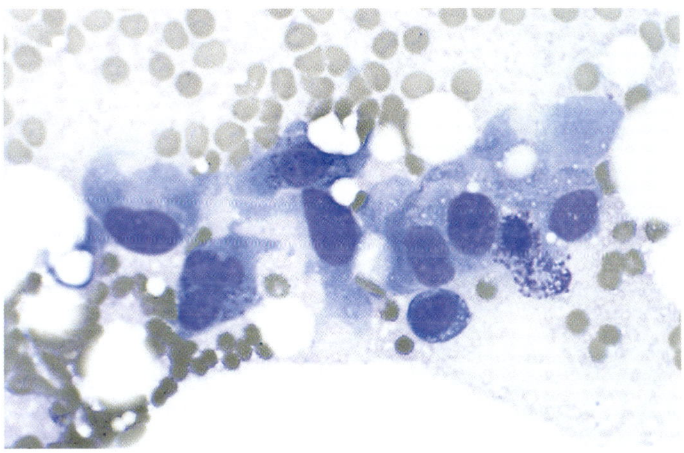

B

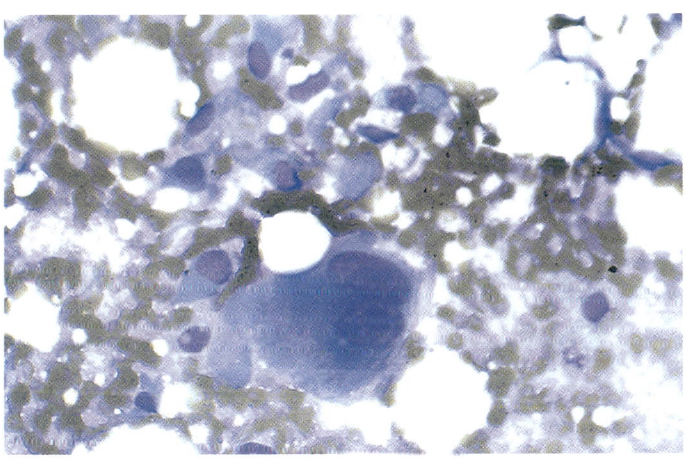

C

Figure 5.6 Nodular fasciitis. **A.** Smears contain myxoid background substance and tufts of fibrillary myxoid material. As a rule, smears are hypercellular (MGG ×400). **B.** Fibroblast-like cells which vary widely from spindle shaped with long cytoplasmic processes to more plump with one or more nuclei with nucleoli. Although there is marked anisokaryosis and prominent nucleoli, the chromatin pattern is finely granular (MGG ×1000). **C.** Binucleated or multinucleated cells are always observed, some of which resemble ganglion cells and are polyhedral or triangular cells with abundant cytoplasm and peripheral nuclei. Cytological appearances of nodular fasciitis are fairly characteristic, making it possible to recognise these lesions in FNAC samples (MGG ×1000).

more nuclei with nucleoli. Although there is marked anisokaryosis and prominent nucleoli, the chromatin pattern is finely granular. Cytological appearances of nodular fasciitis are fairly characteristic, making it possible to recognise these lesions in FNAC samples.[4,5]

Benign nerve sheath tumour (neurilemmoma, Schwannoma)

Benign nerve sheath tumour can occur anywhere in the head and neck and is associated with nerves.[6] Intraparotid facial nerve Schwannomas have been documented sporadically throughout the medical literature. These benign tumours of neurogenic origin should be considered in the differential diagnosis of parotid region masses.[7–14]

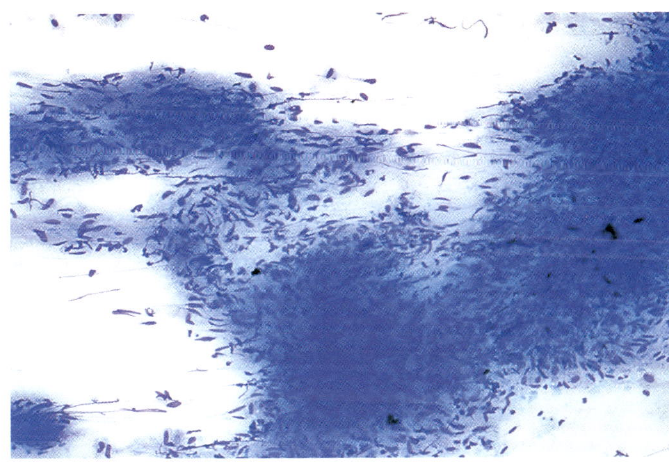

A

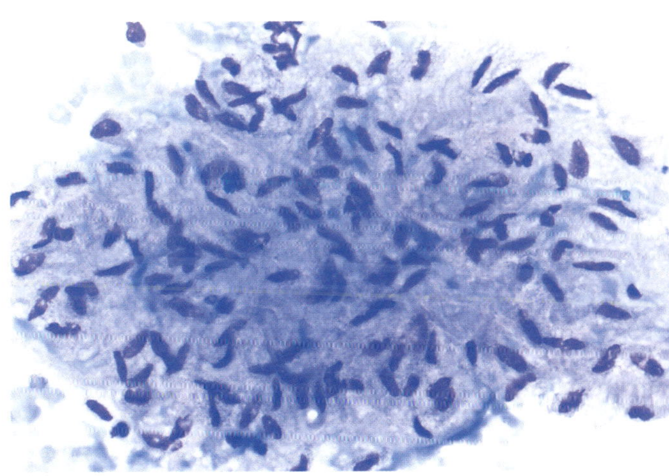

B

Figure 5.7 Benign nerve sheath tumour. **A.** Tumour tissue fragments with sparse dispersed cells and some aggregates against a fibrillary background substance (MGG ×200). **B.** Individual cells have indistinct cell borders, nuclei with pointed ends and occasionally show pallisading (MGG ×600 oil).

Cytological features. Mainly tumour tissue fragments with sparse, dispersed cells and some aggregates against a fibrillary background substance. Smears most often contain a mixture of Antoni A and Antoni B areas and tissue fragments are more common than individual cells. Individual cells have indistinct cell borders, nuclei with pointed ends, occasionally pallisading alternating with more rounded (lymphocytoid) nuclei. Sometimes Verocay body-like structures are seen. Mitoses are not seen[1] (Fig. 5.7).

A most important diagnostic pitfall in the diagnosis of neurilemmoma is leiomyosarcoma. The latter can be misdiagnosed in cases of ancient neurilemmoma. There may be marked cell pleomorphism with large hyperchromatic and bizarre nuclei containing prominent nucleoli. There are no mitoses and intranuclear vacuoles may be seen in ancient neurilemmoma. In the cases of intraparotid neurilemmomas, myoepithelioma of the salivary gland (see Chapter 2) is a differential diagnosis.

CYSTS OF THE HEAD AND NECK

Thyroglossal cyst

Thyroglossal cyst is a congenital cyst. It arises typically in the midline of the neck, close to the hyoid bone, to which it is usually attached. It arises from the remnants of the thyroglossal duct. It is lined with either squamous or columnar epithelium. Clinically, patients present with midline swelling. FNAC yields a small amount of fluid, which contains proteinaceous background, macrophages, cholesterol crystals and sparse epithelium (Fig. 5.8).

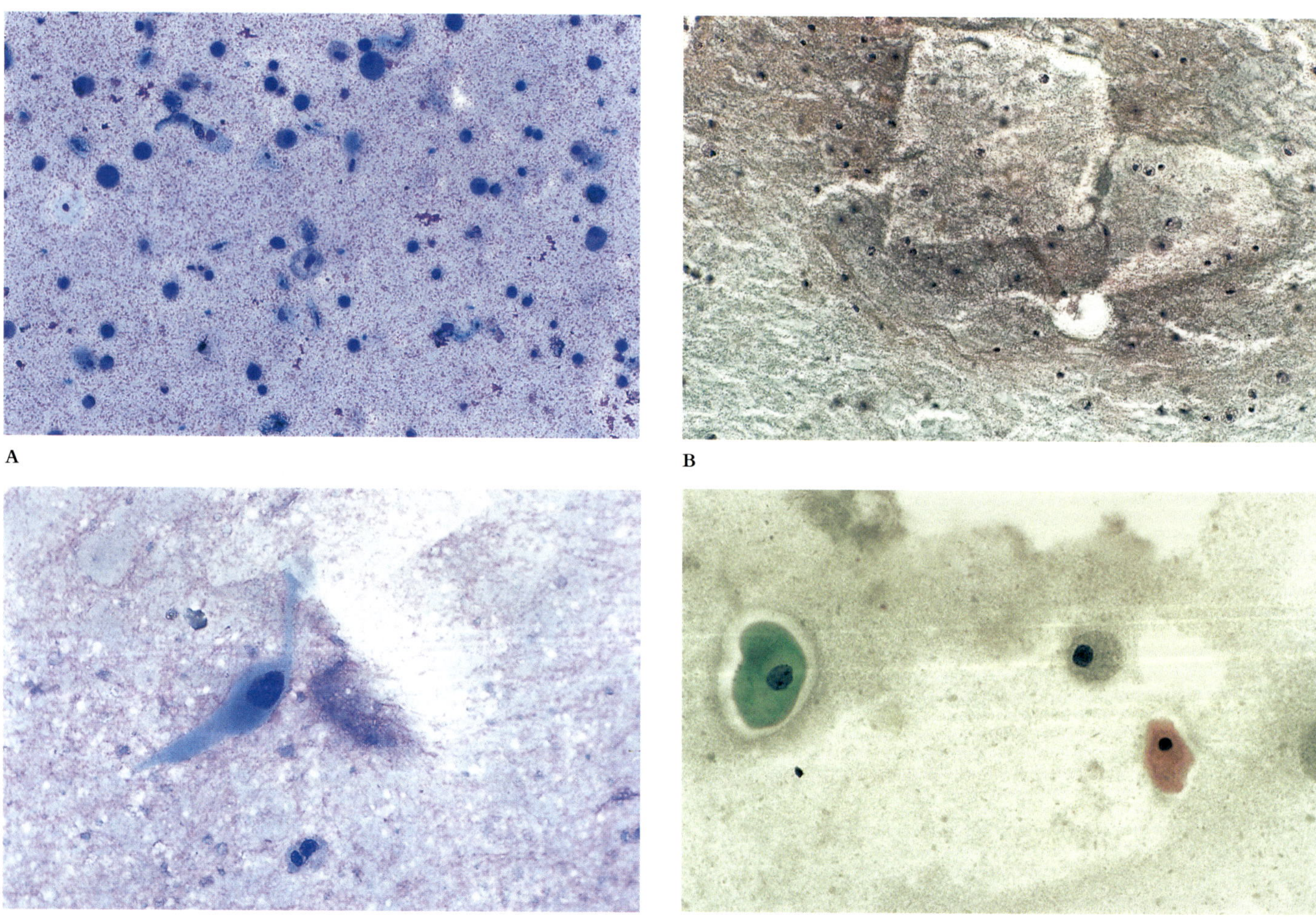

Figure 5.8 Thyroglossal cyst. **A, B.** Fluid from the cyst contains proteinaceous background, debris, macrophages, cholesterol crystals and sparse epithelium (MGG, PAP ×200). **C, D.** Epithelium of the thyroglossal cyst is inconspicuous and barely noticeable. It is usually squamoid, showing marked degenerative changes (MGG ×600 oil).

Branchial cyst

Branchial cysts derive from the second branchial cleft. They may appear in different anatomical positions. As a rule, they are more or less covered by the anterior border of the sternocleidomastoid muscle, but they can occur below and above this position (Figs 5.9A and 5.10A). Clinically, diagnosis of branchial cleft cyst may be more difficult than diagnosis of medial cysts. Lesions of similar appearance in this area include lymph nodes, carotid body tumours, salivary gland tumours, lymphangiomas and lipomas. The reliability of preoperative diagnosis of branchial cleft cyst is between 50% and 60%.[15] Histologically, the inner layer of the cyst is lined by squamous epithelium with lymphoid cells in the wall of the cyst.

Cytological features. Branchial cysts contain epithelial cells and keratinous debris. This is most frequently mature squamous epithelium and anucleate squames[16] (Fig. 5.9B, see also Chapter 2, Fig. 2.10C). Inflamed branchial cysts contain polymorphs, macrophages and may contain epithelial atypia which may be mistaken for squamous cell carcinoma[17] (Fig. 5.10B). The distinction is sometimes difficult because metastases of squamous cell carcinoma may be well differentiated and contain mainly mature squamous epithelial cells (Fig. 5.10D). A thorough search for nuclear atypia is suggested. Failing this, a diagnosis of branchial cyst in any patient over the age of 30 has to be issued with a degree of caution, allowing for the possibility of a metastasis of a well-differentiated squamous cell carcinoma. Excision biopsy, while usually performed on branchial cleft cysts, is not a procedure of choice in cases of metastatic squamous cell carcinoma. The excision is normally part of a radical neck dissection. Accurate preoperative diagnosis is therefore very important.

Mucous retention cyst

Mucous retention cyst is a common submucosal lesion of the oral cavity that, when deeply seated, simulates a neoplasm. Its occurrence within the salivary gland has been described in Chapter 2 (Figs 2.8 and 2.9). Cytological differential diagnosis is from other benign and malignant cystic lesions of the head and neck.[18]

Intraosseous cysts and other lesions

In their experience of FNAC of intraosseous jaw lesions in both children and adults, Gunhan et al[19] found that the most commonly sampled benign lesions are odontogenic cysts, ameloblastomas and fibro-osseous and giant cell lesions[20–23] (Fig. 5.11). FNAC is a useful technique to distinguish between malignant and benign intraosseous jaw lesions. Its simplicity, suitability as an outpatient procedure, rapidity of interpretation and minimal morbidity, potentially make it the diagnostic tool

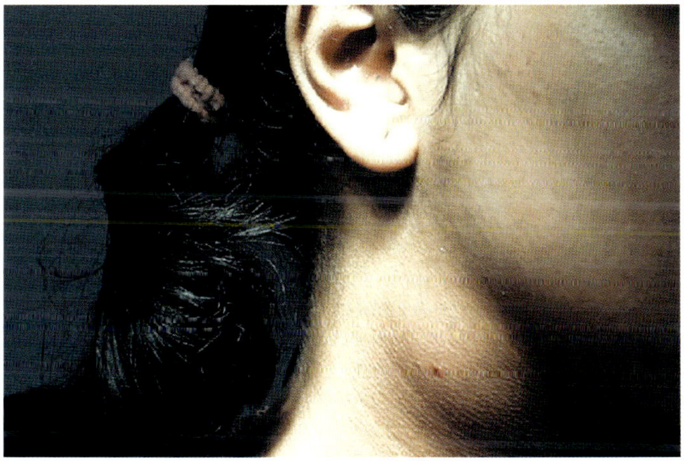

A

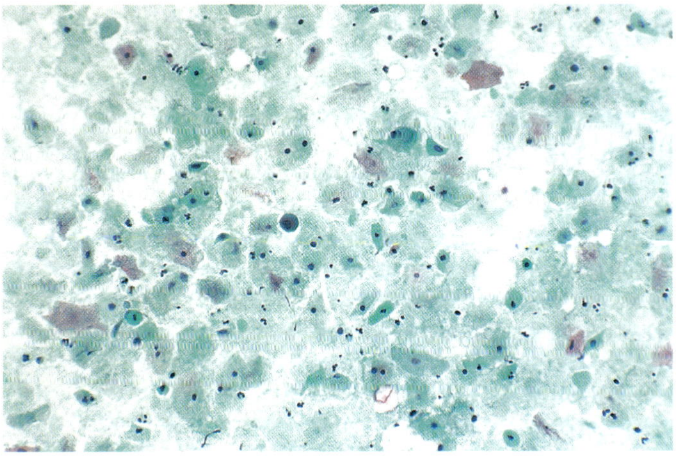

B

Figure 5.9 Branchial cleft cyst. **A.** A 26-year-old patient, referred by the ENT surgeon from an inner city area with high prevalence of tuberculosis, presented with a 6-month history of painless swelling in the neck. Swelling was fairly firm, non-fluctuant. FNAC yielded thick yellow fluid. **B.** Branchial cysts contain epithelial cells and keratinous debris. This is most frequently mature squamous epithelium and anucleate squames (PAP ×200).

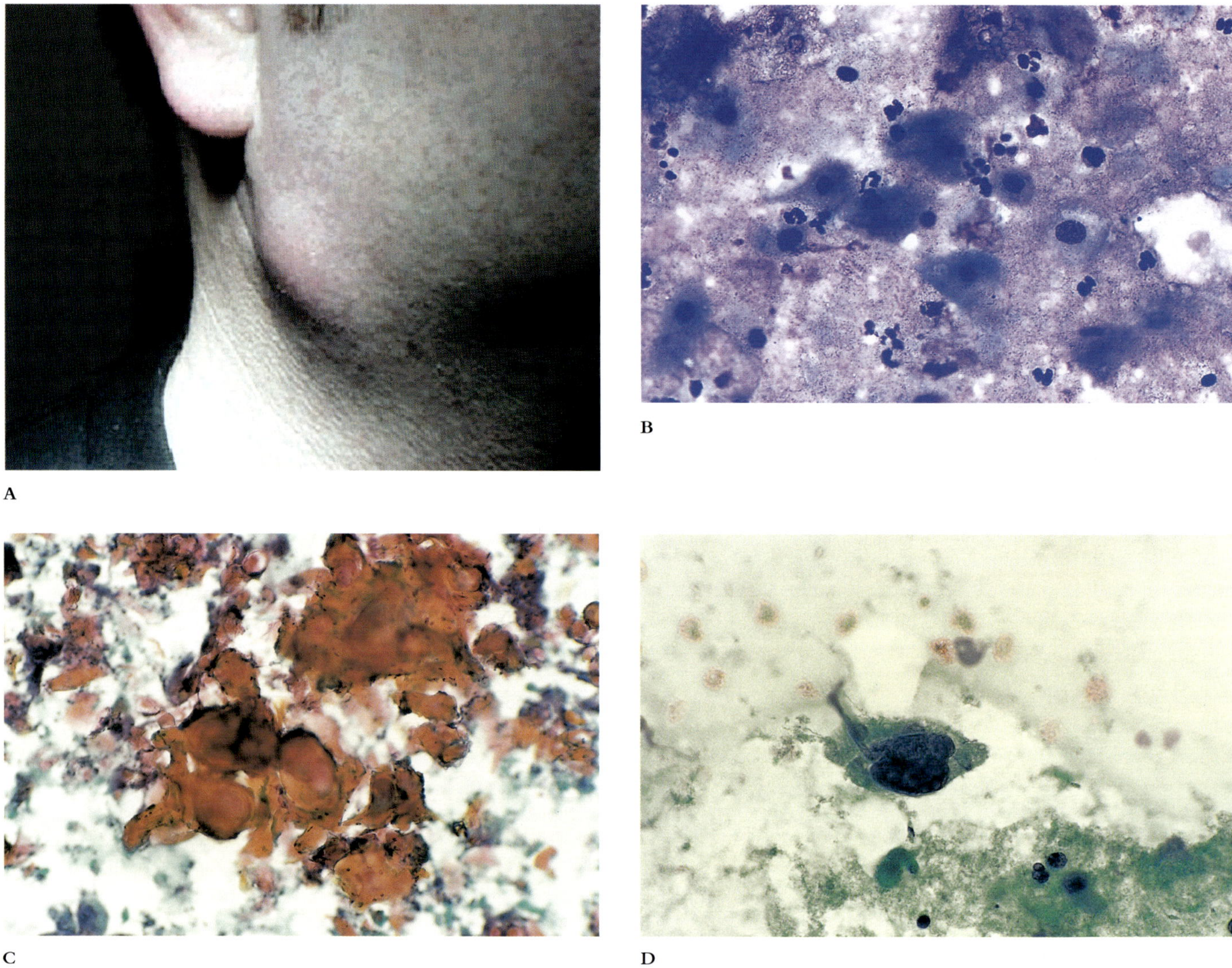

Figure 5.10 Inflamed branchial cleft cyst. **A.** A 37-year-old patient with a painful, red swelling at the side of the neck which had come up suddenly in the last 2 weeks. FNAC yielded thick yellow fluid. **B.** In addition to mature squamous epithelium, numerous polymorphs are seen (MGG, PAP ×600 oil immersion). **C.** Another case, squamous cell carcinoma. Keratinised squamous cells may occasionally be the only finding in the cases of metastatic squamous cell carcinoma. This patient had a primary tumour in the tongue. (PAP x400). **D.** Same case as **C.** A thorough search reveals dyskaryotic nuclei which confirm the diagnosis of squamous cell carcinoma. The abnormal cells may be very sparse. The similarity of the findings with branchial cleft cyst may be misleading. Clinical history and the age of the patient are important when reporting the lesion with squamous epithelium in the neck.

of choice in the hospital setting. The overall accuracy of FNAC in the oral cavity and jawbones is high and is not significantly different from that obtained in other body regions.[24]

Rare cysts and differential diagnosis of cystic lesions of the head and neck

Parathyroid,[25,26] *cervical thymic*[27] and other rare cystic lesions occasionally can be encountered in the head and neck area.[28] *Epidermoid cyst* of the skin may be mistaken for another lesion (Fig. 5.12).

Apart from the above cysts, which are mainly congenital, other cystic lesions in the neck include: lymphoepithelial cyst of the salivary gland, pleomorphic adenoma with cystic change, Warthin's tumour, mucoepidermoid carcinoma, squamous cell carcinoma and metastatic papillary carcinoma.[29]

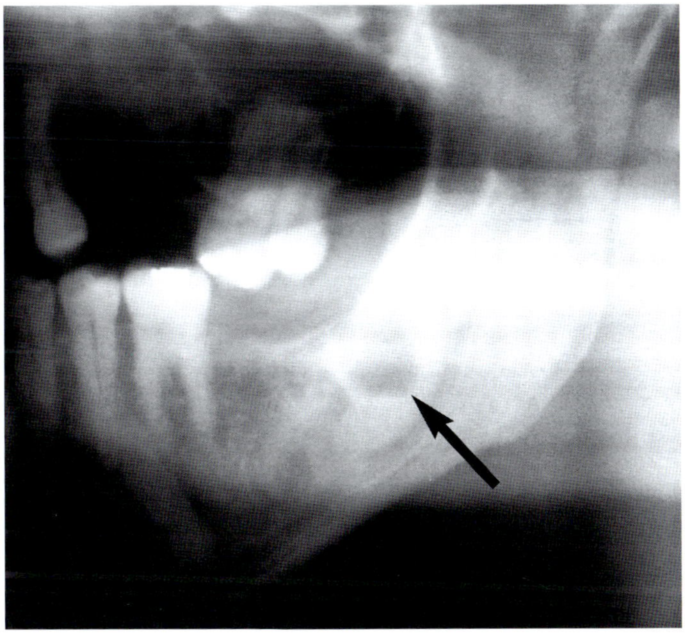

A

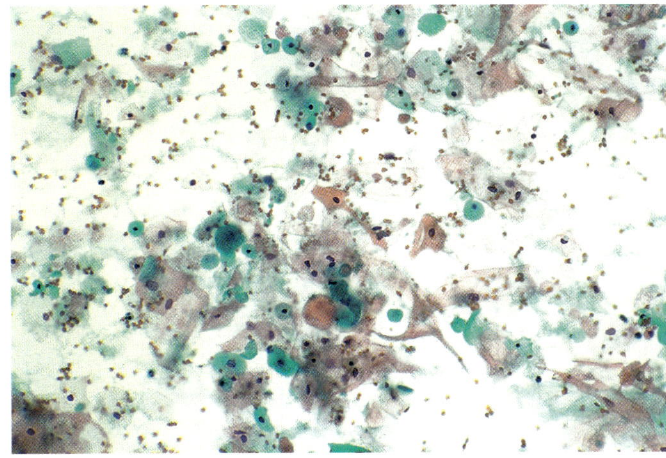

B

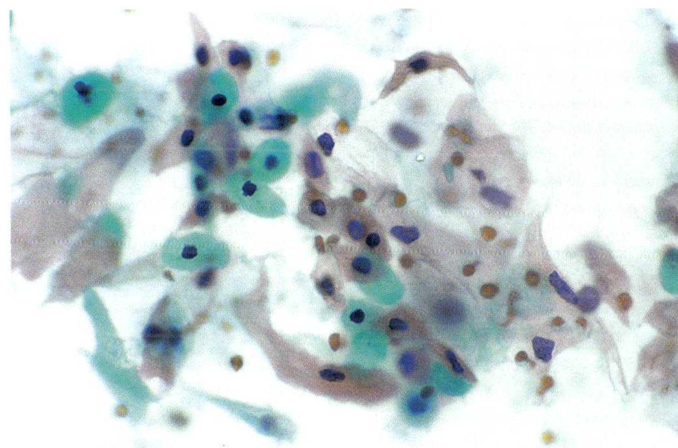

C

Figure 5.11 Keratocyst. **A.** X-ray appearances of the ramus of mandible showing intraosseous cyst (arrow). **B, C.** FNAC material from cyst contains karatinised squamous epithelium. Nuclei appear benign. No other features are seen (PAP ×200, ×600 oil).

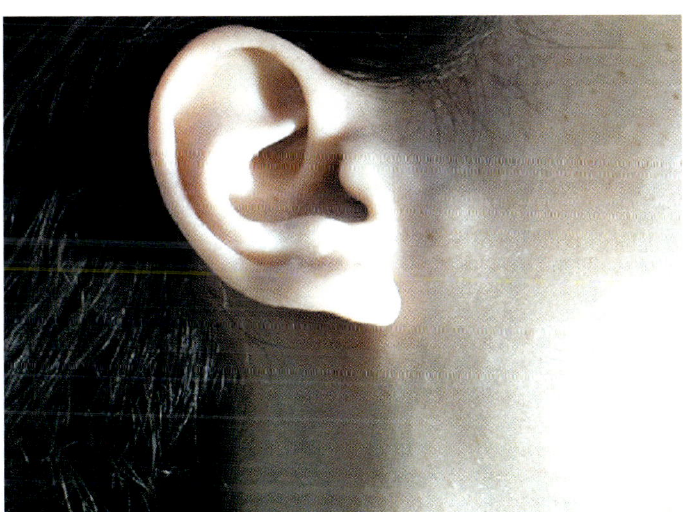

Figure 5.12 A 20-year-old patient presented with a small mobile painless pre-auricular swelling clinically thought to be a lymph node. Microscopy revealed an epidermoid cyst composed of flakes of keratinous debris. No lymphoid cells were seen.

SMALL ROUND CELL TUMOURS

A group of malignancies that share similar morphological features are known as small round cell tumours. They commonly occur in childhood and adolescence and include embryonal and alveolar rhabdomyosarcoma, neuroblastoma, Ewing's sarcoma/peripheral neuroectodermal tumour (ES/PNET) and lymphoma (usually lymphoblastic). All of these tumours may occur in the head and neck, either as primary tumours or as metastases. Accurate diagnosis in either of these situations is important to ensure appropriate treatment. Biopsies, particularly in the case of secondary deposits, may not be necessary or feasible. FNAC therefore aims to be as diagnostically useful as possible.[30–34]

Rhabdomyosarcoma

The head and neck region, including the eye, is one of the most common locations of rhabdomyosarcoma.[35,36] The tumour is common in children and adolescents. Clinically, the enlargements may appear to be inflammatory, and they are usually treated unsuccessfully with antibiotics.

Cytological features. Uniform population of primitive, small round cells with scant cytoplasm, arranged as single cells and cohesive aggregates. The cells are predominantly round/polygonal, with uniform nuclei (Fig. 5.13, Fig. 2.62, p. 67). The nuclear chromatin is finely granular and hyperchromatic, while nucleoli are inconspicuous. Binucleated and multinucleated cells are found in the majority of cases. Intracytoplasmic vacuoles may be present. The presence of bi/multinucleated cells is an important clue for the diagnosis of rhabdomyosarcoma on fine needle aspiration cytology.[37–41] Tumour cells are often enclosed in a background of mucosubstances. The lack of cytological features proving rhabdomyoblastic differentiation, such as cross-striation, requires use of additional methods in the cytological diagnosis.[42–44] An immunoperoxidase stain for the demonstration of intracellular desmin in FNAC smears shows a positive reaction of variable intensity in some of the undifferentiated round cells and in the more mature bipolar sarcomatous elements.[45]

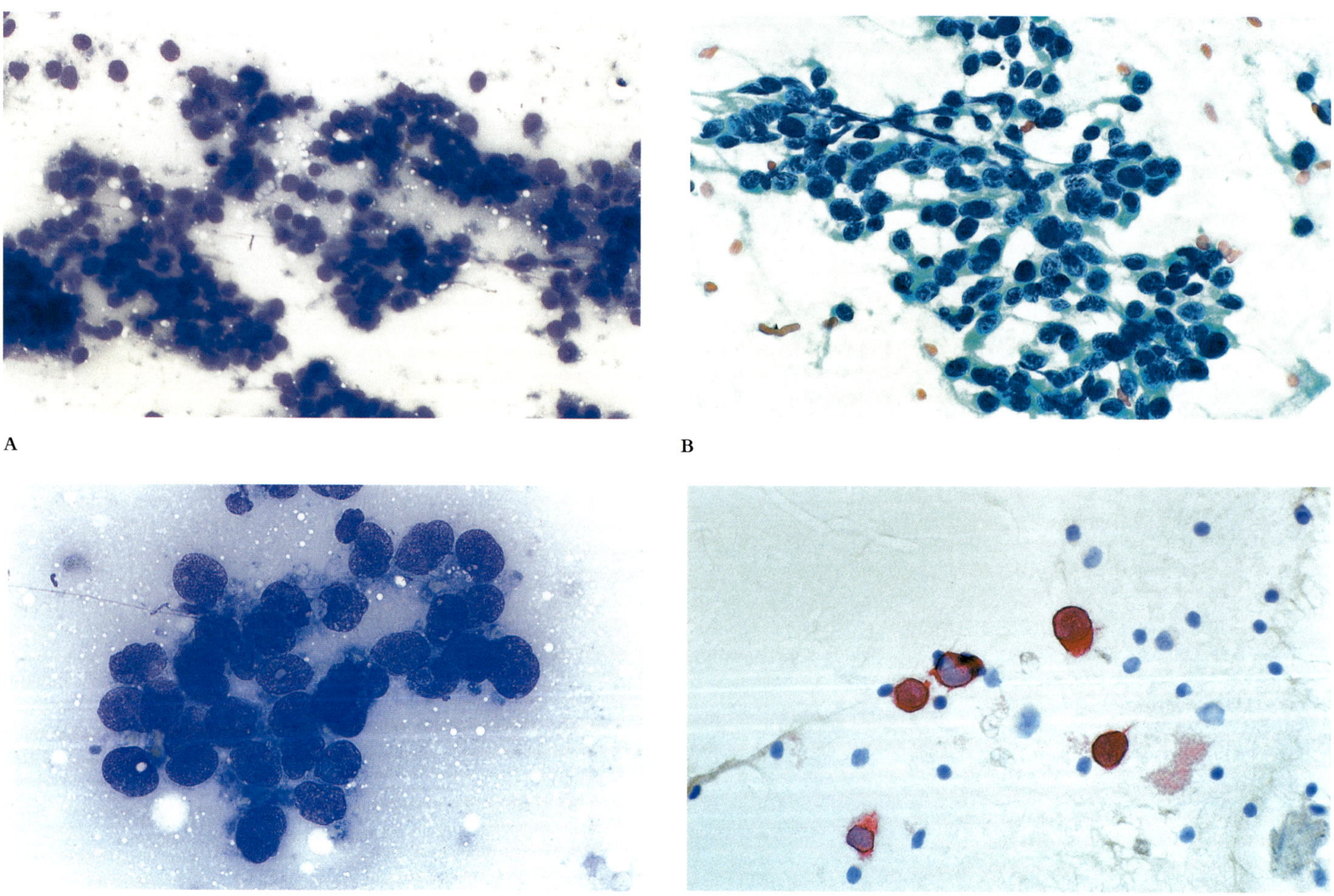

A B C D

Figure 5.13 Rhabdomyosarcoma. A case of embryonal rhabdomyosarcoma in a submandibular area of a 9-year-old child. **A, B.** Uniform population of primitive, small round cells with scant cytoplasm, arranged as single cells and cohesive aggregates (MGG, PAP ×200). **C.** Nuclear chromatin is finely granular and hyperchromatic, while nucleoli are inconspicuous. Binucleated and multinucleated cells are found in the majority of cases. Intracytoplasmic vacuoles may be present (MGG ×600). **D.** An immunoperoxide stain for the demonstration of intracellular desmin in FNAC smears shows positive reaction in some of the undifferentiated round cells (desmin, APAAP ×600 oil).

Rhabdomyosarcomas are a heterogeneous group of tumours with respect to their molecular basis, degree of differentiation, histology and clinical behaviour. Because of the wide variation of tumour morphology, it is often difficult to distinguish between the distinct subtypes. Differentiation between alveolar and embryonal rhabdomyosarcoma is not possible on cytology alone and yet this distinction may be important for further management.[46] The advances in therapeutic approach stress the importance of including molecular diagnostic studies in the routine evaluation of paediatric solid tumours. Reverse transcriptase polymerase chain reaction (RT-PCR) is used to detect chimaeric transcripts specific for major paediatric solid tumours, including peripheral primitive neuroectodermal tumour (pPNET), alveolar rhabdomyosarcoma (ARMS) and desmoplastic small round cell tumour (DSRCT).[47] Dias et al[48] found that a strong immunohistochemical expression of myogenin in histological sections of rhabdomyosarcoma is associated with alveolar cell type. In contrast, most embryonal rhabdomyosarcomas are either negative or show a low level of staining for myogenin. Alveolar rhabdomyosarcomas that stain strongly for myogenin are also positive for Pax3-7/Forkhead (FKHR) by RT-PCR.[49] Staining for myogenin may become a simple, rapid and accurate adjunct for distinguishing between alveolar and embryonal rhabdomyosarcomas.[48]

Extraskeletal Ewing's sarcoma/peripheral neuroectodermal tumour (ES/PNET)

Extraskeletal Ewing's sarcoma (EES) is a round cell malignancy that manifests most commonly in the paravertebral and intercostal regions. It occurs predominantly in adolescents and young adults, between the ages of 10 and 30 years, and follows an aggressive course with a high recurrence rate. Distant metastases are common (Fig. 5.14). The tumour is often confused with other round, small cell neoplasms, including neuroblastoma, embryonal rhabdomyosarcoma and lymphoma.[50] The purpose of FNAC is to diagnose these tumours and evaluate metastases in patients with known Ewing's sarcoma.[51]

Cytological features. FNAC smears from ES/PNET show cellular smears with many single cells and focal clustering. Numerous naked nuclei and focal crush artefacts are seen. Mitoses and necrosis are rare. Cells are small with fine chromatin, small, inconspicuous but distinct basophilic nucleoli, scanty cytoplasm, cytoplasmic

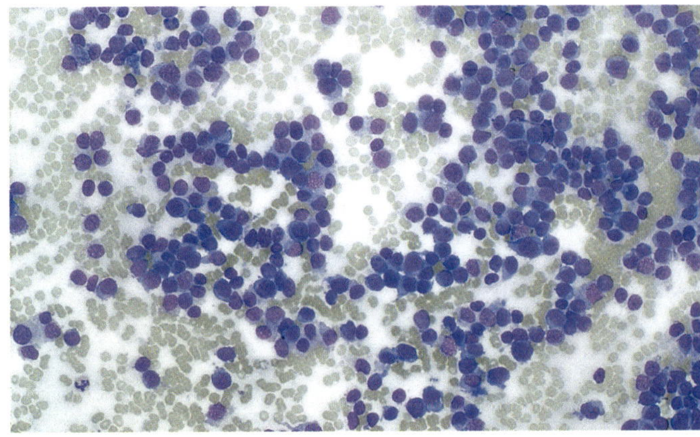

A

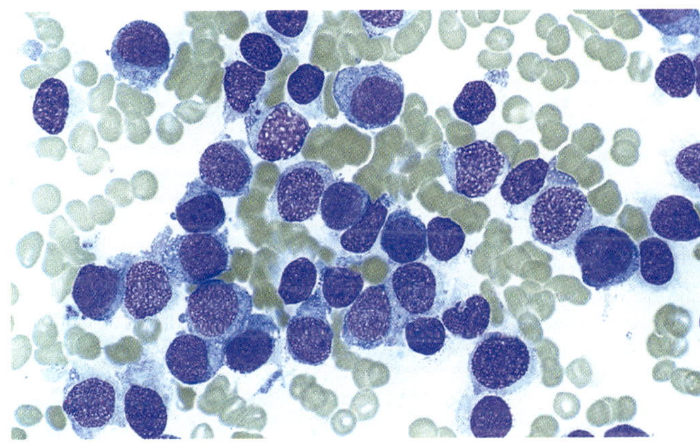

B

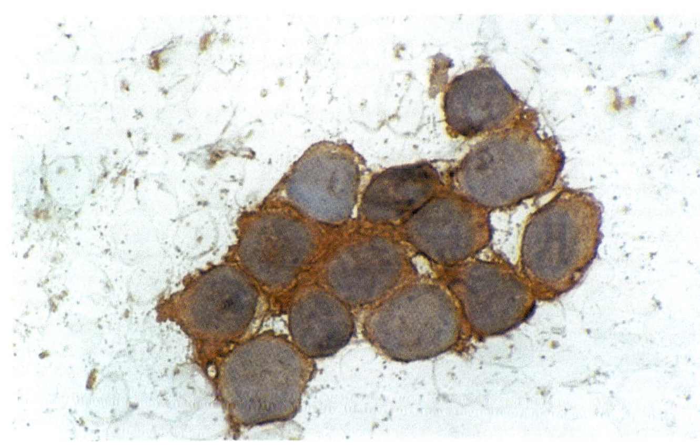

C

Figure 5.14 Ewing's sarcoma. The patient is a 14-year-old boy with a subcutaneous deposit of tumour in the scalp and a previous history of Ewing's sarcoma in the forearm. **A.** FNAC shows cellular smears with many single cells and focal clustering. Numerous naked nuclei and focal crush artefacts may be seen (MGG ×200). **B.** Cells are small with fine chromatin, small inconspicuous but distinct basophilic nucleoli, scanty cytoplasm, cytoplasmic vacuoles and nuclear moulding (the so-called typical variant). Less common are tumours with cells having abundant eosinophilic cytoplasm, large nuclei and large eosinophilic nucleoli (atypical or large eosinophilic nucleoli; atypical or large cell variant). Tumours with features in between, with cells showing abundant cytoplasm, nuclear grooves and medium-sized nucleoli, represent the intermediate variant (MGG ×600 oil immersion). **C.** Immunocytochemistry (CD 99/013) shows strong membranous reactivity (Mic 2, IP ×1000 oil).

vacuoles and nuclear moulding (the so-called typical variant)[52] (Fig. 5.14). Less common are tumours with cells having abundant eosinophilic cytoplasm, large nuclei and large eosinophilic nucleoli (atypical or large cell variant). Tumours with features in between, with cells showing abundant cytoplasm, nuclear grooves and medium-sized nucleoli, represent the intermediate variant. Immunocytochemistry (CD99/O13) shows strong membranous reactivity. In addition, cytogenetic [t(11;22)(q24;q12)] and/or molecular evidence of ES/PNET specific chromosomal translocation is demonstrated in histological or cytological material.[51,53–58] Immunocytochemistry with [MIC2 (CD99)] in FNAC smears can provide initial diagnosis and supportive evidence of ES/PNET in patients with known disease.

Olfactory neuroblastoma

Oesthesioneuroblastoma (olfactory neuroblastoma) is a rare malignant neoplasm derived from the olfactory epithelium.[59] Although a rare tumour, it is important to recognise it because it has a better prognosis than the more commonly encountered malignancies of the nose.[60]

Cytomorphological features show a predominance of single cells with intermixed small, loosely cohesive, three-

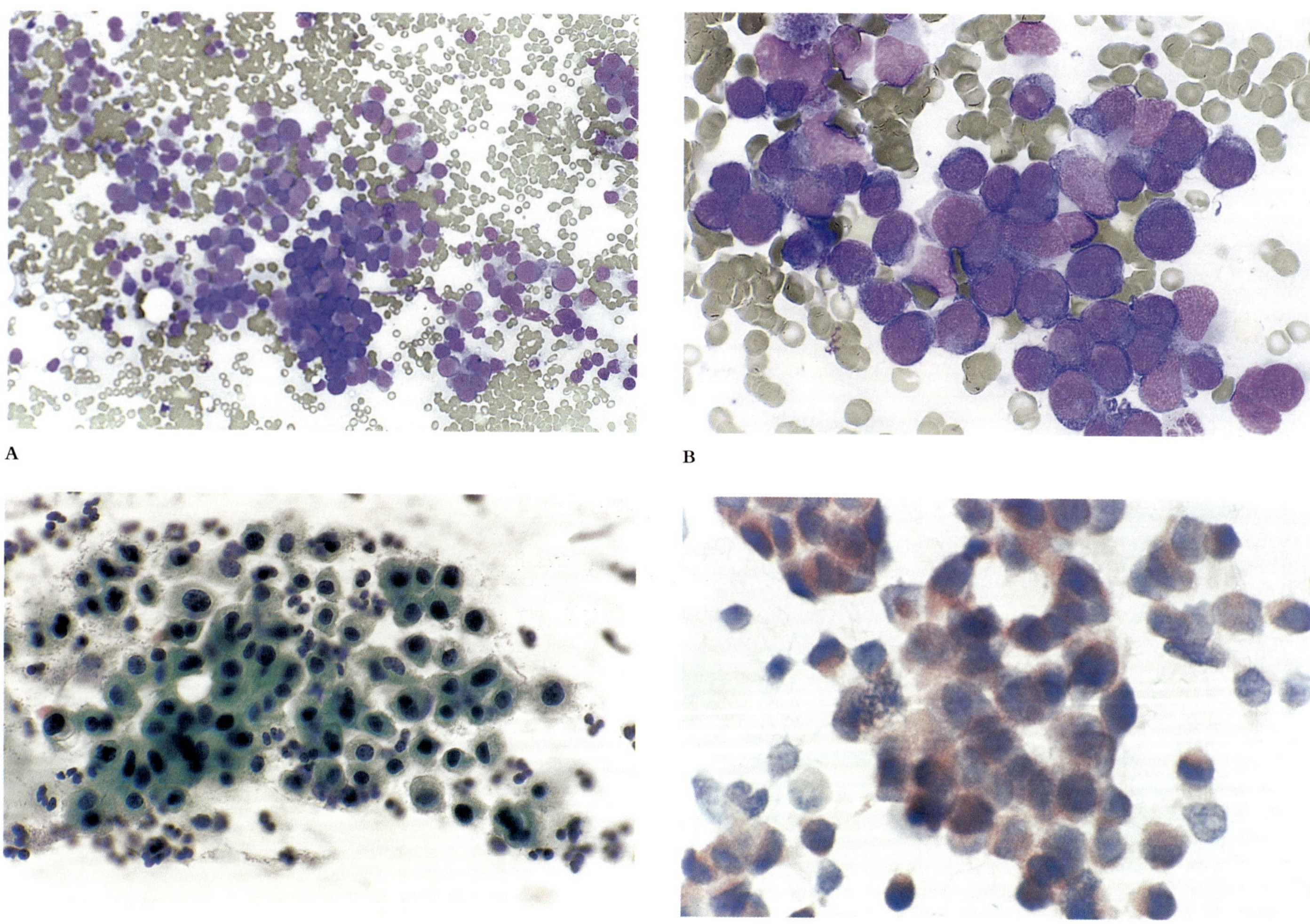

A

B

C

D

Figure 5.15 Olfactory neuroblastoma. **A.** Smears show predominance of single cells with intermixed small, loosely cohesive, three-dimensional cell groups (MGG ×200). **B, C.** Cell size is small to intermediate, with round nuclei. There is an overall monomorphic appearance with minimal nuclear pleomorphism. Chromatin is finely granular and stippled with multiple, small chromocentres. Cytoplasm in the cell groups has a fibrillary quality and is moderate in amount. Single bare nuclei are seen. Occasional pseudorosettes are noted (MGG, PAP ×600 oil immersion). **D.** Immunocytochemical stains are positive for chromogranin (chromogranin, IP ×600).

dimensional cell groups (Fig. 5.15). Cell size is small to intermediate, with round nuclei. There is an overall monomorphic appearance with minimal nuclear pleomorphism. Chromatin is finely granular and stippled, with multiple small chromocentres. Cytoplasm in the cell groups has a fibrillary quality and is moderate in amount. Single bare nuclei are seen. Occasional pseudorosettes are noted.[61] Immunocytochemical stains are positive for chromogranin and synaptophysin. Ultrastructural examination shows neuritic cell processes with neurosecretory, membrane-bound, dense-core granules and microtubules. Immunoelectron microscopy shows positive labelling of neurosecretory granules by chromogranin. FNAC morphology, in combination with ancillary studies, can provide an accurate diagnosis of metastatic olfactory neuroblastoma.[62]

Lymphoma

Lymphoma may present as a tumour of the head and neck and its small round cell features may mimic other similar tumours already described. Cytological and clinical features of lymphomas have been presented in Chapter 4. Occasionally, patients with a known history of lymphoma present with a new mass which needs investigating to exclude other pathology or transformation of the tumour (Fig. 5.16, Fig. 4.44).

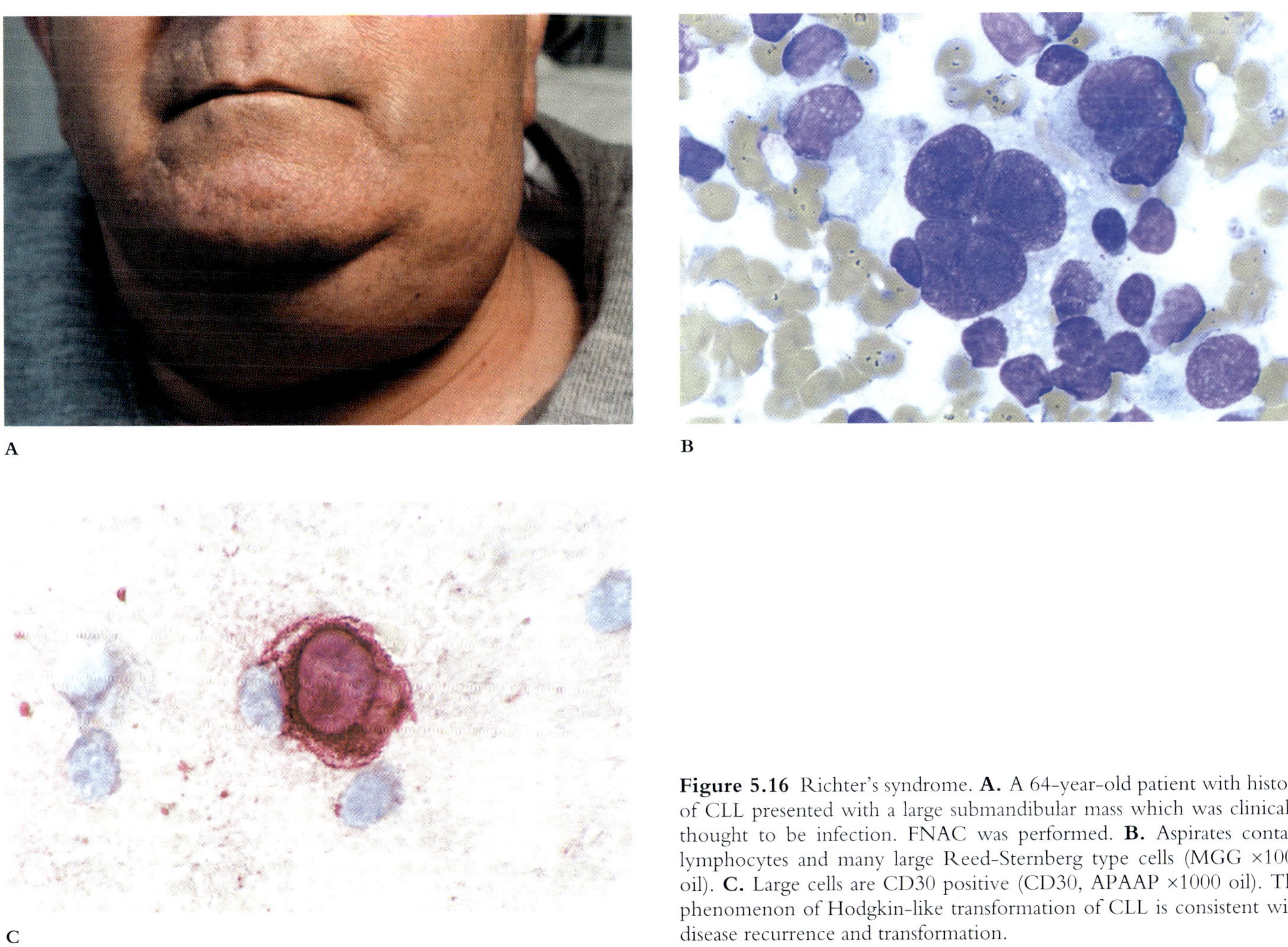

Figure 5.16 Richter's syndrome. **A.** A 64-year-old patient with history of CLL presented with a large submandibular mass which was clinically thought to be infection. FNAC was performed. **B.** Aspirates contain lymphocytes and many large Reed-Sternberg type cells (MGG ×1000 oil). **C.** Large cells are CD30 positive (CD30, APAAP ×1000 oil). The phenomenon of Hodgkin-like transformation of CLL is consistent with disease recurrence and transformation.

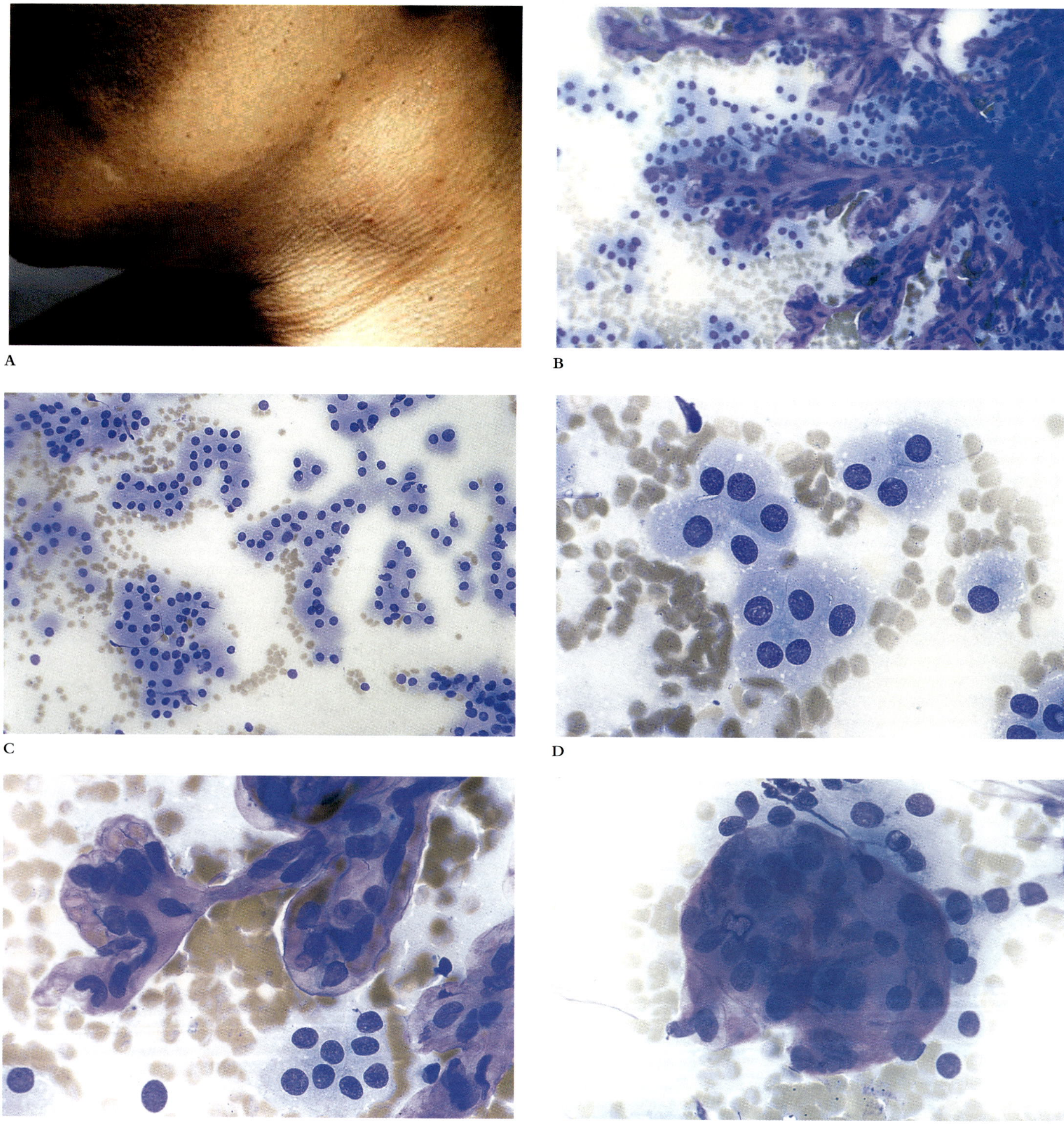

A B C D E F

Figure 5.17 Carotid body tumour. **A.** A 27-year-old woman presented with a 6-month history of swelling in the anterior triangle. The swelling was slow growing, mobile in a horizontal direction, non-tender and did not vary in size. The patient suffered no night sweats, temperatures or any other generalised symptoms. **B.** A strikingly vascular lesion with branching capillary meshwork and delicate pale staining oncocytic cells (MGG ×200). **C.** Oncocytic-type cells in cords and nests look monotonously uniform (MGG ×200). **D.** Cell detail shows round, centrally placed nuclei and abundant dense cytoplasm (MGG ×600 oil). **E.** Detail of capillaries in close proximity to neuroendocrine cells (MGG ×600 oil immersion). **F.** 'Zellballen', aggregate of neuroendocrine cells wrapped in sustentacular cells (MGG ×600 oil immersion).

LOCALLY ARISING MISCELLANEOUS TUMOURS

Carotid body tumours

Carotid body tumours develop from a chemoreceptor organ which is most often located on the medial aspect of the internal carotid artery close to the bifurcation and is embedded in perivascular connective and fatty tissue. It consists of collections of neuroendocrine cells associated with parasympathetic paraganglion. Clinically, carotid body tumours can be moved horizontally but not vertically; they are vascular and may pulsate. They can be found at any age, predominantly in females, and may be bilateral. Patients present with a mass in the neck which may cause symptoms of compression. The tumours are benign generally, although malignant ones have been described. Histologically they are composed of cell nests ('zellballen') surrounded by sustentacular cells and stromal septae. The cells contain neurosecretory granules, are argyrophil, but non-chromaffin and only weakly argentaffin.[63] They stain positively with neuroendocrine markers (synaptophysin, chromogranin).

Cytological features. Aspirates contain clusters and discretely scattered cells, with occasional acinar/rosette configuration. Cells have round to oval nuclei with moderate to marked anisonucleosis, prominent nucleoli, intranuclear inclusions and abundant, delicate, poorly defined, vacuolated, slightly basophilic cytoplasm. Fine, reddish, intracytoplasmic granules are also noted[64–73] (Figs 5.17 and 5.18). A

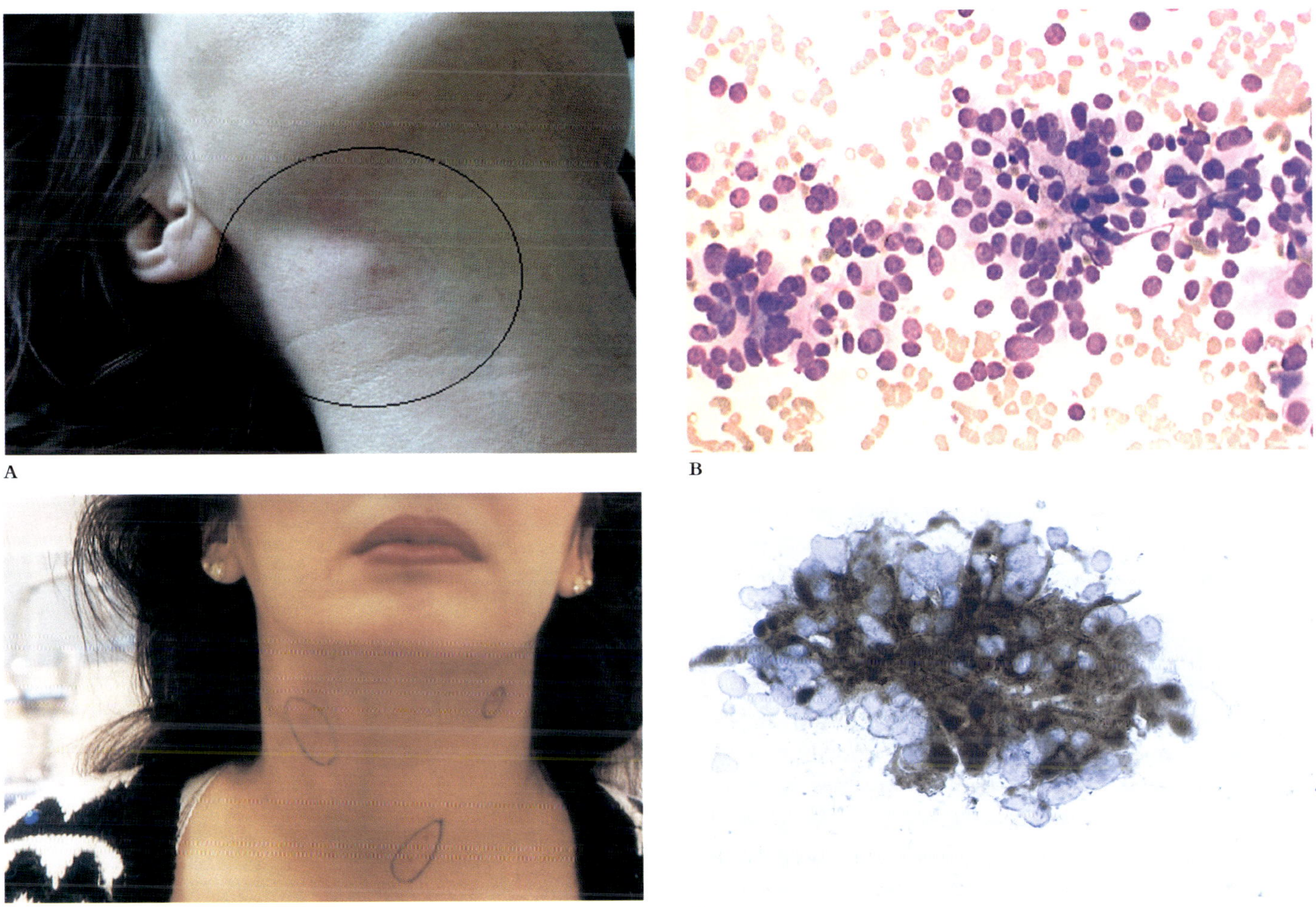

Figure 5.18 Carotid body tumour. **A.** A 34-year-old woman presented with a painless swelling in the right side of the neck. **B.** FNAC revealed clusters and discretely scattered cells, with occasional acinar/rosette configuration. Cells have round to oval nuclei with moderate to marked anisonucleosis, prominent nucleoli, intranuclear inclusions and abundant, delicate, poorly defined, vacuolated, slightly basophilic cytoplasm (MGG ×400, ×600 oil immersion). Examination of the material with rapid stain in the clinic raised the suspicions of an endocrine tumour, in a young woman, possibly metastatic from thyroid. A thorough examination of the neck was performed. **C.** Further examination of the patient revealed enlarged right lobe of thyroid and left jugulodigastric lymph node. Thyroid aspirate showed lymphocytic thyroiditis. Jugulodigastric node was diagnosed as reactive. **D.** Synaptophysin positivity in carotid body tumour cells (IP, ×600 oil).

striking feature of some carotid body tumours may be the presence of capillary endothelium with many spindle-shaped cells mixed and wrapping around the epithelium. Cell pleomorphism, which can be striking and may be misleading, does not imply malignancy. On initial morphological diagnosis, 5 of the 7 paragangliomas diagnosed by Kapila et al[74] were considered malignant (4 undifferentiated and 1 adenocarcinoma) (Fig. 5.19). Malignant carotid body tumours have been found, and the presence of mitoses and necrosis is suspicious of malignancy, but their rarity justifies reporting all carotid body tumours without suggestion of malignancy.[64,75]

Differential diagnosis of aspirates of cervical paragangliomas, which may be difficult to interpret due to poor cellularity especially when intranuclear vacuoles are found, is papillary thyroid carcinoma[76] (see Chapter 3, Figs 3.24 and 3.25).

Angiosarcoma

Angiosarcomas of the head and neck are rare lesions, but they are becoming more common in association with HIV infection. They are usually diagnosed clinically and biopsied for obtaining histological diagnosis. FNAC is likely to be requested to exclude a possible recurrence or metastases in the regional nodes (see Chapter 4, Fig 4.71).

Cytological features. Oval, round and spindle shaped, mainly discohesive malignant cells of variable size ranging from 2 to 9 times the size of red cells (Fig. 5.20). Nuclei are eccentric, round to spindle shaped with large nucleoli or macronucleoli. Cytoplasm is moderate to abundant pale grey and vacuolated (intracytoplasmic lumina). Microacinar structures lined with abnormal spindle-shaped to polygonal cells are noted. Immunohistochemical markers, including

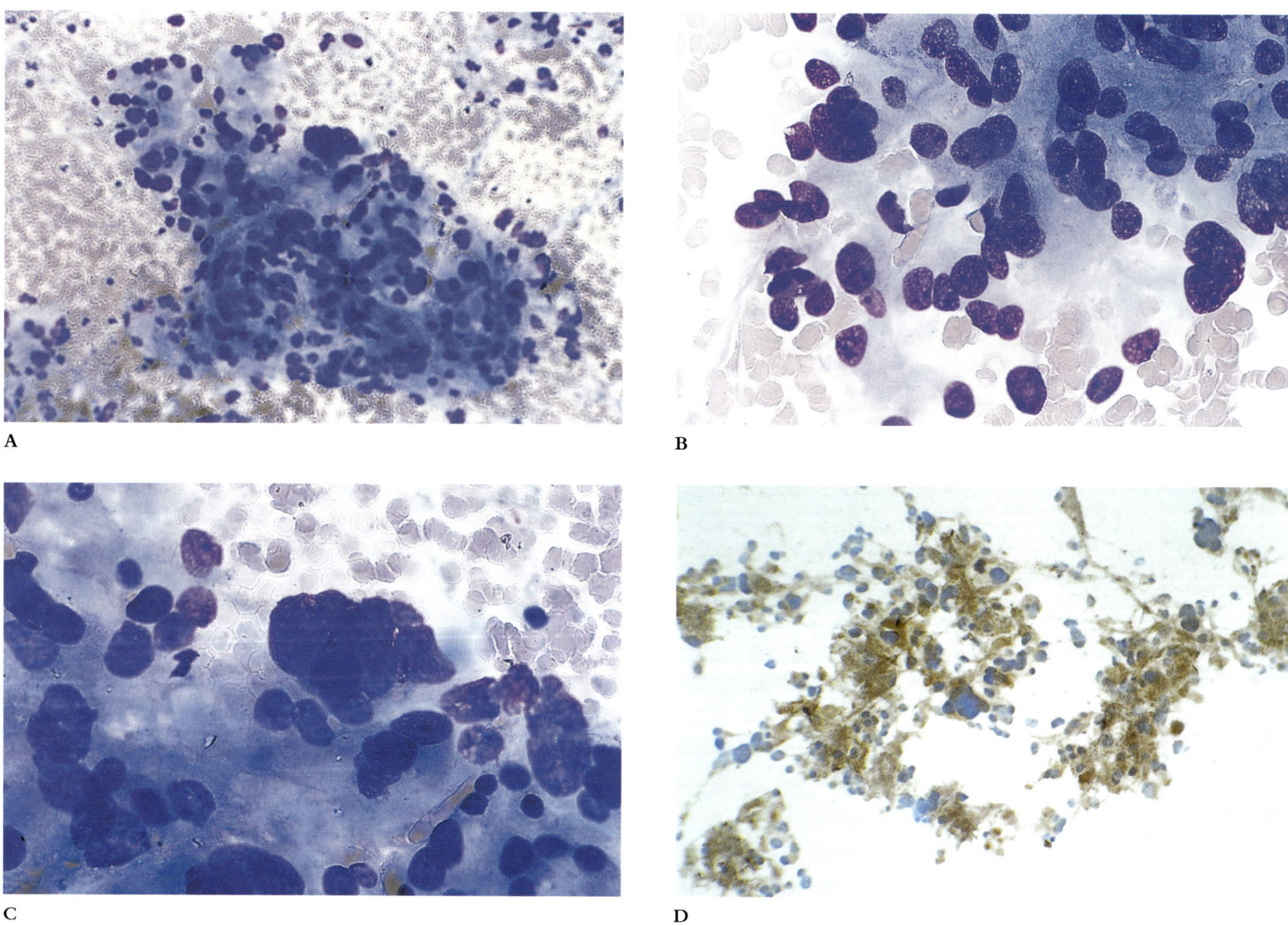

A B C D

Figure 5.19 Carotid body tumour. **A, B, C.** In carotid body tumours, cell pleomorphism, which can be striking and may be misleading, does not imply malignancy. Malignant carotid body tumours have been described; presence of mitoses and necrosis is suspicious, but extremely rare (MGG ×400, ×600, ×1000 oil immersion). **D.** Chromogranin shows strong cytoplasmic staining confirming the neuroendocrine nature of the atypical cells (IP ×400).

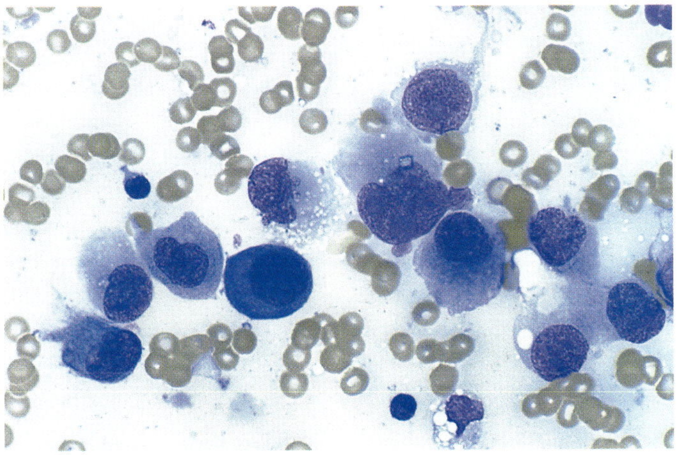

A

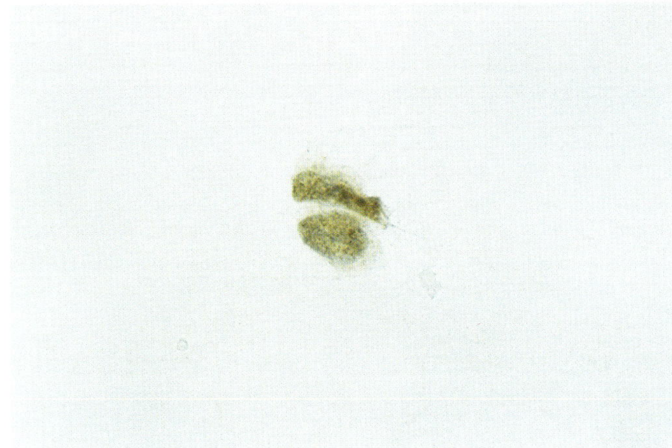

B

Figure 5.20 Angiosarcoma. Patient with a history of angiosarcoma of the scalp treated with radiotherapy. Now, a possibility of further tumour outside the radiation field had to be investigated by FNAC (see Figure. 4.71). **A.** Oval, round and spindle, mainly discohesive malignant cells of variable size ranging from 2–9 times the size of red cells. Nuclei are eccentric, round to spindle shaped with large nucleoli or macronucleoli. Cytoplasm is moderate to abundant pale grey and vacuolated (intracytoplasmic lumina). Microacinar structures lined with abnormal spindle to polygonal cells are noted (MGG ×600 oil). **B.** Immunocytochemistry for KSHV is positive (KS 99 IP ×600 oil).

factor VIII antigen, CD31, CD34 and KSHV, are positive, confirming the vascular origin of the tumour. CAM 5.2 and HMB 45 are negative, ruling out carcinoma and melanoma.[77–84]

Meningioma

Extracranial extension of meningioma, although rare, is an important differential diagnosis of head and neck masses. The cytological appearance of meningioma in smears is very characteristic[85] (Fig. 5.21). Cellular smears present a uniform appearance with cells appearing as cohesive groups and single discohesive cells in a clean background. Cells have round and oval nuclei and poorly outlined cytoplasm. Nuclei have intranuclear vacuoles.[86,87] Chromatin is evenly distributed and nucleoli are not prominent. Psammoma bodies, although characteristic, are not always seen.[88] A specific type of meningioma that produces a highly specific appearance on smear is *secretory meningioma*, which is characterised by numerous large, round cytoplasmic inclusions that dominate the smear. These inclusions are positive for carcinoembryonic antigen (CEA).[89,90] Meningiomas frequently show degenerative changes, usually xanthomatous degeneration, and may contain foamy macrophages. *Fibroblastic meningiomas* may show collagen fibres in the background, which may resemble cell processes. *Atypical meningiomas* are characterised by marked pleomorphism of cells with hyperchromasia and a background of necrosis and haemorrhage.[86,91,92] In difficult cases, intranuclear inclusions help to differentiate meningioma from other tumours and this is a helpful diagnostic feature. Meningiomas are positive for epithelial markers and negative for GFAP (glial fibrillary acid protein). Differential diagnosis in the neck includes soft tissue tumours and metastatic carcinoma.[93,94]

Ethmoid sinus adenocarcinoma

Among malignant neoplasms of the sinonasal tract, tumours of the nasal vault have special features: their higher incidence in woodworkers; their frequent local recurrence; and their invasiveness in the skull base. Histologically, too, they are peculiar by the predominance of the adenocarcinomas, especially of colonic or enteric type. Squamous carcinoma and adenoid cystic carcinoma are less frequent than in other parts of the sinonasal tract. Rare other tumours, often undifferentiated, include esthesioneuroblastomas, malignant melanomas, neuroendocrine carcinomas, malignant lymphomas or sarcomas.[95]

Ethmoid sinus adenocarcinomas have a tendency for extensive local invasion but a low propensity for lymphatic and haematogenous spread. Hence, local recurrence is the main cause of cancer-related death.[96–98] Direct leptomeningeal spread may occur through the cribriform plate to the

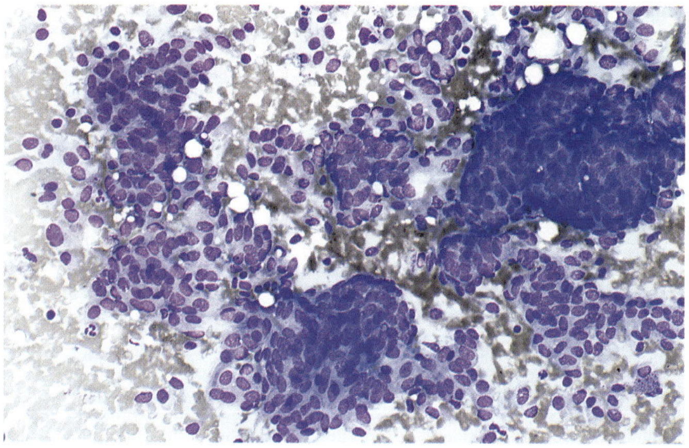

A

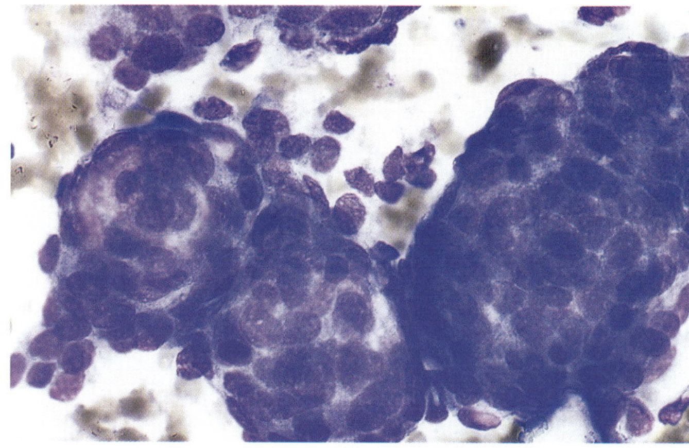

B

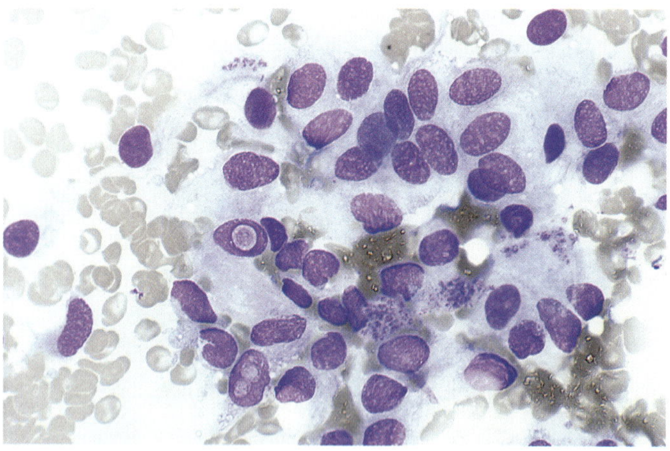

C

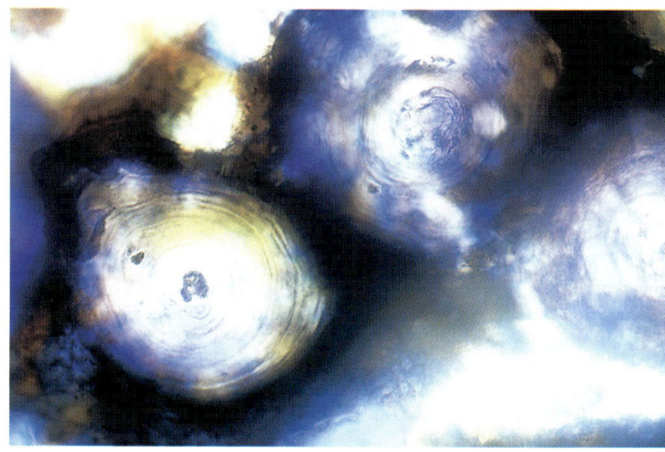

D

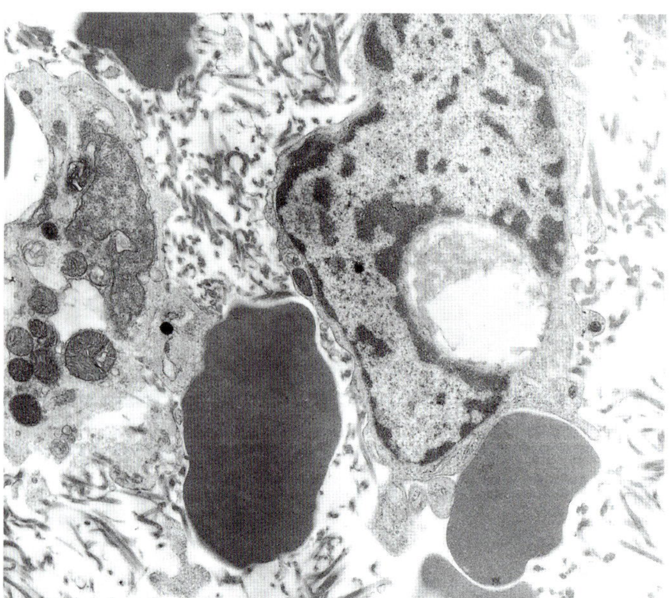

E

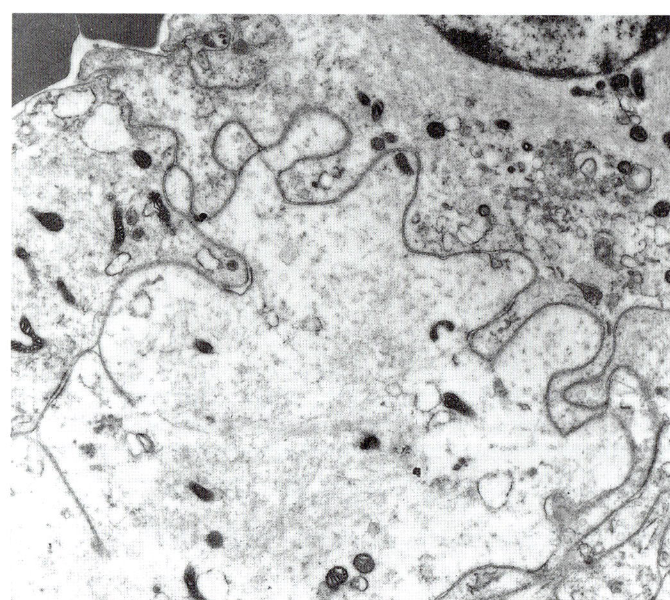

F

Figure 5.21 Meningeoma. A 55-year-old woman with a diffuse hard swelling in the right occipital region and right neck. Hard on palpation. Needle aspirate yields relatively little material which is very cellular. **A.** Cellular smears present a uniform appearance with cells appearing as cohesive groups and single discohesive cells in a clean background (×200, MGG). **B.** Cells appear to form whorls (MGG ×600). **C.** Intranuclear vacuoles are characteristic (MGG ×600, oil). (See **E.**) **D.** Concentric laminations of psammoma bodies. Psammoma bodies, although characteristic, are not always seen (MGG ×600). **E, F.** EM appearances of meningioma show intranuclear vacuoles and numerous cytoplasmic interdigitating process between cells which are attached by desmosomes (×11 200).

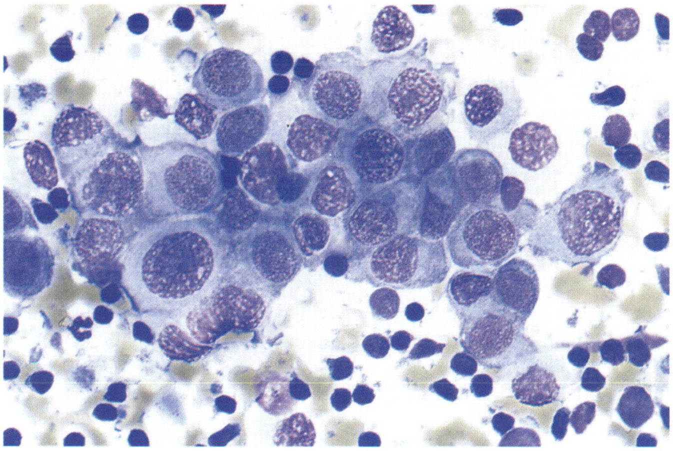

A

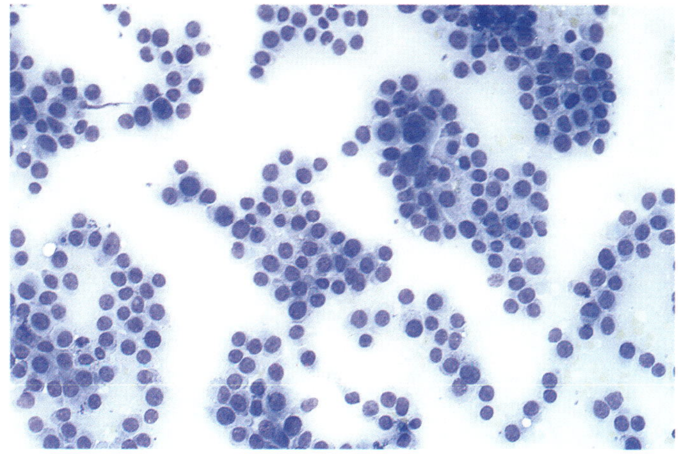

B

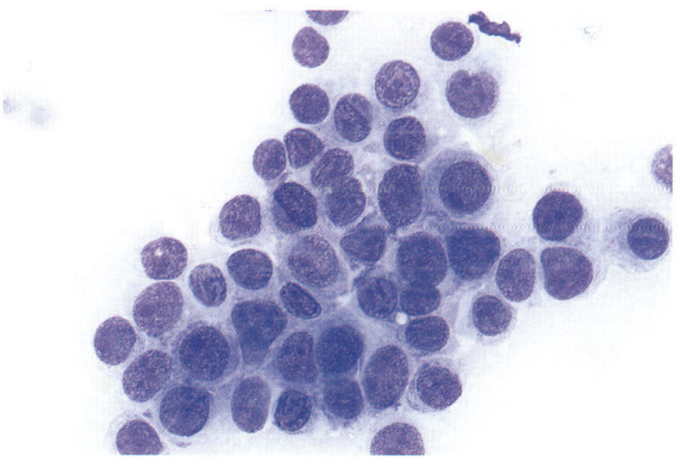

C

Figure 5.22 Ethmoid sinus adenocarcinoma. A 27 year old man presented with a diffuse hard swelling of the cheek. FNAC revealed inflammatory changes only. Biopsy proved an ethmoid sinus carcinoma. Some time later he presented with a submandibular node which was aspirated. **A** Lymph node FNAC showed relatively uniform large cells arranged in aggregates or singly, with medium-sized, eccentric nuclei, prominent nucleoli and a moderate amount of well-defined cytoplasm against a background of lymphocytes (MGG ×600 oil immersion). **B.** Another case. Tumour cells appear arranged in aggregates and chords (MGG ×400). **C.** High-power view of the same tumour. Epithelial cells have high nuclei:cytoplasmic ratio, eccentric nuclei and prominent nucleoli (MGG ×600 oil immersion).

cerebrospinal fluid.[99] Histologically, the low-grade lesions have a well-developed glandular pattern throughout, very uniform nuclei and minimal mitotic activity. The high-grade tumours have a less uniform glandular pattern, commonly with solid or sheet-like areas, manifested nuclear pleomorphism, and generally a higher mitotic rate. The low-grade group has a markedly better prognosis than the high-grade group. Since the literature tends to consider all sinonasal adenocarcinomas as relentlessly progressive neoplasms with poor prognosis, it is important to recognise this category of low-grade neoplasm so that treatment and prognosis can be better related to their behaviour.[100]

Cytological features. Low-grade tumours have relatively uniform large cells arranged in aggregates or singly, with medium-sized eccentric nuclei, prominent nucleoli and a moderate amount of well-defined cytoplasm (Fig. 5.22). Cytological diagnosis is usually made from cervical lymph node metastases in cases of a known primary tumour. Otherwise, differential diagnosis may include any metastatic adenocarcinoma.

REFERENCES

1. Akerman M. *Fine Needle Aspiration Cytopathology*. Oxford: Blackwell Scientific, 1993.
2. Raab SS, Silverman JF, McLeod DL, Benning TL, Geisinger KR. Fine needle aspiration biopsy of fibromatoses. *Acta Cytol* 1993; 37(3): 323–8.
3. Anglo-Henry MR, Seaquist MB, Marsh WL Jr. Fine needle aspiration of proliferative fasciitis. A case report. *Acta Cytol* 1985; 29(5): 882–6.
4. Stanley MW, Skoog L, Tani EM, Horwitz CA. Nodular fasciitis: spontaneous resolution following diagnosis by fine-needle aspiration. *Diagn Cytopathol* 1993; 9(3): 322–4.

5. Dahl I, Akerman M. Nodular fasciitis a correlative cytologic and histologic study of 13 cases. *Acta Cytol* 1981; 25(3): 215–23.

6. Samet A, Podoshin L, Fradis M, Simon J, Lazarov N, Boss H. Unusual sites of schwannoma in the head and neck. *J Laryngol Otol* 1985; 99(5): 523–8.

7. Bianchini E, Mazzolari MG, Squillaci S, Pascale M, Reale D, Micoli G. [Benign intraparotid schwannoma]. *Pathologica* 1990; 82(1079): 303–7.

8. Helidonis E, Dokianakis G, Pantazopoulos P. A schwannoma of the parotid gland. Report of a case. *J Laryngol Otol* 1978; 92(9): 833–8.

9. Kuczkowski J, Jagielski J. [A case of schwannoma in the parotid gland]. *Otolaryngol Pol* 1997; 51(3): 324–7.

10. Jayaraj SM, Levine T, Frosh AC, Almeyda JS. Ancient schwannoma masquerading as parotid pleomorphic adenoma. *J Laryngol Otol* 1997; 111(11): 1088–90.

11. Shah HK, Kantharia C, Shenoy AS. Intraparotid facial nerve schwannoma. *J Postgrad Med* 1997; 43(1): 14–5.

12. Elahi MM, Audet N, Rochon L, Black MJ. Intraparotid facial nerve schwannoma. *J Otolaryngol* 1995; 24(6): 364–7.

13. Avery AP, Sprinkle PM. Benign intraparotid schwannomas. *Laryngoscope* 1972; 82(2): 199–203.

14. Claros P, Knaster J, Weinberg P, Claros A. [Parotid schwannoma]. *Acta Otorrinolaringol Esp* 1994; 45(4): 295–8.

15. Zajicek J. *Aspiration Biopsy Cytology*. Stockholm, Sweden, 1974.

16. Ramos-Gabatin A, Watzinger W. Fine needle aspiration and cytology in the preoperative diagnosis of branchial cyst. *South Med J* 1984; 77(9): 1187–9.

17. Warson F, Blommaert D, De Roy G. Inflamed branchial cyst: a potential pitfall in aspiration cytology [letter]. *Acta Cytol* 1986; 30(2): 201–2.

18. De Las Casas LE, Bardales RH. Fine-needle aspiration cytology of mucous retention cyst of the tongue: distinction from other cystic lesions of the tongue. *Diagn* Cytopathol 2000; 22(5): 308–12.

19. August M, Faquin WC, Ferraro NF, Kaban LB. Fine-needle aspiration biopsy of intraosseous jaw lesions. *J Oral Maxillofac Surg* 1999; 57(11): 1282–6; discussion 1287.

20. Gunhan O, Demirel D, Sengun O, Celasun B, Finci R. Cementifying fibroma diagnosed by fine needle aspiration cytology. A case report. *Acta Cytol* 1992; 36(1): 98–100.

21. Carrillo R, Cuesta C, Rodriguez-Peralto JL, Marin J. Ameloblastic fibroma. Report of a case with fine needle aspiration cytologic findings. *Acta Cytol* 1992; 36(4): 537–40.

22. Gunhan O, Finci R, Celasun B, Demiriz M. A case of ameloblastoma diagnosed by fine-needle aspiration cytology. *J Nihon Univ Sch Dent* 1989; 31(4): 565–9.

23. Layfield LJ, Ferreiro JA. Fine-needle aspiration cytology of chondromyxoid fibroma: a case report. *Diagn Cytopathol* 1988; 4(2): 148–51.

24. Gunhan O, Dogan N, Celasun B, Sengun O, Onder T, Finci R. Fine needle aspiration cytology of oral cavity and jaw bone lesions. A report of 102 cases. *Acta Cytol* 1993; 37(2): 135–41.

25. DeRaimo AJ, Kane RA, Katz JF, Rolla AP. Parathyroid cyst: diagnosis by sonography and needle aspiration. *AJR Am J Roentgenol* 1984; 142(6): 1227–8.

26. Patel KD, Rege JD, Varthakavi PK, Desai SA, Nihalani KD. Fine needle aspiration of an unsuspected parathyroid cyst. *J Assoc Physicians India* 1995; 43(11): 791.

27. Shepard KA, Miller JD. Cervical thymic cyst. A consideration in the differential diagnosis of neck masses. *J Maine Med Assoc* 1973; 64(1): 3–4.

28. Engzell U, Zajicek J. Aspiration biopsy of tumors of the neck. I. Aspiration biopsy and cytologic findings in 100 cases of congenital cysts. *Acta Cytol* 1970; 14(2): 51–7.

29. Frierson HF Jr. Cysts of the head and neck sampled by fine-needle aspiration: sources of diagnostic difficulty [editorial, comment]. *Am J Clin Pathol* 1996; 106(5): 559–60.

30. Ravinsky E, Safneck JR, Quinonez G, Yazdi HM. Fine needle aspiration biopsy of a small round cell tumor exhibiting both neural and myogenic differentiation. A case report. *Acta Cytol* 1997; 41(4 suppl): 1320–4.

31. Kilpatrick SE, Ward WG, Chauvenet AR, Pettenati MJ. The role of fine-needle aspiration biopsy in the initial diagnosis of pediatric bone and soft tissue tumors: an institutional experience. *Mod Pathol* 1998; 11(10): 923–8.

32. Powers CN, Berardo MD, Frable WJ. Fine-needle aspiration biopsy: pitfalls in the diagnosis of spindle-cell lesions. *Diagn Cytopathol* 1994; 10(3): 232–40, discussion 241.

33. BJ OH, Ehya H, Shields JA, Augsburger JJ, Shields CL, Eagle RC Jr. Fine needle aspiration biopsy in pediatric ophthalmic tumors and pseudotumors. *Acta Cytol* 1993; 37(2): 125–30.

34. Akhtar M, Ali MA, Sabbah R, Bakry M, Nash JE. Fine-needle aspiration biopsy diagnosis of round cell malignant tumors of childhood. A combined light and electron microscopic approach. *Cancer* 1985; 55(8): 1805–17.

35. De Lutiis MA, Pizzicannella G, Artese L. Embryonal rhabdomyosarcoma of the eye: cytological diagnosis by fine needle aspiration. *Pathologica* 1991; 83(1083): 75–9.

36. Salomao DR, Sigman JD, Greenebaum E, Cohen MB. Rhabdomyosarcoma presenting as a parotid gland mass in pediatric patients: fine-needle aspiration biopsy findings. *Cancer* 1998; 84(4): 245–51.

37. de Almeida M, Stastny JF, Wakely PE Jr, Frable WJ. Fine-needle aspiration biopsy of childhood rhabdomyosarcoma: reevaluation of the cytologic criteria for diagnosis. *Diagn Cytopathol* 1994; 11(3): 231–6.

38. Akhtar M, Ali MA, Bakry M, Hug M, Sackey K. Fine-needle aspiration biopsy diagnosis of rhabdomyosarcoma: cytologic, histologic, and ultrastructural correlations. *Diagn Cytopathol* 1992; 8(5): 465–74.

39. Henkes DN, Stein N. Fine-needle aspiration cytology of prostatic embryonal rhabdomyosarcoma: a case report. *Diagn Cytopathol* 1987; 3(2): 163–5.

40. Mazzoleni S, Stellini E, Infantolino D, Favero GA. A case of embryonal rhabdomyosarcoma of the cheek in adolescence. Its cytological diagnosis by fine-needle aspiration via the gingival fornix. *Minerva Stomatol* 1994; 43(1–2): 43–7.

41. Kumar PV, Kazemi H, Khezri A. Testicular embryonal rhabdomyosarcoma diagnosed by fine needle aspiration cytology. A report of two cases. *Acta Cytol* 1994; 38(4): 573–6.

42. Seidal T, Walaas L, Kindblom LG, Angervall L. Cytology of embryonal rhabdomyosarcoma: a cytologic, light microscopic, electron microscopic, and immunohistochemical study of seven cases. *Diagn Cytopathol* 1988; 4(4): 292–9.

43. Agarwal PK, Srivastava A, Mathur N, Pant MC, Agarwal S. Fine needle aspiration of poorly differentiated rhabdomyosarcoma presenting with quadriparesis. A case report. *Acta Cytol* 1996; 40(5): 985–8.

44. Nishikawa A, Tanaka T, Kanai N, Kato K, Mori H, Takahashi M. Exfoliative cytopathology of alveolar rhabdomyosarcoma. *Acta Pathol Jpn* 1987; 37(6): 1003–7.

45. Torres V, Ferrer R. Cytology of fine needle aspiration biopsy of primary breast rhabdomyosarcoma in an adolescent girl. *Acta Cytol* 1985; 29(3): 430–4.

46. Atahan S, Aksu O, Ekinci C. Cytologic diagnosis and subtyping of rhabdomyosarcoma. *Cytopathology* 1998; 9(6): 389–97.

47. Kushner BH, LaQuaglia MP, Cheung NK et al. Clinically critical impact of molecular genetic studies in pediatric solid tumors. *Med Pediatr Oncol* 1999; 33(6): 530–5.

48. Dias P, Chen B, Dilday B et al. Strong immunostaining for myogenin in rhabdomyosarcoma is significantly associated with tumors of the alveolar subclass. *Am J Pathol* 2000; 156(2): 399–408.

49. Kempf BE, Vogt PK. A genetic analysis of PAX3-FKHR, the oncogene of alveolar rhabdomyosarcoma. *Cell Growth Differ* 1999; 10(12): 813–8.

50. Bakhos R, Andrey J, Bhoopalam N, Jensen J, Reyes CV. Fine-needle aspiration cytology of extraskeletal Ewing's sarcoma. *Diagn Cytopathol* 1998; 18(2): 137–40.

51. Collins BT, Cramer HM, Frain BE, Davis MM. Fine-needle aspiration biopsy of metastatic Ewing's sarcoma with MIC2 (CD99) immunocytochemistry. *Diagn Cytopathol* 1998; 19(5): 382–4.

52. Cohen MC, Pollono D, Tomarchio SA, Drut R. Cytologic characteristics of peripheral neuroectodermal tumors in fine-needle aspiration smears: a retrospective study of three pediatric cases. *Diagn Cytopathol* 1997; 16(6): 513–7.

53. Guiter GE, Gamboni MM, Zakowski MF. The cytology of extraskeletal Ewing sarcoma. *Cancer* 1999; 87(3): 141–8.

54. Renshaw AA, Perez-Atayde AR, Fletcher JA, Granter SR. Cytology of typical and atypical Ewing's sarcoma/PNET. *Am J Clin Pathol* 1996; 106(5): 620–4.

55. Kontozoglou T, Krakauer K, Qizilbash AH. Ewing's sarcoma. Cytologic features in fine needle aspirates in two cases. *Acta Cytol* 1986; 30(5): 513–18.

56. Dahl I, Akerman M, Angervall L. Ewing's sarcoma of bone. A correlative cytological and histological study of 14 cases. *Acta Pathol Microbiol Immunol Scand [A]* 1986; 94(6): 363–9.

57. Brehaut LE, Anderson LH, Taylor DA. Extraskeletal Ewing's sarcoma. Diagnosis of a case by fine needle aspiration cytology. *Acta Cytol* 1986; 30(6): 683–7.

58. Meister P, Gokel JM. Extraskeletal Ewing's sarcoma. *Virchows Arch A Pathol Anat Histopathol* 1978; 378(2): 173–9.

59. Jelen M, Wozniak Z, Rak J. Cytologic appearance of esthesioneuroblastoma in a fine needle aspirate. *Acta Cytol* 1988; 32(3): 377–80.

60. Jobst SB, Ljung BM, Gilkey FN, Rosenthal DL. Cytologic diagnosis of olfactory neuroblastoma. Report of a case with multiple diagnostic parameters. *Acta Cytol* 1983; 27(3): 299–305.

61. Collins BT, Cramer HM, Hearn SA. Fine needle aspiration cytology of metastatic olfactory neuroblastoma. *Acta Cytol* 1997; 41(3): 802–10.

62. Logrono R, Futoran RM, Hartig G, Inhorn SL. Olfactory neuroblastoma (esthesioneuroblastoma): appearance on fine-needle aspiration: report of a case. *Diagn Cytopathol* 1997; 17(3): 205–8.

63. Buley I. *Diagnostic Cytopathology*. London: Churchill Livingstone, 1995.

64. Fleming MV, Oertel YC, Rodriguez ER, Fidler WJ. Fine-needle aspiration of six carotid body paragangliomas. *Diagn Cytopathol* 1993; 9(5): 510–15.

65. Mincione GP, Urso C. Carotid body paraganglioma (chemodectoma): cytologic remarks. *Pathologica* 1989; 81(1072): 179–83.

66. Engzell U, Franzen S, Zajicek J. Aspiration biopsy of tumors of the neck. II. Cytologic findings in 13 cases of carotid body tumor. *Acta Cytol* 1971; 15(1): 25–30.

67. Papanicolaou S, Daskalopoulos Z. Carotid body tumor: report of a case. *J Oral Med* 1986; 41(3): 204–6, 209.

68. Nickel AA Jr, Roser SM. Carotid body tumors. *J Oral Med* 1977; 32(3): 64–6.

69. Krishnamurthy SC, Gopinath KS, Rao RS, Talvalkar GV. Carotid body tumour – a clinicopathologic study of 10 cases. *Indian J Cancer* 1981; 18(4): 245–9.

70. Kapoor R, Saha MM, Das DK, Gupta AK, Tyagi S. Carotid body tumor initially diagnosed by fine needle aspiration cytology [letter]. *Acta Cytol* 1989; 33(5): 682–3.

71. Chen LT, Hwang WS. Fine needle aspiration of carotid body paraganglioma [letter]. *Acta Cytol* 1989; 33(5): 681–2.

72. Mincione G, Urso C. Fine needle aspiration cytologic findings in a case of carotid body paraganglioma (chemodectoma) [letter]. *Acta Cytol* 1989; 33(5): 679–81.

73. Rana RS, Dey P, Das A. Fine needle aspiration (FNA) cytology of extra-adrenal paragangliomas. *Cytopathology* 1997; 8(2): 108–13.

74. Kapila K, Tewari MC, Verma K. Paragangliomas – a diagnostic dilemma on fine needle aspirates. *Indian J Cancer* 1993; 30(4). 152–7.

75. Rao KS, Prasad AS, Rao AS. Malignant carotid body tumour. *Indian J Pathol Bacteriol* 1968; 11(3): 207–9.

76. Jacobs DM, Waisman J. Cervical paraganglioma with intranuclear vacuoles in a fine needle aspirate. *Acta Cytol* 1987; 31(1): 29–32.

77. Gupta RK, Naran S, Dowle C. Needle aspiration cytology and immunocytochemical study in a case of angiosarcoma of the breast. *Diagn Cytopathol* 1991; 7(4): 363–5.

78. Liu K, Layfield LJ. Cytomorphologic features of angiosarcoma on fine needle aspiration biopsy. *Acta Cytol* 1999; 43(3): 407–15.

79. Cho NH, Lee KG, Jeong MG. Cytologic evaluation of primary malignant vascular tumors of the liver. One case each of angiosarcoma and epithelioid hemangioendothelioma. *Acta Cytol* 1997; 41(5): 1468–76.

80. Vesoulis Z, Cunliffe C. Fine-needle aspiration biopsy of postradiation epithelioid angiosarcoma of breast. *Diagn Cytopathol* 2000; 22(3): 172–5.

81. Carson KF, Hirschowitz SL, Nieberg RK, Sadeghi S. Pitfalls in the cytologic diagnosis of angiosarcoma of the breast by fine-needle aspiration: a case report. *Diagn Cytopathol* 1994; 11(3): 297–9, discussion 299–300.

82. Layfield LJ, Dodd LG. Cytologic findings in a case of postirradiation angiosarcoma of the breast [letter]. *Acta Cytol* 1997; 41(2): 612–14.

83. Parsi B, Dilhuydy MH, Leger F et al. [Cytologic diagnosis of breast angiosarcoma]. *Arch Anat Cytol Pathol* 1989; 37(5–6): 231–4.

84. Nguyen GK, McHattie JD, Jeannot A. Cytomorphologic aspects of hepatic angiosarcoma. Fine needle aspiration biopsy of a case. *Acta Cytol* 1982; 26(4): 527–31.

85. Nguyen GK, Johnson ES, Mielke BW. Cytology of meningiomas and neurilemomas in crush preparations. A useful adjunct to frozen section diagnosis. *Acta Cytol* 1988; 32(3): 362–6.

86. Vogelsang PJ, Nguyen GK, Mielke BW. Cytology of atypical and malignant meningiomas in intraoperative crush preparations. *Acta Cytol* 1993; 37(6): 884–8.

87. Janisch W, Schreiber D. Morphological findings in the cell nuclei of meningiomas and neurinomas. *Zentralbl Allg Pathol* 1965; 108(3): 268–76.

88. Cerda-Nicolas M, Piquer J, Peydro A, Barcia C, Barcia JL. Cytology of meningiomas. Morphological study of 23 cases. Correlation with the histopathology. *Arch Neurobiol (Madr)* 1988; 51(6): 342–8.

89. Hinton DR, Kovacs K, Chandrasoma PT. Cytologic features of secretory meningioma. *Acta Cytol* 1999; 43(2): 121–5.

90. Imlay SP, Snider TE, Raab SS. Clear-cell meningioma: diagnosis by fine-needle aspiration biopsy. *Diagn Cytopathol* 1998; 18(2): 131–6.

91. Maier H, Ofner D, Hittmair A, Kitz K, Budka H. Classic, atypical, and anaplastic meningioma: three histopathological subtypes of clinical relevance. *J Neurosurg* 1992; 77(4): 616–23.

92. Riazmontazer N, Bedayat G. Cytodiagnosis of meningioma with atypical cytologic features. *Acta Cytol* 1991; 35(5): 501–4.

93. Kobayashi S. Meningioma, neurilemmoma and astrocytoma specimens obtained with the squash method for cytodiagnosis. A cytologic and immunochemical study [see comments]. *Acta Cytol* 1993; 37(6): 913–22.

94. Kudo M, Mikami T, Maeda Y. Reticulin fiber staining of crush preparations for the rapid differentiation between schwannomas and meningiomas. *Acta Cytol* 1991; 35(5): 521–3.

95. Carnot F. [Histological aspects of naso-ethmoidal tumours]. *Neurochirurgie* 1997; 43(2): 64–7.

96. Gaillard J, Haguenauer JP, Pignat JC, Long C. Plurifocality and concept of recurrence in ethmoido-nasal glandular cancers. *Rev Laryngol Otol Rhinol (Bord)* 1988; 109(1): 31–3.

97. Jiang GL, Morrison WH, Garden AS et al. Ethmoid sinus carcinomas: natural history and treatment results. *Radiother Oncol* 1998; 49(1): 21–7.

98. Harbo G, Grau C, Bundgaard T et al. Cancer of the nasal cavity and paranasal sinuses. A clinico-pathological study of 277 patients. *Acta Oncol* 1997; 36(1): 45–50.

99. Devos A, Lemmerling M, Vanrietvelde F et al. Leptomeningeal metastases from ethmoid sinus adenocarcinoma: clinico-radiological correlation. *JBR-BTR* 1999; 82(6): 285–7.

100. Heffner DK, Hyams VJ, Hauck KW, Lingeman C. Low-grade adenocarcinoma of the nasal cavity and paranasal sinuses. *Cancer* 1982; 50(2): 312–22.

Index

A

acinic cell carcinoma 45–7
  cytological features 45, 46
  diagnostic difficulties 13
  differential diagnosis 45, 47
  paediatric lesions 69
adenocarcinoma not otherwise specified, salivary gland 62
adenoid cystic carcinoma, salivary gland 50–4
  basal cell adenoma differentiation 40–1
  cytological features 50, 51, 52, 53
  diagnostic difficulties 13
  differential diagnosis 52–3
  FNAC diagnostic accuracy 54
  myoepithelial differentiation 53
  pleomorphic adenoma differentiation 50–2
adenolymphoma, salivary gland (Warthin's tumour) 12, 31, 37–40
  crystalloid structures 25
  cytological features 37–9
  incidence 15
  lymphoid cells 39–40
  malignant transformation 40
  oncocytic change 39
  squamous metaplasia 39
AIDS *see* HIV infection/AIDS
alpha-1-antichymotrypsin 127
alpha-lactalbumin 61
alpha-smooth muscle actin 53, 54, 61
alveolar rhabdomyosarcoma 193
anaplastic carcinoma, thyroid gland 84, 109–10
  immunohistochemistry 110
anaplastic large cell lymphoma 122, 149, 167–70
  cutaneous type 167, 169
  cytological features 168, 169
  immunophenotype 169–70
  systemic type 167, 169
ancillary techniques
  lymphoma 149–50
  salivary gland lesions 15
angiosarcoma 198–9
anticonvulsant drug-related lymphadenopathy 138
antimalarials, hypersensitive lymphadenopathy 138
artefacts 6
aspiration technique 4
atypical meningioma 199
atypical mycobacterial infection 128, 129, 138

B

B-cell lymphoma 122, 152–64
  clonality 122, 123
  comparative cytomorphology 153
  molecular genetic analysis 123
  small lymphocytic 152–3
bacterial culture 6
basal cell adenocarcinoma, salivary gland 56–8
basal cell adenoma, salivary gland 40
  adenoid cystic carcinoma differentiation 40–1
bcl-1 123, 155
bcl-2 123, 156
bcl-6 156
benign mixed salivary gland tumour 15
benign nerve sheath tumour 187–8
  salivary gland 66, 67
benign soft tissue lesions 185–8
Ber-EP4 61
berylliosis 129
Birbeck granules 143
branchial cyst 3, 189, 190
  salivary gland 20
brucellosis 129
Burkitt's lymphoma 149, 162–4
  cytological features 163
  immunophenotype 163–4

C

C-cell hyperplasia, thyroid medullary carcinoma differentiation 109
C-erbB2 61
calcitonin 99, 109
CALLA *see* CD10
calponin 53, 54, 61
Cameco syringe 5, 14
Candida sialadenitis 26
capillary sampling technique 4
carbamazepine-related lymphadenopathy 138
carcinoembryonic antigen 61, 199
carcinoma ex pleomorphic adenoma 37, 62, 64
carcinomatous salivary duct obstruction 25
carotid body tumour 3, 196, 197–8
  neuroendocrine markers 197
Castleman's disease 138, 140, 141
  immunohistochemistry 140
cat scratch disease 129, 131–2
CD1a (leu 6) 143, 165
CD2 165
CD3 152, 165
CD4 165
CD5 123
  diffuse large-cell lymphoma 159
  lymphocytic lymphoma 152, 153
  mantle zone lymphoma 154, 155
  T cell lymphoma 165
CD7 165
CD8 165
CD10 (CALLA) 123
  Burkitt's lymphoma 163
  diffuse large-cell lymphoma 159
  follicular lymphoma 156
  lymphoblastic leukaemia/lymphoma 152
CD15
  Hodgkin's cells 147
  Reed-Sternberg cells 145
CD19
  Burkitt's lymphoma 163
  diffuse large-cell lymphoma 159
  follicular lymphoma 156
  lymphoblastic leukaemia/lymphoma 152
  lymphocytic lymphoma 152
  lymphoplasmacytic lymphoma (immunocytoma) 153
  mantle zone lymphoma 155
CD20
  Burkitt's lymphoma 163
  diffuse large-cell lymphoma 159
  follicular lymphoma 156
  Hodgkin's cells 147
  L&H cells 148
  lymphoblastic leukaemia/lymphoma 152
  lymphocytic lymphoma 152
  lymphoplasmacytic lymphoma (immunocytoma) 153
  mantle zone lymphoma 155
CD21 124, 125
CD22
  Burkitt's lymphoma 163
  diffuse large-cell lymphoma 159
  follicular lymphoma 156
  lymphoplasmacytic lymphoma (immunocytoma) 153
  mantle zone lymphoma 155
CD23 123
  lymphocytic lymphoma 152, 153
CD30
  anaplastic large cell lymphoma 167, 168, 169
  Hodgkin's cells 147
  L&H cells 146, 148
  Reed-Sternberg cells 145

CD30-positive lymphoproliferative conditions of skin 167
CD31 199
CD34 199
CD44 86, 105
CD45 (LCA)
  anaplastic large cell lymphoma 169
  diffuse large-cell lymphoma 159
  Hodgkin's cells 147
  L&H cells 146, 148
  lymphoblastic leukaemia/lymphoma 152
CD57 (HNK-1)
  L&H cells 148
  thyroid papillary carcinoma 105
CD79a
  Burkitt's lymphoma 163
  diffuse large-cell lymphoma 159
  follicular lymphoma 156
  lymphocytic lymphoma 152
  lymphoplasmacytic lymphoma (immunocytoma) 153
  mantle zone lymphoma 155
CD99/O13 194
CDw75 (LN1) 146
centroblastic lymphoma *see* diffuse large-cell lymphoma
cervical thymic cyst 190
chromogranin 109, 197
clinic organisation 7
clinical history 3
cMYC 164
collagenous fibroma, salivary gland 44
colloid (multinodular non-toxic) goitre 84, 85, 87–90
  adenoma/adenomatous nodule 88
  cysts 90, 91
  cytological features 88–9, 90
  degenerative changes 89, 90, 91, 92
  diagnostic evaluation 87
  management strategy 87–8
  psammoma bodies 89, 90
composite lymphoma 149
consulting room 3
cost effectiveness 14, 84, 85
cryptococcosis 132, 133, 138
cutaneous B-cell lymphoma 159, 160
cutaneous T-cell lymphoma 167
cyclin D1 155
cystadenoma, salivary gland 44
cystic lesions
  goitre 84, 85
  head and neck 188–91
  salivary gland 12, 17–22, 27
cystic lymphoid hyperplasia, salivary gland 27
cytomegalovirus sialadenitis 26
cytopathologist 7, 8
cytopathology report 7

D

De Quervain's thyroiditis 93
dermatopathic lymphadenopathy 127
dermoid cyst, salivary gland 22
diffuse large-cell lymphoma 149, 159, 160, 161
  cytological features 159, 160, 161
  immunophenotype 159
  WHO classification 159
DNA content evaluation
  lymphoma 150
  salivary gland tumours 44–5
    basal cell adenocarcinoma 58
drug-related lymphadenopathy 138
Dutcher bodies 153

E

embryonal rhabdomyosarcoma 192, 193
emperipolesis (lymphophagocytosis) 127
eosinophilic granuloma 141
epidermoid cyst 3, 190, 191
epithelial membrane antigen 61, 146, 169
epithelial-myoepithelial carcinoma, salivary gland 54–6
  cytological features 54, 55, 56
  differential diagnosis 56
  smooth muscle-specific protein immunohistochemistry 53, 54
Epstein-Barr virus 66, 136, 143, 147, 161
ethmoid sinus adenocarcinoma 199, 201
extraskeletal Ewing's sarcoma 193–4
  immunohistochemistry 194

F

factor VIII antigen 199
fibroblastic meningioma 199
fibromatosis colli 186
fine needle aspiration cytology 3–8
  clinical history 3
  material preparation 5–6
  physical examination 3–4
  procedure 4–5
flow cytometry 3
  Castleman's disease 140
  lymphoma 122–3, 149
    clonality analysis 122–3
  post-transplant lymphoproliferative disorder 143–4
  salivary gland tumours 44–5
  thyroid papillary carcinoma 105
follicle centre lymphoma 149
follicular adenoma, thyroid gland 96, 97–8
  atypical 97
  cytological features 98
follicular carcinoma, thyroid gland 106–7
  clear cell variant 106
  cytological features 106–7
  Hürthle cell variant 106
  insular variant 107
follicular hyperplasia, lymph node 124–6
  cytological features 124, 125, 126
  immunohistochemistry 124, 125
  lymphoma differentiation 124, 126
  progressive transformation of germinal centres 124
follicular lymphoma 123, 148, 156, 157
  immunophenotype 156
  WHO classification 155
frozen section histology
  salivary gland lesions 13–14
  thyroid lesions 86
fungal lymphadenitis 129, 132

G

galectin-3 86
GCDFP-15 61
glandular fever (infectious mononucleosis) 136–7
goitre 87–93
  colloid (multinodular non-toxic) 84, 85, 87–90
  hyperactive 90, 92, 93, 94
granulocytic sarcoma, salivary gland 68
granulomatous lymphadenitis 127–35
  mycobacterial infection 127–9
granulomatous sialadenitis 25–6
granulomatous thyroiditis 93, 94
Grave's disease 90

H

haemangioma, salivary gland 69
haemangiopericytoma, salivary gland 68
Hand Schüller-Christian syndrome 141
Hashimoto's thyroiditis *see* lymphocytic thyroiditis
HBME-1 86, 105
heavy chain gene rearrangements 123, 124
  diffuse large-cell lymphoma 159
  marginal zone (MALT type) lymphoma 159
  post-transplant lymphoproliferative disorder 144
hepatitis C 27
histiocytosis X *see* Langerhans' cell histiocytosis
histoplasmosis 132, 138
  sialadenitis 26
HIV infection/AIDS
  angiosarcoma association 198
  FNAC-detected infections 138
  lymph node mass FNAC 138
  mycobacterial granulomatous lymphadenitis 128–9
  persistent generalised lymphadenopathy 136–8, 139
  salivary gland pathology 22
  salivary lymphoepithelial cyst 18, 20, 27
    p24 marker 19
HLA DR 143
HNK-1 *see* CD57
Hodgkin's cells 146, 147
Hodgkin's lymphoma 122, 145–8
  cell phenotype 145
  classification 145
  cytological diagnosis 147
  diagnostic difficulties 147–8
  granulomatous reactions 129
  Hodgkin's cells 146, 147
  L&H (lymphocytic and histiocytic) cells 145–6, 148
  lymphocyte depletion type 145
  lymphocyte-rich type 145
  mixed cellularity type 145
  nodular lymphocyte predominance type 145–6, 148
  nodular sclerosis type 145, 148
  Reed-Sternberg cells 145, 146, 147
  role of FNAC in management 149
human herpesvirus-8 140, 161, 170
human T-lymphotropic virus-1 (HTLV-1)-associated T cell lymphoma 165, 166

Hürthle cell tumour 85
adenoma 98
carcinoma 98
papillary with lymphoplasmacytic stroma 103–4
hyalinising trabecular adenoma, thyroid gland 84, 97, 98–9
immunohistochemistry 99
hydantoin-induced lymphadenopathy 138, 140
hyperthyroidism, hyperactive goitre 90

I

immunocytochemistry 3, 6
immunocytoma *see* lymphoplasmacytic lymphoma
immunoglobulin-negative malignant lymphoma 149
immunohistochemistry
anaplastic thyroid carcinoma 110
Castleman's disease 140
follicular hyperplasia 124, 125
lymphomas 122
medullary thyroid carcinoma 109
mucoepidermoid salivary gland carcinoma 50
myoepithelial differentiation in salivary gland tumours 53
myoepithelioma, salivary gland 44
oncocytoma 41
papillary thyroid carcinoma 105
salivary duct carcinoma 61
salivary gland lesions 15
tumour malignancy 44
sinus histiocytosis with massive lymphadenopathy (Rosai Dorfman) 127
thyroid lesions 86–7
undifferentiated salivary gland carcinoma 66
see also immunophenotype
immunophenotype 122
anaplastic large cell lymphoma 169–70
Burkitt's lymphoma 163–4
diffuse large-cell lymphoma 159
follicular lymphoma 156
lymphoblastic leukaemia/lymphoma 152
lymphocytic lymphoma 152–3
lymphoplasmacytic lymphoma (immunocytoma) 153
MALT lymphoma 158–9
mantle zone lymphoma 155–6
peripheral T cell lymphoma 165
reactive lymphoid hyperplasia 122
sinus histiocytosis with massive lymphadenopathy (Rosai Dorfman) 127
immunosuppression
fungal lymphadenitis 132
Mycobacterium avium intracellulare lymphadenitis 128
in situ hybridisation 124
Epstein-Barr virus demonstration 143
infectious mononucleosis (glandular fever) 136–7
intraductal papillary adenocarcinoma, salivary gland 44
intraductal papilloma, salivary gland 44
intraosseous cyst 189–90, 191
iodine deficiency 87

K

Kaposi's sarcoma 124
keratin 61, 109
Ki-67 (MIB-1)
Burkitt's lymphoma 163
hyalinising trabecular adenoma, thyroid gland 99
lymphomas 122
salivary gland lesions 15
tumour malignancy 44
Kikuchi's lymphadenitis 135–6
Kimura's disease 144–5
Kuttner's tumour *see* sialadenitis, chronic

L

L&H (lymphocytic and histiocytic) cells 145–6, 148
Langerhans' cell histiocytosis (histiocytosis X) 140–3
immunohistochemistry 143
large cell T-cell lymphoma 166
laser scanning cytometer 150
LCA *see* CD45
leiomyosarcoma, salivary gland 68
Leishman-Donovan bodies 135
leishmaniasis 129, 135
leprosy 129
Letterer-Siwe syndrome 141
leu 6 (CD1a) 143, 165
light chain gene rearrangements 159
light chain ratio (LCR) 123
lipoma 185–6
LN1 (CDw75) 146
local anaesthesia 3, 4
needle-free system 4, 5
lymph node 121–75
accuracy of FNAC diagnosis 121
diagnostic difficulties 122
distribution of pathology 121
lymphoma *see* lymphoma
metastatic carcinoma 121, 170–5
reactive/inflammatory lesions 121
role of FNAC 121
lymph node follicular hyperplasia 121–6
lymphadenitis, chronic infective 135–8
lymphadenopathy
drug reactions 138
post-transplant 143–4
lymphoblastic leukaemia/lymphoma 151–2
immunophenotype 152
lymphocyte-predominant Hodgkin's disease 122
lymphocytic lymphoma (B-cell small lymphocytic lymphoma) 122, 123, 152–3
immunophenotype 152–3
role of FNAC in management 149
transformation to high-grade lymphoma (Richter syndrome) 152, 195
lymphocytic thyroiditis (Hashimoto's thyroiditis) 84, 93
cytological features 93, 94, 95, 97
diagnostic problems 84
differential diagnosis 97
lymphoma association 110, 112
lymphoepithelial cyst, salivary gland 18–22
differential diagnosis 20
lymphoepithelial (nasopharyngeal) carcinoma, salivary gland 66–7
lymphoepithelial sialadenitis (benign lymphoepithelial lesion; myoepithelial sialadenitis) 12, 27
cytological features 28–9
MALT lymphoma 27–8
lymphogranuloma venereum 129
lymphoid proliferations, salivary gland 26–30
neoplastic 27–30
reactive 27
lymphoma (non-Hodgkin's lymphoma) 3, 121, 148–70, 195
anaplastic large cell 149, 167–70
ancillary techniques 149–50
B-cell 152–64
cutaneous 159, 160
Burkitt's 149, 162–4
composite 149
diagnosis 121
accuracy of FNAC 148, 149
difficulties 13, 122
flow cytometry 122–3
immunohistochemistry 122
molecular techniques 122, 123–4
role of FNAC 148
diffuse large-cell 149, 159, 160, 161
follicle centre 149
follicular 148, 155, 156, 157
frequency 150
granulomatous reactions 129
handling FNAC material 150
immunoglobulin negative 149
immunophenotyping 122
lymphocytic (B-cell small lymphocytic) 149, 152–3
lymphoplasmacytic (immunocytoma) 153
MALT *see* MALT lymphoma
mantle zone 149, 153–6
marginal zone 148, 149, 156, 158–9
peripheral T-cell 149, 164–5
precursor lesions 151–2
primary effusion 161–2
REAL classification 150–1
role of FNAC in management 149, 151
salivary gland 12, 13, 27, 69, 70
HIV-positive patient 22
T-cell rich B-cell 149
T/NK-cell 164–70
thyroid gland 110–12
WHO classification 145, 148, 150
see also Hodgkin's lymphoma
lymphomatoid papulosis 167
lymphophagocytosis (emperipolesis) 127
lymphoplasmacytic lymphoma (immunocytoma)
cytological features 153, 154
immunophenotype 153
lymphoproliferative disorders 3
non-neoplastic 124–45
salivary gland 13

M

malignant haemangiopericytoma, salivary gland 68
MALT lymphoma 156, 158–9
  accuracy of FNAC diagnosis 148–9
  immunophenotype 158–9
  salivary gland 27–8, 29–30, 31, 69
  thyroid gland 110
mantle zone lymphoma 122, 123, 149, 153–6
  blastic variant 154–5
  immunophenotype 155–6
marginal zone lymphoma 122, 148, 149
  see also MALT lymphoma
material preparation 5–6
medullary carcinoma, thyroid gland 107–9
  C-cell hyperplasia differentiation 109
  cytological features 108, 109
  immunohistochemistry 109
  variants 107
meningioma 199, 200
  atypical 199
  fibroblastic 199
  secretory 199
metastatic carcinoma 3
  lymph node 121, 170–5
  salivary gland 71–2
    HIV-positive patient 22
  thyroid gland 112
    renal cell carcinoma 84
metastatising pleomorphic adenoma 37
methicillin-resistant staphylococcal infection, AIDS patients 138
MIB-1 *see* Ki-67
microsatellite instability (MSI) 86–7
minor salivary gland tumours
  incidence 15
  pleomorphic adenoma 31
molecular techniques 3, 6
  lymphoma 122, 123–4
  papillary thyroid carcinoma 105
  rhabdomyosarcoma 193
monomorphic adenoma, salivary gland 40
mucinous adenocarcinoma, salivary gland 59
mucocele, salivary gland 17, 19
mucoepidermoid carcinoma, salivary gland 47–8
  cytological features 47, 48, 49
  diagnostic difficulties 13
  differential diagnosis 48
  ex pleomorphic adenoma 49–50
  immunohistochemistry 50
  paediatric lesions 69
mucous retention cyst 189
multinodular goitre
  diagnostic problems 84
  non-toxic *see* colloid goitre
  toxic *see* toxic goitre
multiple endocrine neoplasia (MEN) syndrome 107
multiple oncocytic cyst, salivary gland 22
mycobacterial granulomatous lymphadenitis 127–9
Mycobacterium avium intracellulare lymphadenitis 128, 129
mycotic sialadenitis 26
myoepithelial differentiation, salivary tumour immunohistochemistry 53
myoepithelioma, salivary gland 41, 43, 44
myogenin 193

N

neurilemmoma *see* benign nerve sheath tumour
nodular fasciitis 186–7
  salivary gland 44
non-aspiration technique, salivary gland lesions 14
non-steroidal anti-inflammatory drugs, hypersensitive lymphadenopathy 138
nuclear grooves 101–2, 103, 105

O

odontogenic keratocyst, salivary gland 22
oesthesioneuroblastoma *see* olfactory neuroblastoma
olfactory neuroblastoma 3, 194–5
oncocytic change 39
  thyroid lesions 84
    colloid goitre 88
    lymphocytic (Hashimoto's) thyroiditis 93, 95
oncocytic neoplasms
  salivary gland crystalline structures 25
  thyroid gland 84
oncocytoma, salivary gland 41, 42
  malignant (oncocytic carcinoma) 59, 60
oncogene alterations
  non-Hodgkin's lymphoma 124
  papillary thyroid carcinoma 105

P

p16 61
p27Kip1 86
p53 44, 156
p161NK4a 156
paediatric lesions
  salivary gland 69
  thyroid nodule 85
papillary carcinoma, thyroid gland 84, 85, 86, 99–106
  cutaneous needle track metastasis 87
  cytological features 100, 101–2
  differential diagnosis 105–6
  FNAC in management 99, 101
  immunohistochemistry 105
  molecular genetics 105
  nuclear grooves 101–2, 103, 105
  psammoma bodies 99, 101, 103, 105
  variants 99, 102–5
    columnar cell 102–3
    diffuse sclerosing 104
    follicular 101, 102
    macrofollicular 102
    nodular fasciitis-like stromal component 104–5
    oxyphil cell 103, 104
    papillary Hürthle cell carcinoma with lymphoplasmacytic stroma 103–4
    tall cell 102, 103
papillary cystadenocarcinoma, salivary gland 58, 59
papillary Hürthle cell carcinoma with lymphoplasmacytic stroma 103–4
parathyroid cyst 190
parotid lesions, FNAC-related histological changes 15
parotid tumours 12, 13, 31, 41, 44
  incidence 15
  paediatric lesions 69
Pax3-7/Forkhead 193
PC10 *see* proliferating cell nuclear antigen (PCNA)
penicillin, hypersensitive lymphadenopathy 138
peripheral neuroectodermal tumour (PNET) 193–4
peripheral T-cell lymphoma 149, 164–5
  cutaneous 167
  cytological features 164, 165
  human T-lymphotropic virus-1 (HTLV-1)-associated 165, 166
  immunophenotype 165
  large cell 166
persistent generalised lymphadenopathy 136–8
phenytoin-induced lymphadenopathy 140
physical examination 3–4
pleomorphic adenoma 30, 31–6, 63
  adenoid cystic carcinoma differentiation 50–2
  atypical cells 12
  benign-metastatising 37
  cystic change 34
  cytological features 32–6
  diagnostic difficulties 12, 13
  differential diagnosis 35–6
  epithelial atypia 34, 36, 37
  malignant change
    carcinoma ex pleomorphic adenoma 37, 62, 64
    mucoepidermoid carcinoma ex pleomorphic adenoma 49–50
  paediatric lesions 69
  preoperative diagnosis 31–2
  presentation 31, 32, 34, 36
  salivary gland crystalloid structures 25
pleomorphic lipoma, salivary gland 44
Plummer's disease *see* toxic goitre
polymerase chain reaction (PCR)
  Epstein-Barr virus demonstration 143
  human herpesvirus-8 detection 124
  lymphoma 123, 124, 150
  post-transplant lymphoproliferative disorder 143–4
  see also reverse transcriptase polymerase chain reaction (RT-PCR)
polymorphous low-grade adenocarcinoma, salivary gland 54
post-transplant lymphoproliferative disorder 143–4
postirradiation salivary gland changes 13
PRAD-1 155
primary effusion lymphoma 161–2
  human herpesvirus-8 association 161
primitive neuroectodermal tumour, salivary gland 70–1
procedure 4–5
  salivary gland lesions 14
  thyroid lesions 81, 82, 83

progressive transformation of lymph nodes 122
proliferating cell nuclear antigen (PCNA; PC10) 15, 44, 50
proliferative fasciitis 186
psammoma bodies
colloid (multinodular non-toxic) goitre 89, 90
meningioma 199
papillary thyroid carcinoma 99, 101, 103, 105

R

rapid reporting system, salivary gland lesions 14
reactive lymphoid hyperplasia
clonality analysis 122, 123
immunophenotyping 122
role of FNAC in management 149
reactive lymphoid proliferations, salivary gland 27
reactive/inflammatory lesions 3
lymph node 121
Reed-Sternberg cells 145, 146, 147
referrals 3
retention cyst, salivary gland 18, 20
reverse transcriptase polymerase chain reaction (RT-PCR), rhabdomyosarcoma 193
rhabdomyosarcoma 3, 192–3
alveolar 193
embryonal 192, 193
molecular diagnostic studies 193
salivary gland 67–8
rheumatoid arthritis, granulomatous lymphadenitis 129, 130
Richter's syndrome 152, 195
Riedel's thyroiditis 97
Rosai Dorfman disorder *see* sinus histiocytosis with massive lymphadenopathy

S

S-100 protein 127, 143
S-phase fraction 44–5
salivary duct carcinoma 59
cytological features 61, 62
differential diagnosis 61
FNAC diagnostic accuracy 61–2
immunohistochemistry 61
salivary gland adenocarcinoma 62, 63
salivary gland crystalloid structures 23, 25
salivary gland cysts 12, 17–22
branchial cleft 20
dermoid 22
lymphoepithelial 18–22
mucocele 17, 19
multiple oncocytic 22
odontogenic keratocysts 22
retention 18, 20
salivary gland lesions 9–72
cystic *see* salivary gland cysts
diagnosis 11
accuracy 11–12
ancillary techniques 15
difficulties 12–13
FNAC cost effectiveness 14
rapid reporting 14
FNAC complications 14–15
FNAC procedure 14
FNAC-related histological changes 15
neoplastic *see* salivary gland tumours
non-neoplastic/inflammatory 11, 12, 17–30
paediatric 69
salivary gland lymphoid proliferations 26–30
salivary gland lymphoma 27
salivary gland, normal cytology 15, 16
acinar cells 15, 16
ductal cells 15, 16
salivary gland tumours 3, 11, 12
benign 11, 12, 30–44
diagnosis 12
difficulties 12–13
FNAC versus frozen section 13–14
incidence 15
malignant 11, 12, 44–66, 67–72
flow cytometry 44–5
immunohistochemical markers 44
p53 overexpression marker 44
smooth muscle-specific proteins 53
metastatic 71–2
WHO classification 12, 13
sampling performance 6–7
sarcoidosis 25, 26, 129
sarcoma, salivary gland 67–8
schwannoma *see* benign nerve sheath tumour
sebaceous adenoma, salivary gland 44
secretory meningioma 199
sensitivity
non-Hodgkin's lymphoma diagnosis 148, 149
salivary gland lesions
FNAC 11
frozen section 14
thyroid malignancy diagnosis 83, 84
service organisation 7
sialadenitis 22–6
acute 22, 23
chronic (Kuttner's tumour) 13, 23, 24
crystalloid formation 23, 25
cytomegalovirus 26
granulomatous 25–6
lymphoepithelial of Sjögren's syndrome 27
MALT lymphoma 27–8
mycotic 26
sialadenosis 17, 18
silicone, granulomatous lymphadenitis 129, 130
sinus histiocytosis with massive lymphadenopathy (Rosai Dorfman) 126–7
differential diagnosis 127
histiocyte immunophenotype 127
Sjögren's syndrome, lymphoepithelial sialadenitis 27
MALT lymphoma 27–8
small cell carcinoma, salivary gland 65
small round cell tumours 191–6
smear preparation 5–6
smooth muscle myosin heavy chains 53, 54, 61
smooth muscle-specific proteins 53
soft tissue lesions, benign 185–8
Southern blot analysis 124
Epstein-Barr virus demonstration 143
lymphoma 150
specificity
non-Hodgkin's lymphoma diagnosis 148, 149
salivary gland lesions
FNAC 11
frozen section 14
thyroid malignancy diagnosis 83, 84
squamous cell carcinoma, primary of salivary gland 64–5
cytological features 65
differential diagnosis 64
staining methods 6
sublingual gland tumours
incidence 15
pleomorphic adenoma 31
submandibular gland tumours
incidence 15
oncocytoma 41
pleomorphic adenoma 31
sulphonamide hypersensitive lymphadenopathy 138
surface Ig
Burkitt's lymphoma 163
diffuse large-cell lymphoma 159
follicular lymphoma 156
lymphocytic lymphoma 152
lymphoplasmacytic lymphoma (immunocytoma) 153
mantle zone lymphoma 155
marginal zone lymphoma (MALT type) 158
synaptophysin 197
synovial sarcoma, salivary gland 68
syphilis 129
syringes 4, 5

T

t(2;5)(p23;q35), anaplastic large cell lymphoma 170
t(8;14), Burkitt's lymphoma 164
t(11;14), mantle zone lymphoma 155
t(11;22)(q24;q12), extraskeletal Ewing's sarcoma/peripheral neuroectodermal tumour (PNET) 194
t(14;18)
diffuse large-cell lymphoma 159
follicular lymphoma 156
T-cell lymphoma 122
T-cell receptor gene rearrangements 123, 127, 165
T-cell rich B-cell lymphoma 149
T/NK-cell lymphoma 164–70
TdT 152
telomerase assay 86, 105
thymic cyst 190
thyroglobulin 99
thyroglossal cyst 188
thyroid cyst 90, 91
thyroid hyperplasia (goitre) 87–93
see also colloid goitre
thyroid lesions 3, 81–112
complications of FNAC 87
cost-effectiveness of FNAC 84, 85

thyroid lesions – (*contd*)
  diagnosis
    accuracy 83–4
    frozen section histology comparison 86
    problems 84
  immunohistochemistry 86–7
  multinucleate giant cells 93
  neoplasms 97–112
  non-neoplastic/inflammatory 87–97
  paediatric 85
  post-FNAC infarction 87
  procedure 81, 82, 83
    ultrasound guidance 82, 83
  role of FNAC 84–6, 97
  sampling technique 4–5
thyroid metastatic tumours 112
thyroid peroxidase (TPO) 86
thyroiditis 84, 85, 93–7
  acute (purulent) 93
  De Quervain's 93
  granulomatous 93, 94
  lymphocytic (Hashimoto's) 93, 94, 95, 97
  Riedel's 97
  subacute 93
thyrotoxicosis, hyperactive goitre 90, 93
toxic goitre 87, 90, 92, 94
  management 87
toxoplasmosis 129, 132–5
  granulomatous lymphadenitis 129
  HIV infection/AIDS 138
  lymphadenopathy 133–5
training in FNAC interpretation 12
trisomies, lymphocytic lymphoma 153
tuberculosis 11
  granulomatous lymphadenitis 127–9
  granulomatous sialadenitis 25
  HIV infection/AIDS 138
tularaemia 129

U

ultrasound guidance, thyroid lesions 82, 83
undifferentiated carcinoma, salivary gland 65–6
  immunohistochemistry 66

V

vimentin 110

W

Waldenström's macroglobulinaemia 153
Warthin's tumour *see* adenolymphoma, salivary gland

Z

zellballen 197